A NEW BEGINNING

AN ANTIDOTE TO CIVILIZATION

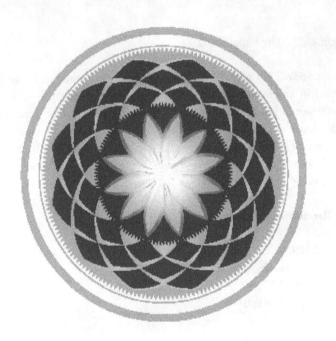

BLAKE SINCLAIR

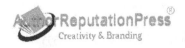
Author ReputationPress ®
Creativity & Branding

Author Reputation Press LLC
45 Dan Road Suite 5
Canton MA 02021
www.authorreputationpress.com
Hotline: 1(800) 220-7660
Fax: 1(855) 752-6001

Ordering Information:
Quantity sales. Special discounts are available on quantity purchases by corporations, associations, and others. For details, contact the publisher at the address above.

Printed in the United States of America.

ISBN-13:   Softcover   978-1-64961-037-9
           eBook   978-1-64961-038-6

Library of Congress Control Number: 2020913555

Cover Design: Mardi Coeur de Lion

Cover, spine and back cover Digital Artist: Airi Beltran

Editors: Dr. Mikaelah Cordeo, Ph.D., Stephen G. Lew and Kathryn Shanti Ariel

TABLE OF CONTENTS

ACKNOWLEDGEMENTS

To My Heavenly Father, Divine Mother and Friend
Thank you for your love, support, protection and guidance throughout my life! Special thanks for guiding me to all the experts that contributed to my book and those who have helped me find my way home. Thank you for allowing me to incarnate during this turbulent time period in the history of humanity so that I may fulfill thy mission and my dharma to help humankind bring an end to much of its suffering. Thank you for giving me the tools to share with humanity on how they too can find their way back home to you and their true and Divine Nature.

To all the Ascended Masters who have been a part of my life, including but not limited to the following: Gautama Buddha, Venerable Ācariya Mun Būridatta Thera, Venerable Ajahn Lee, the Maha Chohan, Saint Germain, the Violet Tara, El Morya, Kuthumi, Master Lady Pearl, Kwan Yin, Jesus, Mother Mary, Paramahansa Yogananda, Babji, Sathya Sai Baba, Babaji, Lord Krishna, Guru Nanak, the Great Divine Director, Djwal Khul, Padmasambhava and all of those who have come in and out of my life at various times.

Thank you for your great wisdom, teachings, and ongoing guidance and support with my book and spiritual life. Thank you for your ongoing guidance with increasing my consciousness during U.U.M.M. and continued guidance to me on the path that transcends the laws of karma that leads to oneness with my Father who art in Heaven, Mother Earth and all of humanity and all creatures great and small.

To Amma or Mātā Amritānandamayī Devī

Thank you for always being that Divine Mother who reminds me
of what true spirituality is all about! Thank you for being such
an exemplary spiritual leader and figure. Thank you for all your
love, compassion and kindness to humanity. How I love thee!
You have my eternal love and gratitude!

To Shree Ma

Thank you for inspiring me to continue to live in communion
with God. You are such a luminary but yet so humble,
loving, giving, compassionate and Divine. Thank you for
welcoming me in your Divine Presence and Love!
You have my deepest love and gratitude!

To Amma Sri Karunamayi

Thank you for taking time to learn about my dream and vision
for helping humanity. Thank you for your blessings to support
me in the fulfillment of my dream through your Darshan.
You have my deepest love and gratitude!

To Masami Saionji and family (Maki, Rika and Yuka)

Thank you for all you and your family have done in promoting peace on
this planet. You and your daughters have truly inspired me to do my utmost
to promote world peace. After meeting with your daughters in Tokyo, I
was further inspired to work on more ways of promoting world peace. I
look forward to ongoing support of your organizations (Byakko Shinko
Kai, the World Peace Prayer Society, and the Goi Peace Foundation) in
promoting world peace.
May Peace Prevail on Earth!

To Peter Mt. Shasta

Thank you for guiding me to the Ascended Masters and teaching me about
the sacred I AM teachings. Thank you for all your support, guidance, love
and compassion throughout the years. Your wisdom and Light have guided
me in discovering the path of enlightenment which has led to me finding
the great Guru within. You are truly an inspirational spiritual master,

teacher, guru, and bodhisattva. Thank you for inspiring me to write the "I AM" Wellness Method. Thank you for leading me to the Masters especially the Maha Chohan, Saint Germain, Kwan Yin, the Violet Tara, Kuthumi, Master Lantos and El Morya.

You have my deepest love, respect and gratitude!

To Master Yuanming Zhang

Thank you for your kindness, wisdom, compassion, love and generosity. Thank you for allowing my wife and I to experience the mystical, mythical and magical Dragon Pearl. You also have our deepest love and gratitude for joining our souls and consciousness together as one which gave birth to us being new Twin Flames. I had no idea how one mystical evening could change our lives forever. Thank you for your openness to a lifelong friendship. Thank you for the blessings you have given to our lives and this sacred book.

You have our eternal love, respect and gratitude.

To Venerable Panyavro Vachira

Thank you for always taking the time to guide me in your Dharma teachings. Thank you for reminding me about the four elements that we are all comprised of. You planted a seed of wisdom that later gave birth to a new version of the Element Theory of wellness within my "I AM" Wellness Method. I appreciate your authenticity, kindness, compassion, wisdom, insights and openness. Your smile is quite healing and refreshing.

You have my deepest respect and gratitude!

To Master Relica

Thank you for reaching out to me and helping me to remember who I AM. Thank you for connecting me back to Buddha, Master Mun and Master Lee and sharing your mystical world of the sacred relics. Thank you for introducing me to Master Panyavro Vachira. He is an extraordinary Buddhist Master.

You have my eternal love, friendship and gratitude!

To my wife

Thank you for all your love, support and patience with me despite all the long hours I spent writing endlessly. Thank you for believing in me when many others did not. Thank you for joining me in my amazing journey in life and spirituality that has led you to finding the path that leads you back home. I am very proud of all the gains you have made with your U.U.M.M. practice and how connected you are now with your I AM Presence. You are destined for spiritual greatness! Thank you for your love. It is so powerful that no matter how dark it is or how murky the sea of life is, your love will always guide me back home to your arms and the arms of God and the Masters. Thank you so much for your ongoing support with my spirituality! I love, admire and adore you! I am also so proud of you! Thank you for showing me what real love looks and feels like.

I love you beyond the depth of the Universe!

To my kids

Thank you for stepping up and allowing love and compassion to fill your hearts, minds and souls. It was God's Love that guided your thoughts and actions when the going got tough. Sometimes life throws us spiritual curve balls but when we unite in love, support and compassion, we could make it through the darkest night and weather through any seasons in life and become an even more loving family. I love both of you so much and so proud of both of you!

To Stephen Lew and Diane Tong

You have my deepest love and gratitude for your patience,
dedication and committed help with my book!!!

To Ryu Okada, Joycelyne Lew, Wendy Schulte, Vladimir Beltran, Claudia Umanzor, Silvia, Karen, Mary Ann Liu, David Pryce, Elizabeth Lee and all those special souls who shared their wisdom and or testimonials

Thank you for your openness and generosity with sharing information to help others live a higher quality of life. May your wisdom help others live well and help end some of their sufferings.

To Mardi Coeur de Lion

Thank you for your friendship and support! Thank you for believing in me and sharing my vision with helping the word create more peace. You have my deepest gratitude for designing the cover of my book and sharing your magnificent talent with me and the world. You are truly one of the most extraordinary and amazing women I have ever met, and you are definitely a true artistic genius, humanitarian and beautiful soul in so many ways.

To Airi Beltran

Thank you for bringing Mardi's art design into paperback reality that truly reflect her vision. Thank you for sharing your artistic abilities with bringing my book to a whole new level. You are truly amazing! You have my deepest gratitude!

To Tai Monique

Thank you for your ongoing friendship and support with my spirituality! Thank you for your support with my third literary Baby. Always be that extraordinary and beautiful woman that you are. So proud of you and all your achievements!

To Kathryn Shanti Ariel

Thank you for all your assistance and contributions with making this sacred book into a reality. You have me deepest gratitude!

To my Dream Team of Healers and Enlightened Beings:

Dr. Alex Feng, Traditional Chinese Medicine Practitioner, Taoist Priest, Grandmaster of Martial Arts, and Licensed Acupuncturist (voted as one of the top Acupuncturists in the Bay Area), Dr. Paul Hannah, MD, Psychiatrist, Intuitive Professional Speaker, author and Licensed Acupuncturist, Dr. Sonia Badreshia-Bansal, World-Class Plastic Surgery and dermatologist, Elitemdspa, Dr. Hector Oksenendler, DC and Physical Therapist, Flenje Oaferina, Registered Physical Therapist, Janet Doer, Intuitive Nutritionista, David Granovsky, Stem Cell advisor and expert, Andrei Volhonttseff, Nutritionist, Marian Brandenburg, a body healer, an intuitive massage therapist, Chi Nei Tsang Practitioner, and Ajna and Neuro Light Practitioner, Romarishi Siddha and Tara Leela, authors of *Herbs for*

Spiritual Development, spiritual teachers, Tea Masters and founders of the Universal Fellowship of Light, Darshan Baba, Yogi, Author, Spiritual Mentor, Subtle Energy Healer, and Teacher of Online Subtle Energy and Meditation Courses, Lisa De Witt, Healer, Felix Fojas, a veteran spiritual warrior, Mystic, lecturer, teacher, Reiki master and healer, Joanna Marie Fojas, Reiki master, Star Santos (Stargazer), a famous psychic, radio show host at ABS-CBN, exorcist and paranormal expert, Lori Guidinglight, LCSW and Intuitive Healer, Savannah Brooke, Ascension Guide, Shaman, Pranic Healer, writer and speaker, Yumiko Yoga, a Yoga Teacher, Reiki Teacher, Sound and Voice Healer, and Neo Healer, Rebecca-Danbi Kim, Feng Shui Practitioner, Personal Energy Clearing Expert and Face Reading Expert, Dr. Steve Jackowicz, Mac, Lac, PhD, Dr. Paul Wang, Doctor of Acupuncture and Chinese Medicine and Wu Shu Master, Bella, CEO and Founder of Metaphysical Medium, Master Hypnotherapist, Life Coach, and Reiki Master, Dr. Mikaelah Cordeo, Ph.D., Spiritual Teacher, Healer and Messenger for the Ascended Hosts of Light, Patti Gee, Massage Therapist and Holistic Health Practitioner, Lou Corona, President and founder of Puradyme and many other great healers that contributed to the success of this book.

Thank you for sharing your wisdom, expertise and knowledge in this concerted effort to help bring greater health, wellness and harmony to humanity and our planet. Collectively, the wisdom and information you all have shared will help end the suffering of many around the world for many years to come.

You are the great ones that have chosen to make a huge difference in the lives of millions; through this collaborative effort of this dream team, millions if not billions will have their lives impacted in a great and positive way. Your kindness will be blessed and magnified many folds by the Universe and you all are a piece of history in the making that will change the shape the future of our planet. I salute all of you and you all have my most profound gratitude and love. God bless you!!!! Wishing you infinite love and blessings! Your kindness will burn an indelible mark in the Universe of love, hope, kindness and compassion!

INTRODUCTION

Humanity has suffered from various illnesses throughout the centuries while also being aware of various degrees of help from shamans, healers and doctors of eastern and western medicine. However, during our modern industrialization age, a new type of suffering was born and has wreaked havoc on millions of people worldwide and if not corrected has the potential of destroying Earth, our amazing homeland.

Many enlightened beings and health conscientious individuals have been observing our chaos and global suffering with much sadness for the past few decades. Due to many calls and prayers to the Heavens for Divine intervention, Divine guidance is being offered worldwide to help awaken the masses to each one's true Divine Nature. Humanity is awakening from a spiritual coma, a coma that has crippled and rendered us ignorant or oblivious to our true and Divine Nature for millennia. This coupled with the modern industrialization has given birth to many chronic illnesses, diseases, and suffering of different kinds. It has even resulted in the premature death of millions all around the world. We have in essence co-created our current health crisis due to our ego perpetuated civilization.

Now, however, many great beings of Light, Love and Wisdom are coming forth to give guidance on how we can navigate our way through the layers of disharmony, illness, pain and suffering that so many of us are experiencing so that we may experience the fullness of life we were meant to live. A life that is full of love, peace, happiness, gratitude, bliss and joy; a life that is enlightened, empowered and Divine. It is through making this choice and embracing the dedication to make it a reality that we can begin to heal ourselves and Mother Earth. Despite the damages that were done in the past which have escalated during 60 – 70 years through our ego-perpetuated system, we can begin to reverse all the damages by starting A New Beginning. We can begin to create heaven within our inner Universe as well as on Earth. Before we can do that, it will help us to put things in perspective by more clearly understanding our origins.

In the beginning before time, space and matter, there was the so-called great Void. I like to refer to it as the Womb of Love that is full of Nurturance, Divine Feminine Energy and the Nutrients (the chemicals, gases and energetic imprints, sacred geometric patterns for creation of matter to create and sustain life) of life. I see it as a Zen state of Consciousness that is in perfect sublime bliss.

When it was time for space and matter to be given birth, a big bang of the awakening of the consciousness occurred and expressed itself in its fully awakened and God-Realized creative nature. A transmission of love, creation and self- sustaining systems (creation, destruction, integration and balance) were born out of the Great Void and gave birth to the Cosmic sound of AUM. Although many think it is only a word, it is more than that. It is a frequency, energy, creative force – the Consciousness and Love of God. Nonetheless, AUM, the word, energy, frequency, love and consciousness all represent God, Source or Creator.

In the beginning was the Word,
and the Word was with God,
and the Word was God. (John: 1:1) (R 1)

That sacred primordial Word was AUM. It has a creative energy of manifestation full of God's Love, Light (full spectrum), and Consciousness. The Light (the idea), Force, and Energy is Love in action of manifesting physical, energetic, conscious, emotional and spiritual energies (Qi, astral, causal and auric). **Aum (ॐ) is the vibration by which the Supreme Spirit brings all things into manifestation.** Paramahansa Yogananda has explained that everything—all matter, all energy, all thoughts—exists in Aum.

AUM can be further broken down and understood by the following: "A (Akaar)" represents the vibration that brings into manifestation the created universe; "U (Ukaar)" represents the vibration that preserves the creation, and "M (Makaar)" represents the destructive vibration that dissolves the manifested universe back into the Infinite Spirit." (**R 2**)

I see AUM as Source Energy and chant it at each chakra during my meditation as I allow myself to become one with God's Consciousness, the Universe and Mother Earth.

I AM That I AM

The Bible tells of Moses' encounter with God's Presence in a burning bush near Mt. Sinai. Moses said to God, "Suppose I go to the Israelites and say to them, 'the God of your fathers has sent me to you', and they ask me, 'What is his name?' then what shall I tell them?" God said to Moses, "I AM That I AM. This is what you are to say to the Israelites: I AM has sent me to you." (Exodus 3:14) (**R 3**) This communication with Moses and God was in a sense a Divine teaching and transmission. Those who understood it, embraced it, integrated it into their life and became the enlightened and empowered ones.

Another common translation of I AM THAT I AM is from the Sanskrit mantra HUM SA or So Ham – which calls on your personal I AM. Each individual human is connected to a personal I Am Presence. All of the personal I AM Presences exist in a field of Oneness with all others. It is said the at the sound of the inhale is HUM and the sound of the exhale is SA. As we breathe in and exhale, we are unconsciously saying the name of God. It anchors the God Self in the heart and fosters oneness with that God Presence or what I call the Great I AM.

In the beginning of time, God's Pure Love, Light, Energy and Consciousness manifested all of creation and reality. Everything was made holy, pure and perfect. We were initially made as beings of Light before we incarnated into our various physical forms to experience the diversity of life. All of God's creations were created as a Torus or self-sustaining system and were planted with a seed of Divine Presence. This is the Spark of Divine Light, Love and Christ Consciousness, or the I AM within. When the I AM is in unity with the entire being, it regulates, guides, supports and monitors each system of consciousness. The spark of the I AM Presence within each person is the individualized aspect of God that is always in Oneness with all the other I AM of each individual and with all of Life.

In the beginning, we were Beings of Light and Love with a direct link or connection with Source, God or Creator because the I AM Presence was in its pure and full expression within us. We were essential immortal beings that manifested and created our reality through our loving thoughts, intentions, visualizations coupled with our hearts desire. In this place of origin everyone was fully awake and enlightened. Everyone was able to live in their bodies as long as was necessary for them to achieve the mastery level they came to experience in accordance with the Divine Plan.

The Cycle after the Fall from Grace

However, as we began to relate more with the material world, the ego and the things we created, the I AM Presence within us withdrew leaving its Divine spark anchored within the heart of each individual. Those early enlightened ones who chose to stay connected with God could still do so by listening to the promptings of their I AM Presence. In so doing, they paved the way for the reawakening of humanity.

In the beginning of civilization, there was harmony with all of creation. Humankind, all creation - great and small, Mother Nature, Mother Earth and God co-existed in great harmony and unity. All our food and water supply were equally created with perfect harmony. The food that was consumed and the pure water we drank were designed to support the harmony in our bodies. They gave us the proper hydration, minerals, trace minerals and fuel for our bodies to enable it to thrive and heal. This was understood, and all life thrived in gratitude, health, love and joy.

Even after the Fall from Grace, those who were very enlightened or awakened beings lived quite long lives and even attained immortality or ascension through their mastery in living in alignment with God's original plan for us to live in harmony with God, Mother Earth and all creatures great and small. They were astute at discovering which food, plants and herbs were able to create the optimal environment for harmony, wellness and longevity. They also engaged in spiritual practices that allowed them to experience that oneness with their Creator. These included meditation, yogic breathing, conscious connection and communication with the

Divine realms, activation of the Amrita (spiritual nectar from the pineal gland) and energy work.

However, as the fall continued, much of humanities' collective ego began to identify more with the material world instead of its true Divine nature. As this occurred, their individual I AM Presence withdrew leaving the ego to run the show. The ego through its state of fear began to go awry taking control of our embodiments through fear thus resulting in life became a journey of the survival of the fittest. Instead of hungering for Truth, Love and Harmony, the ego of humanity began to hunger for power, fame, lust, desires and attachment to the material matters that it created. It began to see itself differently (as though they were superior) from others, both human and other species.

This separation or duality broke a vital link of wholeness, wellness and harmony- the link that connects to Spirit or the I AM Presence. Eventually the ego began guiding many to eat for pleasure and indulgence versus eating with harmony, balance and reverence for all creatures great and small.

Humanity's disconnect from their Divine Nature affected their ability to heal and live a long life. Eventually many had forgotten how to live in alignment with the original Divine Plan of Love and began to experience illnesses, diseases and even death. Many had forgotten their Divine and immortal nature and became bounded by the law of karmic energies they had created by their ego perpetuated life. This began the endless suffering of humanity and much of Creation on Earth.

Despite the pain and suffering of sickness and death that was created by our ego perpetuated life, God planted seeds of wisdom and love in the water, air, plant kingdom, crystals and mineral kingdoms and animals to assist us in remembering the Divine Truth of who we are. As God (the Divine) is in all things, they contain the secrets to supporting the Divine Presence within each and every one of us to restore harmony and wellness. Individuals such as shamans, medicine people, and healers are connected to this Divine Presence within themselves and all of Nature.

They were guided to discover the great healing powers of the various kingdoms that would bring us to wellness again. This knowledge has been formalized in many models of wellness that have been passed down from generation to generation like Traditional Chinese Medicine, Ayurvedic Medicine, herbology and indigenous healing wisdom.

Yet, due to the predominant greed of humanity and its ego, more and more people suffered, as did Earth and her kingdoms of life. Over time, prayers and calls from people on Earth were made to end much of the suffering it had co-created and repeatedly Mother/Father/God and the Company of Heaven attempted to assist humanity out of separation and back into our True Divine Nature and Unity. Many great Saints, Avatars and Enlightened Ones have come to guide us back to our true nature including Babaji, Buddha, Kwan Yin, Padmasambhava, Paramahansa Yogananda, Jesus, Mother Mary, Sathya Sai Baba, Saint Germain, and Amma (the hugging saint).

However, due to free will many of us continued to live in an illusion instead of following the teachings of many great masters that were sent here to bridge that gap between God and humankind. Hence, many have continued to perpetuate our sufferings.

While on one hand the awakening of humanity had begun, the gap between humanity and this divine and natural wisdom continued to broaden – especially during the modern industrialization period. Along with this, our ability to heal, thrive and flourish began to be severely compromised. Through the recent industrialization period of humanity, corporations were born. They found ways to make material things in huge quantities, and eventually it found ways to make things faster and faster, to grow their profits exponentially to keep up with the demands of the exploding population. Corporate marketers began using industrial psychology to better understand how to weave and manufacture the perfect plan or package to persuade and manipulate the average citizen to purchase its products.

Many were led to believe that by purchasing their products, they would simultaneously purchase happiness, joy, power and ultimately the American Dream. This was all part of the illusion that life in separation can actually be fulfilling.

As science began to advance, companies started to manipulate our food supply in order to sell things faster and faster. Hormones, antibiotics and other chemicals began to be added to our food to improve shelf-life and thus increase profits and protect its assets. As the soils were overly burdened to keep up with the demand of mono-cropping, crops began being sprayed with herbicides and pesticides. Furthermore, grains in many countries were even genetically altered to increase profits.

Preservatives, additives and artificial sweeteners were also added to make things taste better and last longer on the shelf for the purpose of profits. Meanwhile, the size of the people in our country began to grow significantly compared to other countries. Many types of addictions began to take place including food and shopping addictions when our appetites became uncontrollable. We have become a consumer society in America. However, this has also affected many other countries to varying degrees.

All of this is a result of our attempting to be fulfilled through the outer world, rather than renewing our deep inner connection with the God within us and in all of life. Instead, most of humanity are unconsciously being driven by their ego to fulfill their needs through material satisfaction and greed.

As an outcome of the universal law of attraction, what you focus on is what you create, humanity has given its power away to an ego perpetuated reality - or matrix - that until recently has kept the populace happy and content at perpetuating its system or prison.

The many side effects of this system have included the suffering of Mother Earth such as: deforestation, pollution, contamination of the oceans and most water supplies, depletion of fossil fuels, etc.

It has also created great suffering of humanity through addictions, obesity, depression, anxiety, and the birth of many illnesses and diseases. This type of ego perpetuated reality lead to disharmony of the body, mind and spirit which if left unresolved will only create more and more suffering in the future and premature deaths.

So, who is responsible? Are the corporations to blame? I think that they are partly responsible, but we must take responsibility as well. We fuel the system that they created by our choice of purchases and by pursuing an elusive dream that has kept us trapped in the matrix of illusion. When we wake up from this illusion or Maya, we will begin to truly live, thrive and heal, finally breaking free from it.

As we change our thoughts, ideas and purchasing habits to those that are healthier, companies are beginning to follow our new habits and they are/ will be changing how they do business. Examples of this include the high demand for organic fruits and vegetables, an ever-increasing demand for vegan or plant-based foods, and biodegradable, eco-friendly cleaning and home care products. In addition, more companies are selling products that do not contain gluten, GMO and soy because of our collective concerns about those products in our foods.

Despite all of the progress towards healthier eating, many people are still getting sick. Have you ever noticed that there is a trend towards an increase incidence and prevalence of diseases and illnesses in the past two decades? Even some health-oriented people are getting sick. Few appear to be immune to getting some form of illness or disease including priests, nuns, gurus, Yogis, spiritual masters, and an acupuncturist and nutritionist I have met or heard about.

Illnesses range from a common cold, to mental illness, to diabetes, to depression, to heart failure, to botulism, to having Parkinson's disease, to suffering a debilitating stroke. If these great ones are getting sick, is there no hope for us?

Yes, there is! I am quite optimistic about how we can achieve a great deal of harmony in our lives by changing how we eat, drink, pray and meditate. This new inner harmony will significantly support our health and well-being. Although we cannot be a bulletproof monk to all the toxins, illnesses and diseases, we can definitely decrease our risk of being severely ill or debilitated. This can be done by shifting our lifestyle to be more harmonious with that of our Creator or Source.

We were originally created in a state of unity consciousness (Christ Consciousness) with our Divine Nature. There was no disease, hunger or war, only Divine Love and Light. We lived in perfect harmony with ourselves, others, all of Creation, the Universe and God. There was a Ying and Yang in our life and a reverence for all life on Earth. Our body was designed to heal itself and received support from the healing fruits and vegetables that were gifted to us that contain much of the Light, pranic nutrients, phytonutrients and micronutrients that our bodies require for optimal health.

God created us to live in harmony. Those who truly follow the path of harmony that leads to God are spiritual and Divine Beings. Gratefully, this path is open for everyone to choose and heal through harmlessness.

Spirituality is not just about awakening, enlightenment and following a path or guru. It is really a way of life that creates harmony within us, our family, society, planet and Universe. True harmony (living without harm) contributes to our collective health and well-being. It is not a Hippy or New Age thing that so many people think it is. It is much more than that and, ultimately, it is a way back home through which we can re-establish our communion and oneness with God as it was when we first came to Earth.

When we remember how to realize and embody our True Divine Nature and live in a constant state of Divine Light and Love, we can contribute to creating greater harmony, peace and love between ourselves and all Life on Gaia. When enough of us have achieved this state of harmony (critical mass), we will see the end the suffering that life on Earth has endured for way too long. We have the potential to co-create Heaven on Earth on our planet and within our bodies.

We can do this by being more conscious with what we drink, eat and put into our bodies. Becoming educated regarding how and where to find the best sources of nutrients to allow out bodies to have the optimal ability to create harmony is a wonderful first step.

Additionally, becoming aware that besides eating the right foods, drinking the best water and doing some exercises, it can also be highly beneficial to detoxify our bodies regularly through fasting, juicing or taking certain supplements.

Overall, it is necessary to ensure we are getting enough vitamins and minerals from our daily diet, with great emphasis on fruits and vegetables. If we are not, then adding vitamins, minerals and supplements that we are deficient in to attain wellness and allow our bodies to heal more effectively can be highly beneficial.

Finding out where to start and what choices to make can be a daunting task. In this book, I have taken the liberty to share some of the most cutting-edge information I have learned that has helped me, my family or people I have met or assisted with their health. Light workers such as I am and many others have incarnated into this physical reality to help contribute to ending the suffering that so many of God's children have endured for so long.

Through *A New Beginning*, I will guide you on a journey of wellness that will lead you to realizing that at the core of your health and wellness issues is a balance between your body, mind, emotion and spirit that requires your attention, awareness and focus. I will teach you how to reconnect with your Divine or I AM Presence; it is your link to God and the Divine Realm that has been disconnected for so long. It is your compass that will lead you to God and to your ultimate freedom. Aligning with it fully will allow you to become a God-Realized Being. This is our true nature and it is what it will take to help transform and heal ourselves, families, communities, and Mother Earth and beyond.

The many great masters who have come to Earth throughout the ages, have been sharing this message to us but many times politics and our collective egos have edited out this original message from the Universe. God and the Ascended Masters have guided me in sharing all the following wisdom to empower you to live as a God-Realized Christ Conscious Being that will assist in creating Heaven on Earth as well as within each one of you.

The outcome of this life is peace, happiness, joy, radiant health, bliss, love, compassion, forgiveness, miracles, oneness, longevity and immortality.

I wish you much success in your journey to experiencing harmony and oneness with yourself, Mother Earth, the Universe, God, and all of Creation. Within this and my previous books, I have shared many secrets that I have learned from my own search to ending the suffering in myself, my mother, family, friends, clients and many others. I have gained much knowledge from nutritionists, an herbalist, medical mediums and intuitives, a stem cell expert, healers, doctors of chiropractic and Chinese medicine, a physical therapist, a Mystic, spiritual leaders, Ascended Masters, and many health conscious individuals who were more than willing to share their wisdom in order to empower people in gaining greater health and wellness.

May you gain insights and wisdom from reading this book that will guide you on your journey of rediscovering the Divine Harmony and wellness our Creator desires you to have, and that is truly your birthright and the birthright of all of Life.

May the Divine teachings contained within this book also re-ignite and activate that Divine Spark of Light within you and every sentient being you encounter. As part of reading this book, you will learn how to illuminate that Light throughout your entire being and become a beacon of Light and God-Realized Being that will lead others to the path of Truth that will help end the suffering and re-unite us all as one Divine Mind, Consciousness and Family.

Namaste! Sat Sri Akal!
Om Shanti, shanti, shanti!

~ *Blake Sinclair*

Disclaimer: *The nutritional information the author shares in this book is not meant to be a definitive list of solutions for you but meant to open your eyes and mind to the many possibilities of how the body can be optimized to allow the Divine Presence to do its job to attain peace, harmony and wellness. It is meant to encourage readers to go on their own journey with the partnership of their physician and alternative healthcare practitioner.*

The intent of the author is to offer information on the author's own spiritual and nutritional awakening, with the hope of motivating the reader to discover their hidden and latent potential for living a more productive, happy and peaceful life. The author is not a physician and does not offer medical advice. Any lifestyle change with regard to health needs to be addressed with the reader's physician or appropriate healthcare provider.

"A journey of a thousand miles begins with a single step."

~

Lao Tzu

CHAPTER 1

CREATING HEAVEN ON EARTH FROM WITHIN

I n the beginning Heaven and Earth were One. Every life form upon Earth (Gaia) was completely and consciously connected with Mother/Father/God/Creator. All life was in a state of thriving and mastery. However, it was through identification with the material world, its collective ego and its disconnection from Source that eventually led to what we know as the fall from grace. Now, however, Gaia is choosing to ascend back into the 5th dimension of harmony and all who are currently embodied upon here are being given the opportunity to ascend with her, A new beginning is underway.

Heaven is returning to Earth with great Divine Assistance, and through the choices that we as individuals make each and every day – choices for peace, harmony and Divine Love. The journey to stay and ascend with Gaia requires everyone to heal and to release all that is not Love. It is an inside out journey. Yet, as all life is interconnected, as we heal ourselves, the new balance, wholeness and harmony that we become ripples out into the world assisting with building the momentum of a new paradigm of living.

Causes of Suffering - Our Fall from Grace

Many of humanity are asking the question, what is truly the origin of all human suffering? Depending on who you ask, you will get a different answer. The Buddhist answer will be different than a Christian's or New Ager's answer. Regardless of the answer, humanity hasn't seemed to escape the suffering of the human condition which includes sickness, old age and death. Though the origins of suffering may vary from one religion to the next, most seem to suggest we came from a life of harmony, peace and wellness. I believe we were all beautifully created by God's Love and Consciousness and hence were perfect at the onset of Creation. We were Godlike Beings of Love and Light who created and manifested reality like our own Creator

We had an ego of awareness who was aware of itself, others and God. We also had a strong connection with God and knowing that we are One. In the beginning of time, there was harmony with all of Creation. Humankind, all Creation Great and Small, Mother Nature, Mother Earth and God co-existed in great harmony and unity.

However, as we began to identify more with the material world we created, our ego began to go awry. The choices we made began to degrade our Godlike Presence and began to corrupt the harmony we once had inside. No longer was our presence one with harmony and Divinity, but now, it became one of self-indulgence, chaos and disharmony. We began forgetting who we were.

We collectively began losing that strong connection and communication with our Creator and began to follow this new disharmonious ego we had created which hungered and thirsted for power, fame, fortune, desires, lust, etc. (It is important to note that there are and still many enlightened beings who still maintain that Godlike Presence, connection and awareness. Each person has the option at this time to become whole again, fully embodying his or her True Divine Nature (I AM Presence.)

Instead of having a healthy ego awareness of ourselves, Divinity within and Divinity outside of us like we had in the beginning of time. We began forgetting that and began believing that we were more important than our Creator, that God was a mere abstract and obsolete religious thing of the past and that science and technology was the new God.

As civilization began to advance technologically and become more industrialized, it gave birth to many corporations, and they have been growing exponentially every year. They, in general, are totally ego and

2

profit driven with little to no regards to the negative effects of what they are doing to our air, food, water and Mother Earth.

This new age of industrialization has given birth to many sicknesses, illnesses and even all these so-called Mystery Diseases which has resulted in the suffering and deaths of millions on this planet.

However, those who live away from the influences of these corporations and understand the Divine karmic laws of the Universe have been able to attain long and vibrant lives. An example of such a person is Master Lee Qing Yuen, a meditator and herbalist who lived to the ripe age of 256 years old.

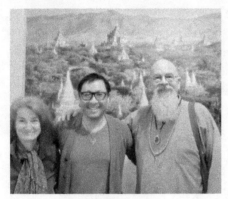

Tara Leela, Blake Sinclair and Romarishi Siddha

Romarishi Siddha (formerly Ganga Nath), Tea Master, spiritual teacher, author and founder of the Universal Fellowship of Light tells of another great Siddha and master meditator, Tapaswiji Maharaj, who lived to be 185 years of age. Those men who lived long and extended lives are quite often spiritual, expressing their own unique Divine nature and living in harmony, love and peace with God and mankind. In fact, Tapaswiji was a Yogi, one who attained oneness with God and became a God-Realized being. **(R 4)**

Our Multibody Systems

Many of these enlightened beings and masters understand how the body functions in quite a holistic way. They realize there is a ying and yang in our system or balance in our intricate system. They are very aware of how the emotions especially negative emotions can affect our body, mind and spirit. They are aware of the various bodies we have: physical, emotional, mental, and etheric and how important it is to ensure that they are balanced and healthy in order for their Spirit Self to live a long and healthy life in its Earth form.

3

In Traditional Chinese Medicine, they see the body as the balance of the five elements - earth, wood, metal, fire and water. It is quite a complex, comprehensive and sophisticated system that has a temporal, emotional, and seasonal component to it. It gets into the relationships between the various organs as well. It is beyond the scope of this book to go over all that, therefore, I will give a simplified system for you to incorporate this into your life.

When I met with Master or Venerable Panyavro Vachira, a Thai Forest Monk, he discussed about how we are comprised of the four elements - earth, air, fire and water. I feel those four elements are very important and essential for our health and wellness, but after analyzing much of the suffering in humanity, I have come to realize that the metal element has a very important role in the harmony or disharmony within our body system. We will explore that further in Chapter 15 where I discuss my interpretation on the Five Elements in my system, which I call "I AM" Wellness Method. The purpose of this system is to allow and support the Divine Presence in creating greater harmony and wellness within.

Regardless of which system we use to regain wellness and harmony, the fact is that our bodies are quite complex and requires a balance of the various bodies and elements that supports the bodies both individually, and as a whole. I resonate with my spin on the Five Elements system and will focus primarily on them in this book, which I feel will be helpful to the reader.

The Elements

- **Earth Element** to me represents our body, muscles, skin, bones, tissues and organs. It also represents that which comes from **Mother Earth** - the food we eat, including the fruits, vegetables, minerals and trace minerals.
- **Air Element** represents our breath, breathing and the air we breathe in and regularly release.
- **Fire Element** represents our kundalini energy, Qi energy and our Divine Spark of Light or I AM Presence anchored within our heart and the electrical impulses from our nerves and muscles.

- **Water Element** represents our blood, urine, cerebral spinal fluids and bodily fluids. It is also the water we drink and the water we get from our fruits and vegetables. Each system needs certain minimum requirements for wellness, but mastery of the five elements may lead to wellness and longevity.
- **Metal Element** represents the good and bad metals that we get into our body. The good metal will support health and wellness but the bad heavy metals like aluminum and mercury can wreak havoc within our system leading to chaos or what we call illness and diseases.

Besides the elements, what is very important and expresses who we truly are is love. **Divine Love** is a necessary component of our lives that creates all the elements and supports all our different bodies (mental, emotional, physical and spiritual, etheric or astral bodies). When we heal with love, it can be so transformative. Speaking, kissing, touching, hugging, praying and meditating with love is the most important part of reestablishing the harmony, peace and well-being of a person. At the core of our being is pure and Divine Love. Allowing it to fill our entire being and being one with it - body, mind and spirit - allows us to be closer to God.

Mastery of elements, body systems and love require spiritual mastery of us being grounded and having mastery of various yogic breathing techniques, meditation and getting the best nutrients, supplements and quality water to drink to support our pineal gland as well as our four lower bodies – the physical, emotional, mental and etheric. It also requires that we practice mindfulness, compassion, unconditional love, mercy, forgiveness and kindness to all creatures great and small. It also requires us to truly understand how to connect with God, Mother Earth and the rest of humanity.

Although many of the previous mentioned great saints, masters or enlightened beings discovered the secret to longevity, they lived in a time period where there was healthy water to drink, unpolluted air to breathe, and fresh organic fruits, vegetables, and herbs to eat or drink.

Nowadays, these same masters and the rest of humanity are faced with a greater challenge. Because of the consequences of our great industrialization and modernization, much of which has poisoned the air

5

we breathe, water we drink, and fruits and vegetables we eat. Many are still eating meat that is also full of antibiotics, hormones, etc.

Industrialization and modernization are not necessarily bad things. Many great inventions and technology have improved the lives of many but due to humanity's collective dysfunctional ego, great suffering has occurred to humanity in epic proportions. This dysfunctional ego is not concerned about the interest and welfare of humanity, or the well-being of Mother Earth. It somehow feels there are no personal consequences to the continued degradation of the health of Life in all forms. Has humankind committed the ultimate Sin against God, Nature and Mother Earth by its greed?

In the Christian and Catholic religions, sin is something we inherited from Adam and Eve. There is a certain shame or judgment that seems to go along with it. But what does sin (S.I.N.) actually mean? I will share with you what the Masters have shared with me about it.

S.I.N.

S" stands for separation from God. This happens when we live an ego-driven life or when the ego has gone awry. "**S**" also stands for the Shadow self that dwells within the subconscious mind. It contains many, if not all, of the most negative, critical and perverse thoughts and emotions of ourselves. These thoughts and emotions have been perpetuated by our society and those around us at an early age of life telling us what is right and wrong. They stay with us and hide within many of our body's organs, our DNA and aura throughout most of our lives until it is acknowledged or finally healed. **"I" stands for Id.** This is a Freudian term describing our basic instinctual human drive. "It is a source of bodily needs, wants, desires, and impulses, particularly sexual or aggressive drives." **"N" stands for negativity,** which can be thought, feeling, action, or deed.

When we have S.I.N. in our lives and allow it to cast a huge shadow and veil over our Divine Self, it disrupts the innate harmony within us resulting in our egos becoming dysfunctional and suffocating our Divinity.

When this continues, it ultimately leads to a person who becomes the center of their own delusional universe where they care only about themselves and are always seeking for what is in it for them. God is no longer important in their lives and they now see themselves as God and may feel superior to all others due to their ability to amass much material things. The ego hungers and desires for power, material things, the flesh, wealth, fame and attention. The ego's appetite is never fully satisfied, and it does what it wants at all cost, including compromising the lives of others. Humanity's out of balance ego has created an ego perpetuated reality that enslaved all of humanity and all of Life. Now, however, the great awakening from this illusion is underway.

It is our collective S.I.N., the greed of the dysfunctional ego and attachment to the things that we have created (also called miscreation due to their negative energy) that creates and perpetuates human suffering, and the subsequent suffering of all Life, especially in this modern day and age. In fact, attachment or addiction to anything or anyone is one of the energies that keeps us a prisoner of misery and perpetuates suffering.

In the past, S.I.N., greed and attachment gave birth to many corporations and industries all around the world in all sectors of life including healthcare, entertainment, technology, social media, the food industry, the oil industry, the power grid industry, etc. Corporations themselves are not bad things. Many of them have given back to society in their donations to schools, churches and other social groups. However, when greed is the driving force of our actions due to corporate shareholders, advancement in technology, industrialization, mass production, and pressing deadlines, we are creating a scenario that will lead to the increased human suffering and the continued destruction of Earth and all of her kingdoms.

Perhaps the corporate world feels that there is just too little time to ponder the harmful effects of what their companies have on the lives of the customers, humanity and Earth overall? Or perhaps they feel it is not cost-effective to discuss and research adverse effects? Or perhaps the bottom line is just more important than the well-being of humanity, Mother Earth and Mother Nature?

We all know that many corporations, industries and we as consumers are depleting the resources of Mother Earth at an alarming rate. We are draining her blood by our voracious appetite for fossil fuel. We have depleted much of the mineral rich soil on our planet. We have destroyed much of the various rainforests and trees which in turn has altered the ecosystems, weather and now her climates. We have contaminated our oceans, sky and water supply with chemicals and toxins from our cars, planes, plastics and industries. Even our food supply is filled with various chemicals, preservatives, dyes, hormones, antibiotics, gluten, GMOs, etc. just for the sake of profits.

What these companies may or may not realize is that there is a price to pay for high profits, mass production, and the raping and polluting of Earth, our home. We reap what we sow, no matter who we are. The actions of our collective population (corporations, industries and us as consumers) has created a karma that all humanity must face. This karma manifests itself as suffering for humanity, all Creatures great and small and Mother Earth.

What types of suffering are there? There are physical, mental, emotional and spiritual forms of suffering. Mental illnesses are on the rise. Many diseases including cancer, heart disease, diabetes, dementia, autoimmune diseases, end stage renal disease, etc. have continued to rise in epic proportions.

It is not a time to blame one another, but a time to heal and change. Although we cannot change all the variables in our lives overnight, every moment we can make positive choices to heal ourselves, Earth and her kingdoms. Choices of what we eat, drink, think, feel, act, and experience, changes both small and large are created from the inside out.

Although there are many external factors (pollution, toxins, radiation, blue light, heavy metals, etc.) around us that contribute to our suffering, we also create our own suffering by what we eat, drink and how we take care of ourselves including our spiritual well-being. Most of us are not hydrated enough and drink poor quality water. Many of us are often on the run, eating either fast or processed foods and too much sugar. On top of that, without the tools of staying in inner peace and balance, most people are experiencing high degrees of stress.

Most illnesses begin with emotional or mental body imbalances or disharmony that over time negatively influence the physical body. Prolonged stress shuts down the immune system. Emotional and mental stresses often result in people making poor choices of diet and self-care. Poor Self-worth and low levels of Self-Love can perpetuate a lack of interest in caring for our body temples. This in turn can result in addictions to food, alcohol, drugs and other activities that further the negative impacts to the whole body resulting in diseases, both acute and chronic.

**Stress → Poor Choices → Poor Self Love →
Imbalances in Multibody System → Illness → Death**

Prolonged stress, poor self-esteem and the poor choices we make with what we eat, drink and do to our bodies lead to imbalance and disharmony within us which may result in diabetes, heart disease, kidney failure, heart attacks, strokes, anxiety disorders, depression, cancer, and many autoimmune diseases.

This will make it extremely difficult to experience our True Divine nature to the fullest. We may be caught in a vicious cycle of disharmony and dysfunction that spirals out of control and lead to our premature demise and we will have to repeat our karmic cycle of rebirth again if we have not attained great spiritual mastery yet.

It is difficult to attain our mastery when our various body systems are out of sync. In order for us to transcend our sufferings including our repeated rebirths, we must review our roots before we incarnated into this physical reality.

Before we incarnated on Earth, we were spiritual beings of Light full of love, harmony and peace, free from pain, sufferings and limitations. We were, in essence, God-Realized beings that created and manifested what we wanted, and we transcended the time and space spectrum and limits. We were able to explore the Universe and embody whatever form we chose in order to experience the different flavors of life so to speak.

We had this incredible oneness with God, Source and I AM Presence in the beginning of time. However, through time, we began to identify more with the things we incarnated into than with God. We delighted more in the material world than the spiritual world or realms. We began to align ourselves and identified ourselves more with the ego and began losing that connection with our I AM Presence. The Collective Ego identification and withdrawal of the I AM Presence is the real fall from grace, and as humanity spiraled out of control, it created the essence of suffering of life on Mother Earth.

Therefore, in order to end the suffering, we must evolve back into that spiritual being of Light that we once were. That can happen if we live in harmony of body, mind and spirit and live in alignment with God's Love instead of our ego gone awry. Our collective dysfunctional ego has caused billions to suffer on Earth as well as cause much suffering to Mother Earth.

The only solution to end all suffering is to end our own sufferings, evolve into a being of Light and evolve further into what I call a Modern-Day Yogi. Anyone can be a Modern-Day Yogi if they are willing to learn, to change the way they live, eat, drink and to embody their I AM Presence.

They must learn to meditate in order to attain God Consciousness and allow their ego to be displaced by God's Consciousness and perfect love for us. Studying yoga is helpful but is not a prerequisite to being one with God (although it does help to make it easier for one to become One with God). It has more to do with expanding one's consciousness to join with God's consciousness through meditation, devotion and spiritual practices. By learning the yogic breathing techniques, visualization and (the meditation system the Ascended Masters taught me) or Kriya Yoga, one can dissolve the ego, the self and experience the Holy Communion and marriage of God Consciousness.

What is a Modern-Day Yogi? It is a term I coined for an individual who is on a path to God Consciousness or Realization but understands the complexities and issues affecting the body systems we have. He or she has an understanding of the elements of how they affect the four lower bodies - physical, mental, emotional, and etheric. He or she has an understanding that we are all part of a whole that is bigger than each of us individually.

Not only is the individual aware of the complexities of Life, in addition, she or he practices harmony in all that he or she does with the body, mind, emotion and spirit. The awareness how our energy ripples out into our world and Universe is constantly in his or her awareness and is a constant guide. The Modern-Day Yogi strives towards mastery of non-attachment to material things and strives towards oneness with Cosmic Light, Love and the Consciousness within all Life.

He or she also sees the patterns of the Universe within and without and realizes that enlightenment, integration of the ego and establishing wellness, harmony and peace within is only a primary level of spiritual evolution. When the individual becomes what I call a Modern-Day Yogi, he or she is involved in a regular meditation practice and works on internal healing and balance as well as sending those healing energies to our Mother Earth as well as into the rest of the Universe. The individual sends healing light and energy to the planet and Universe with no limitation of space and time through the help of the Ascended Masters and God.

These Yogis need not go into spiritual hibernation for months or years but live a relatively normal life that illuminates God's Love and Light in whatever he or she does and in whatever vocation he or she pursues. The goal of the Modern-Day Yogi is being one with God's Consciousness, Love and Light and realizing that all matter and all of creation regardless of how great or small are all a part of the infinite and ever-expanding Consciousness of God.

There are many who will argue with me on what a Yogi is, but if it doesn't resonate with you that is fine. You can call it something else that resonates with you like an Enlightened Being of Light or something else. Names, labels and titles are not as important as being united in Spirit through Divine Love. I just gave a name that represents a way of life that leads to God realization and oneness with our Creator.

Yogis are not limited to those who practice Yoga, are Hindus, or live in India. There are many Tibetan Buddhist Masters who I consider a Yogi. One of the most famous ones includes Milarepa and Padmasambhava. Even Jesus is considered a Yogi. Did Jesus come to be worshipped or did he come to empower humanity to discover their true God nature?

Jesus said, "I have said, 'You are gods; and all of you are children of the Most High'." (John 10:34). "Verily, verily, I say unto you, he that believeth on me, the works that I do shall he do also; *and greater works* than these shall he do, because I go unto my Father." (John 14:12). **(R 5)**

My books will support you in your journey in becoming a Modern Yogi and Being of Light. Becoming a Modern Yogi is crucial for the survival of our civilization and Mother Earth (although she is suffering much and appears to be heading towards destruction, she will always survive beyond us despite our toxic consciousness and behaviors; when she has reached her threshold of toxicity from us, she will find a way to reset herself so to speak and give birth again to a new civilization).

We need Mother Earth more than she needs us. Many awakened and enlightened beings around the world are aware of how much abuse we are doing to Mother Earth and are taking actions to save humanity and her.

If we become a Modern-Day Yogi, we can help even more in a global way. We can send positive healing energy to Mother Earth and into the Universe. Mastery of being a Modern-Day Yogi comes from within first. The first step is to restore unity between our God Self (Presence) and our Earth expression; to become one with God. Then we are able to co-create with God a Universe within that is full of bliss, peace, harmony, balance and have a good flow of energy or Qi. When that happens, and we allow God's Love, Light and Energy to fill our heart, mind and soul, we allowing God to manifest a heaven within our inner Universe. When we allow that Light and Energy to illuminate and radiate to those around us, we begin creating Heaven in our immediate space, Mother Earth and beyond.

Humanity has really made a mess of Earth and all life upon her. It will take a concerted effort between those who are awakened, enlightened and empowered like the Modern-Day Yogis to bring greater balance and harmony to our beloved Mother Earth.

Being a Modern-Day Yogi will accelerate the healing of the planet and neutralize much of the toxic energy on the planet created by our collective consciousness.

Being a Modern-day Yogi is what it will take to truly end the suffering of our self, Earth and all of humanity. Once we attain this, we can transcend the laws of karma and finally end the rebirth cycle unless we choose to come back. Our journey must not stop until we have awakened as many people as we can to end their suffering and teach them how to be set free.

Let me elaborate a little more about the rebirth cycle so that you can understand it more fully as well as about S.I.N. and our spiritual suffering.

When we die, our souls leave our physical bodies and enter the next realm or phase of consciousness or reality. Those who are living in spiritual poverty (those who live an ego driven life), will return to earth by default due to lack of preparation and readiness to move forward on their spiritual evolution. Those individuals are bounded by the laws of karma and will be reincarnated into a new body and for the most part will exist as a clean slate.

Those who are more spiritually evolved often have some memories of their past lives. Lives will repeat over and over until the individual is able to awaken from their spiritual coma, discover their true Divine nature, cultivate and purify themselves until they have attained a high level of spiritual mastery or what I call Cosmic Harmony. This is where the individual remembers that he or she is One with his or her Divine Self and all of Creation, including Mother Earth, the Universe, the Ascended Masters and God.

Until then, each life time of disharmony will create a certain degree of karma that will follow the individual from one life time to the next until the individual finally wakes up and remembers what he or she is supposed to learn in order to move up to the next level spiritual evolution and consciousness. This is a spiritual suffering that can go on for many lifetimes. Such suffering is essentially a repeated death sentence perpetuated by our S.I.N.

According to the Bible, the wages of sin is death. (Romans 6:23). That death is the repetition of the birth and rebirth cycle with no conscious awareness of who we really are as Divine Beings who are One with God. Buddhists call this samsara. This is the real hell we should try to break free from for our own salvation. The other Hell is the one we create from the shadows of our consciousness or from our egos that have gone awry.

That death is also a literal one as well. The sin of our collective consciousness results in the premature death of our bodies; as a result of decades of breathing, drinking and eating toxic chemicals in our air, water and food supply. Our Spirit is indeed eternal, but the body is its temple upon Earth and degrades and reacts adversely to being continuously bombarded by the toxins we have co- created. We must honor and respect our sacred temple of God. The better stewards we are of it, the longer we can stay in that earthly temple and navigate through life much more gracefully.

Although the toxic milieu we have created from our ego perpetuated reality and collective S.I.N. seems so dismal, overwhelming and bleak, there is still hope for us. By stilling or quieting our minds, looking within and opening our hearts to the great messages that are constantly being sent to us from the Universe, from Source, God, the Ascended Masters

13

and other Angelic Beings, we are able to journey deeply into the truth of Life- the truth that we are all interconnected and that we are all One.

When we look within and without, we see a certain harmony, balance, beauty and order that flow so majestically and perfectly. Everything seems to be orchestrated in such a Divine symphony by some incredible and higher intelligence I call Supreme Consciousness, Source or God. He or she connects and animates with all of Creation and Matter in the Universe through its Cosmic Web that penetrates everything at its core with God's Divine Spark of Light, I AM Presence and Cosmic Divine Presence. When we align ourselves with our Divine Presence within and become one with the Cosmos, we become one with God's Consciousness which is full of love, perfection, order, bliss, and harmony. This happens when our human awareness intersects with our awareness of our true Divine Nature and alignment with our I AM Presence.

This way of being leads us to radiant health and well-being. This is the way of life of Mystics, Arahants, Siddhas and Yogis. They do it by way of meditation, yogic breathing techniques, and spiritual practices and by what they ate. Many have achieved long harmonious, vibrant and blissful lives during a time that was free of toxic air, water, food, fruits and vegetables. As mentioned earlier, some lived to be as old as 256 years of age. In this current day and age. One siddha in India is 130 years of age and is full of physical and mental vitality, according to Romarishi who personally knows this saint.

Due to the ego perpetuated illusion we have co-created, modern day Mystics, Yogis and siddhas face a great challenge in achieving the ultimate harmony of body, mind and spirit. The attainment of inner and outer harmony requires that we step out of the illusion of separation, embracing unity and oneness in its stead. We must also relearn how to eat, drink, meditate and pray in a way that is in alignment with our Divine Nature. It helps tremendously for us to tune in to our I AM Presence and follow the Cosmic flow and harmony of life.

In the next few chapters, we will explore how we can gracefully navigate through the obstacles and barriers that are the side effects of an ego-driven civilization. When we allow it, they can limit us from experiencing the inner harmony, peace, bliss and radiance that we were meant to experience. The journey towards achieving inner cosmic harmony requires removing all those obstacles that compromise our physical, emotional and spiritual well-being.

May you allow the words in this book to guide you in your journey to re-establishing that harmony, order and perfection that our Mother and Father who art in Heaven originally created for you. Aligning ourselves to that harmony, God's Consciousness and Love will set you and others free. It will also assist in ending the suffering that so many millions of people and Life as a whole have been enduring needlessly. Let us begin our journey by rethinking how we can eat, drink, pray and meditate our way into being a modern-day Yogi and learning how to create Heaven on Earth and from within.

For the wages of sin is death,
but the gift of God is eternal life
in Christ Jesus our Lord. (Romans 6:23)

"Let food be thy medicine and medicine be thy food."

~

Hippocrates

CHAPTER 2

EATING YOUR WAY INTO HARMONY

Currently, there is much chaos and disharmony within humanity and our planet due to our ego perpetuated reality that humanity has collectively created. We could blame corporations, companies and industries for it, or we can begin to take responsibility for what we have created and take the necessary steps to resolve these global challenges.

Our journey to creating greater harmony begins with what we eat and drink. We are what we eat and drink. If we eat junk food, processed food and fast food all the time, we begin to damage our God-given, innate ability to heal ourselves (our Inner Healer). We may begin to develop high cholesterol or high blood pressure and may accumulate high amounts of plaque in our arteries. Over time, this way of eating may lead also to diabetes which opens the door to many other diseases and illnesses including blindness, stroke, kidney failure or even a heart attack. Eating toxic food makes our bodies more acidic which is an ideal environment for many diseases to thrive within.

Whenever we eat something, we should always ask ourselves if the food is energetically nutritious = supporting our body to function with great harmony and efficiency. We all have our vices, but the key thing is balance. Junk food is intentionally created to be addictive. Once we get started eating it, our gut health becomes imbalanced, creating a type of addiction within our physical body, and also, in time, our mental and emotional ones as well. Then we begin craving it, and begin eating more than we should, and soon we become a slave to our food resulting in disharmony within the body. We may end up gaining an exorbitant amount of weight which puts stress on the heart, digestive system, joints and diaphragm making it hard for us to breathe and move around.

Most junk foods (processed food, fast food, cookies, cakes, candy, chips, fried food and sodas) are filled with either too much sodium, saturated and trans-fats, carbohydrates, sucrose, and high fructose corn syrup. On top of that they are filled with all types of preservatives, dyes and other foreign chemicals which will contribute to the chaos and disharmony within the body; hence the name "junk food". In general, avoid refined sugar, flour, white bread greasy food and unhealthy fats and eat healthy carbohydrates like fruits, vegetables, wholegrain and real food and healthy fats given to us by our Creator and not manufactured by us.

Our bodies were created to be sustained by real food - food that is organic, wholesome and chemical free. The body responds well to fresh fruits and vegetables since they are full of phytonutrients and sun healing energy. The phytonutrients they have from their skin contain antioxidants and helps minimize the inflammation within our bodies that contribute to pain. They also contain fiber which helps with gut health and decreases the bad cholesterol in our bodies like LDL. Fruits are especially important because they are the best source of glucose that our body needs for energy and health. Our body utilizes plant-based protein well. Anthony William, known as the Medical Medium, and author of three best sellers, discourages his readers from consuming animal-based protein due to its negative effects on the digestive system (the liver and spleen).

When something puts more stress on our organs, it is disharmonious to our body and should be avoided or at least minimized. Those that choose to consume meat, chicken or fish, should be mindful and what type they choose. Chicken without hormones would be best. Wild fish is better than farmed fish because farm fish may contain antibiotics that are used to prevent illnesses due to crowded conditions. It must be noted that ocean fish may contain mercury or radiation from the Fukushima nuclear accident. There are methods of removing the mercury in our body that we will be discussing later.

In order to create a world of harmony, humanity must leave behind the killing and consuming animals. They are conscious sentient beings too that have fear, anxiety and suffer when they are caught and butchered. They have as much right to thrive and live as we do. When they are butchered, they suffer and that agony sends an energetic signal that goes throughout the creature as a wave of suffering. Do we really want to consume and perpetuate suffering?

Understanding that we are what we eat, the logical answer is "no". Suffering begets more suffering. Thus, eating and living a vegan or plant-based diet comes with the territory of becoming an enlightened being or a Yogi, as being in a state of harmony is required to achieve the state of enlightenment.

Education Versus Judgement

Although being a vegetarian or vegan is the ultimate path of a Yogi, we should never judge those who are still meat eaters and are not quite ready to make that transition. I have heard about people who were verbally assaulted and called a murderer because they ate meat. When we judge, we begin to regress in our spiritual evolution. Judgement, hate and abomination are some of the lowest level of emotions keeping people prisoners to their egos. Instead of judging others, it is better to enlighten others through educating them about how what they eat affects their well-being and the well-being of our planet. Studies have shown eating a meat diet is not good for our well-being, the well-being of the animals, or of Mother Earth, leading to a host of diseases, destruction and suffering.

Peter Singer, author of **Animal Liberation** and many other great books cited a Harvard study that spanned over 20 years and involved over 100,000 people about how meat was not good for our health. He elaborated on the study during a debate about whether meat should be out of the restaurants or not. The study showed that even a small consumption of red meat would increase the participants of the study chances of dying from a variety of diseases including cardiovascular diseases, cancer and diabetes. **(R 6)**

Peter suggests that we should educate others about the inhumane ways in which animals are crowded together for slaughter, fed antibiotics due

19

to crowdedness and how much their manure and methane disrupts our ecological system affecting climate change. He also reminds us of how animals are also sentient beings who should be respected and treated as such. Countries around the world are now beginning to declare animals as sentient, and are changing their treatment of them accordingly.

There are also other ecological implications of eating meat, chicken, farmed fishes or any animal-based diet. Many natural resources (water, protein and land) are used to farm the food needed to be used to feed the source of our animal-based diet which leads to deforestation. We are literally depleting our planet of our water and land and destroying our rainforests because of our insatiable appetite for meat which will leads to a metaphorical cancer of our planet's lung. Less forest equates to less oxygen produced.

There is also mounting evidence that a plant-based diet offers health benefits across the board for athletes as well as those who have heart disease, diabetes, congestive heart failure, cancer, etc. Moreover, there is much evidence about the harmful effects of an animal-based diet on our energy, health, longevity, endurance and even our libido. The best movie to watch that explains all this objectively, medically as well as scientifically is called *Game Changer.* I highly recommend this outstanding documentary film. I believe it is one of the best and most important films of the decade. It is available on Netflix.

It is also good to show meat eaters videos of how traumatized these animals are when they are awaiting their slaughter or when they are being slaughtered if indicated. Another option is to share the video of an objective debate between those who are pro-meat versus those who are vegan. One such video is entitled "Should Meat Be Off the Menu?". This video is full of facts about health and environmental, which may shift their choices and way of thinking. Visit the link at: **(R 7)**

Before we judge others, please consider and realize that even plants and vegetables have a consciousness. Dr. Jagdish Chandra Bose (India's first biophysicist) proved that plants react to both loving and painful stimuli. Paramahansa Yogananda witnessed this experiment on a plant and wrote about it in his book, *Autobiography of a Yogi.*

Dr. Bose once wrote, "all around us, the plants are communicating. We just do not notice it." He also wrote about how plants grew more quickly when exposed to nice music and gentle whispers, and poorly when exposed to harsh music and loud speech. He even mentioned how plants became depressed. **(R 8)**

Another example of the consciousness of plants was created by Dr. Marcel Vogel who tested plants with his Vogel wand and found that they reacted to his thoughts through his crystal design and invention. When he retired his lab was filled with over $500,000 of equipment donated by IBM at the time of Marcel's retirement. His gadgets included an electron scanning microscope, a Zeiss Ultraphot microscope, an Omega 5 radionic instrument, and a Cary Model 15 spectrophotometer. Within his lab Marcel began a childlike curiosity to discover a new perspective on human-plant communication. Are plants capable of emotions and sensing human thought? Marcel thought so and was able to duplicate **the Backster Effect**, which showed that plants are able to respond to a variety of physical and chemical stimuli including emotions and thoughts. **(R 9)**

Marcel Joseph Vogel (1917-1991) was a research scientist for IBM's San Jose facility for 27 years. He received numerous patents for his inventions during this time. In the 1970's Marcel did some pioneering work in man-plant communication experiments. This led him to the study of quartz crystals and the creation of a faceted crystal that is now known as the Vogel-cut˚ crystal. The Vogel-cut˚ crystal is an instrument that serves to store, amplify, convert, and cohere subtle energies **(R 10)**

What about the good bacteria that thrive in our guts? They too are living and have consciousness. When we eat poorly and have a lot of stress, we create harsh conditions for them and make it hard for them to survive. Are we not in a way contributing to their demise and in so doing compromising our own health? If we take an antibiotic, it is like a nuclear bomb for our gut. It kills the bad bacteria as well as the good ones. We are then in a way responsible for the killings of billions of good bacteria. Think about that before judging others. Instead, have compassion towards others. Be patient and educate others about how all of Creation has consciousness.

With regards to the plants, vegetables, fruits, crystals and the mineral kingdom, they all have some form of consciousness. I consider them very highly advanced expressions of consciousness who incarnate to give of their essence (nutrients and pranic energy) for the betterment of life on Earth. They come to serve us for a noble cause to help us restore the harmony in our bodies, minds and souls.

Changing to Plant-Based Eating

In my experience, being a vegetarian has not been an easy job, but it is well worth the initial challenges. I thought getting enough protein was very hard initially until I understood how much highly available protein fruits, vegetables, nuts and seeds contain. Having adequate protein is very important for our muscles, skin, bones, and for many of our enzymes and hormones. It is important for the healing of our body.

Fortunately, there are many options and methods of getting plant-based protein now. There are plant-based powder mixes. I took Vega myself initially; the one I took contained 20 grams of protein. Eventually I switched to Garden of Life's Raw Organic Protein which contains 22 grams of protein. One of the reasons I switched is because Vega contained soy. The product Raw Organic Protein is USDA Organic, Non- GMO Verified, Vegan, dairy free and soy free. I find it a good healthy source of protein supplement. I am not much of a fan of the taste but a great fan of the product which also contains probiotics and enzymes.

Many body builders take whey protein, but Anthony William, Medical Medium, warns that it is inflammatory to the body because it contains gluten. The much-debated question is how much protein we truly require for optimal health. According to a nutritionist I consulted, we can calculate how much protein per day we need by dividing our weight in half. That will give us the number of grams per day we need for our sustenance. An individual who weighs one hundred pounds would need 50 grams of protein per day or 16 to 17 grams of protein per meal.

On the other hand, my personal trainer, Vladimir Beltran, stated that 80 percent of our weight is what he recommended as the amount of protein we require to eat per day. In this scenario the same person who weighs one hundred pounds should be eating 80 grams of protein per day or 26 to 27 grams per meal. In fact, I followed this method and was able to eat plenty of quality protein and lost 13 pounds of fat which was converted to muscles instead and my hunger pain was minimized.

According to Professor Brian Peskin, BSEE-MIT, there is a minimum amount of protein requirement per day which is 0.8 gm protein/day per kg of body weight. A person one hundred pound would be 45.3592 kg. Multiply that by .8 grams, we get 36.28 grams of protein. However, he quickly points out that this amount would keep you alive, but not provide radiant health. He believes that we need only 30-40 grams of high-quality protein per day. **(R 11)**

I tried both ways and found that eating half my body weight in grams was good but eating eighty percent of my weight per day in grams plus exercise helped me to achieve radiant health and avoid excessive hunger pangs.

When I ate 30-40 grams, I was quite hungry during the end of the day and developed a huge craving. Eating enough protein will allow your body to function properly, lose weight, and heal, but eating too much can cause health related problems with the kidneys. Getting enough protein appears to be related to one's activity level. The higher the level of activity, the more protein one needs. The athlete would need more than a couch potato. Many people are jumping on the bandwagon with high protein diets but how high is high is somewhat debatable.

However, if in doubt, get a blood test and check your creatine level and blood urea nitrogen (BUN) levels, if it is high then consult with your physician and nutritionist on how you could adjust your diet to support your goals while keeping your kidneys healthy. Regular checkups with your physician and getting lab works will help you keep tabs on your protein levels.

On the other hand, many people such as Anthony William, speak quite passionately about protein, but in ways contrary to mainstream knowledge. Anthony believes that there is too much focus on protein and the possibility that we may be consuming too much. He, and other health experts, are concerned that there is too much emphasis on protein and not enough on the many other nutrients our bodies require for radiant health, especially those in seeds, fruits and vegetables. **(R 12)**

Here is a formula I came up with that might help you choose how much protein is best. I feel that it is best to eat somewhere between 30 to 40 grams of protein per day and go up to 50 to 80 percent of our body weight in grams depending on our activity level. An athlete may need much more protein if he or she is body building or working out hard. Your nutritionist or personal trainer can help you calculate more specifically according to the needs of your body and activity level. If we have some health issue, it may behoove us to eat less than 50 grams of protein.

Some experts feel that if we eat 50 grams of protein or more a day every day, it could lead to various illnesses or diseases. It is important that we tune into the needs of our own body based on our nutritional needs, metabolism and life style.

Factors for the proper amount of protein should take into consideration your age, weight, activity level, medical status and overall health. Also, it is deeply important for us to tune into our bodies and see how we are feeling day to day. Those who are quite intuitive or tuned in to their body should take heed of the inner guidance of how much protein you may need. Otherwise, most people should consult a nutritionist or dietician.

Anthony William suggests that three popular sources of protein - eggs, cheese and milk - can be problematic. The first two contain much fat and feed the bugs in our bodies such as the Epstein Barr Virus (EBV). They also grow cysts and tumors. He cautions about milk as well because it feeds the strep and bugs in our body. Instead, he encourages us to eat healthy sources of protein like spinach, nori seaweed and Hawaiian Spirulina. They are noted to contain good amounts of protein as well as micro and macro nutrients and minerals which are necessary for good health.

Anthony William points out that it is really the fat and calories within protein that satisfies our hunger pangs on a high protein diet. Earlier I also believed that it was eating enough protein that helped me get through the day, but Anthony's information makes more sense. Anthony essentially wants us to eat only enough high-quality proteins that our body needs and encourages us to also eat fruits and vegetables for the protein, calories and micronutrients which offer health and healing properties. If you are still eating beef for any reason, he recommends grass fed beef since they do not feed the bugs in our bodies. There are other plant-based options to get much healthier sources of protein.

Other Good Sources of Protein

Other great, plant-based sources of protein include hemp seeds, pumpkin seeds, non-dairy yogurt, nuts, broccoli, beans, legumes, almond butter, avocados, etc. flax and chia seeds also contain some protein. Vegetables like broccoli, spinach, pea, kale, Brussels sprouts, mushrooms, asparagus, artichoke, corn, etc. are also a good source of protein.

Now that you have a general idea of some healthy protein, you can incorporate them into your diet and meal preparation. Those of you who are on the go and have limited time to cook or shop, may be delighted to know that there are many pre-made protein meal options out there that are quite delicious.

Transitional Foods

The company *Beyond Meat* makes an excellent plant-based burger with 20 grams of protein. It is becoming more widely available in stores and restaurants far and wide. Wholefoods and Trader's Joe are great places to get a variety of plant-based protein meals. Even Safeway has a section for them.

However, many of these tasty plant- based protein meals contain added ingredients that may not be good for the body. I call them transitional foods (TF). They are helpful for someone who is transitioning from being an omnivore or flexitarian to a vegetarian or vegan, but the foods are not meant to be a primary source of sustenance over the long-term.

Another T.F. that I have tried is *Hilary's Hemp and Green Burger*. I found it healthier than most of the other transitional foods out there. It is Non-GMO, organic, Certified Gluten- free, Vegan and Kosher. Most of the ingredients are healthy and things I can read and understand. ***Here is a guideline … if you do not know what an ingredient or additive is in your food, do not buy it or eat it!***

Being a vegan or vegetarian requires that we learn even more about our bodies and the nutrients in foods. It may seem difficult to achieve, but millions around the world have successfully achieved it and are thriving being fully plant-based and more are making the shift every day.

Fresh is Best!

Another blessing is that there are more and more great vegan and vegetarian restaurants around. So being a vegetarian and vegan at this time is the perfect time. However, preparing your own organic plant-based foods is the ideal way of creating harmony. Many of the vegetables made to look and taste like meat have many additives added for taste but may not be good for you if consumed long term.

One of the issues of being a vegetarian or vegan is that some people may not be getting enough iron and are anemic. Kathryn Shanti Ariel, The Nature Whisperer, reminds us that "iron deficiencies can be an issue for anybody. Vitamin deficiencies can exist with any diet. One of the steps of mastery of a Yogi is to be aware of the body and what it is telling us."

There are many plant-based foods that contain good levels of iron. According to health line, the following foods contain iron: Black strap molasses, legumes: tofu, tempeh, natto, soybeans, lentils, beans, peas, nuts, seeds, pumpkin, sesame, hemp, flax-seeds. (I prefer non-GMO and organic sources especially for soybeans and tofu as a healthier choice.) Otherwise, eating fresh fruits and vegetables is the best way to go! Fresh is always best!

Interview with Andrei Volhonttseff

Nutritionist and owner of Valley Health Mills in Pleasanton, California. Andrei Volhonttseff, stated that Soy is a source of phytoestrogens called isoflavones. Too many soy isoflavones in the diet can depress thyroid function and cause hypothyroidism, which can lead to other health problems such as, cancer, diabetes, heart disease and depressed immunity.

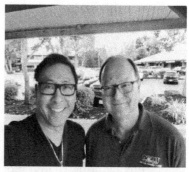

Soy is suspected of increasing risk for breast cancer in at least one study and also thyroid cancer and infertility. (R 13) Several studies appear to show a link with soy products like tofu with cognitive impairment. In a large study *Blake Sinclair with Andrei Volhonttseff* done in Hawaii with Japanese-American seniors. Those who ate soy and tofu more than a couple of times per week had higher rates of senile dementia. (R 14)

Vegetables - Another Source of Iron include leafy greens like spinach, kale, Swiss chard, collard and beet greens. Bitter melon is also a good source of iron. In addition to many vegetables being a good source of iron, they are also a good source of fiber and micronutrients like calcium, Vitamin B-12, and Zinc. According to Onegreenplanet.org, vegetables are important part of healthy eating and provide a source of many nutrients, including potassium, fiber, folate (folic acid) and vitamins A, E and C. **(R 15)**

Besides eating organic plant-based foods, I have found Natures **Plus Hema-Plex*** quite effective for the anemic individual. It contains 85 mg of Elemental Iron. My wife was dangerously low with her iron at one point where her level was 6.8. She was extremely weak, pale and anemic. She quickly went to see her physician who recommended she get I.V. iron immediately, but my wife had an adverse allergic reaction and hence was not a candidate for I.V. iron. Instead, she started to take Hema-plex as well as eating foods and vegetables rich in iron for about a week and noticed that she began to have more energy and felt better. After a few weeks, she was back to her old self. She took another blood test and found that her iron level had improved significantly and was closer to normal range. Natures Hema-plex is available online and various store locations.

Cooking with an iron skillet is also a good way to ingest natural iron. When food that contains iron and is cooked in an iron skillet, it naturally increases the amount of iron in it.

Despite protein being a very important part of our diet and getting enough iron, we need to have other nutrients to create more harmony in our body. We also need fruits' phytonutrients and micronutrients. Many experts write about the importance of getting enough fruits in our diet since they contain a good source of glucose that our body needs for energy, health and the protection of our brain.

Fruits are a delicious and necessary part of our health and well-being because they contain vitamins (vitamin A, vitamin B6, vitamin C, vitamin E and vitamin K), minerals, antioxidants, fiber, potassium, folate acid, magnesium, sodium, etc.

OrganicFacts.net is a wonderful online resource for learning more about fruits and their many body blessings. They also have a focus on particular imbalances that can be assisted. See the link: **(R 16)** Fruits support the healing ability of our bodies, shield and protect us and allow us to have the energy to enjoy life. Without them, it would be difficult for us to thrive.

Vegetables contain many nutrients and are also a good source of prebiotics and fiber. In addition, eating fruits and vegetables on a daily basis can help decrease our risk of heart diseases, diabetes, stroke, chronic diseases and many autoimmune diseases. **(R 17)**

When we talk about non-organic fruits and vegetables, many people are very concerned about the pesticides and how to remove them. Many people use a mixture of water and vinegar to remove the pesticides. The common formula is four parts of water to one-part white vinegar. Some feel that apple cider vinegar or organic white vinegar is better. Some people also add **Essential Oxygen Plus Hydrogen Peroxide 3% Food Grade** as well. It is recommended to soak the fruits or vegetables in the mixture for about 20 to 30 minutes. Thereafter, rinse it thoroughly. I would use filtered water to clean them to reduce ingestion of toxins from the water. Another method is submersing the fruits and vegetables in a pot of water and adding 1 teaspoon to 1 tablespoon of baking soda. Allow it to soak for 15 to 20 minutes then rinse thoroughly.

The Dirty Dozen and Clean 15

There are 12 fruits and vegetables that are known as the **Dirty Dozen.** Eating or growing these organically is important in our health living practice. They include:

- Strawberries
- Spinach
- Kale
- Nectarines
- Apples
- Imported Grapes
- Peaches
- Cherries
- Pears
- Tomatoes
- Celery
- Potatoes

Meanwhile, there are **15 non-organic fruits** and vegetables that are relatively safe to eat due to their skins which are more resistant to absorption.

The current 2020 list includes:

- Avocados
- Sweet corn
- Pineapples
- Onions
- Papayas
- Sweet peas (frozen)
- Eggplant
- Asparagus
- Cauliflower
- Cantaloupe
- Broccoli
- Mushrooms
- Cabbage
- Honeydew melon
- Kiwi

Creating a Rhythm in Your Eating

Besides eating protein, fruits, fats and vegetables, we need to be mindful of the harmony of eating. Binge eating is never good for the body and makes your digestive system work overly hard. Prolonged or extended fasting can also be hard on your body systems unless you are in peak spiritual shape where your body is creating its own nutrients. What does being in peak spiritual shape mean? Some spiritual masters have reportedly been able to produce honey and milk from their pineal gland for sustenance. Other saints and Mystics have been able to live on pranic energy with little to no food at all. Until you have attained such abilities, it is best to eat in a way that creates harmony within.

Being mindful of the calories, nutrients and macros of our diet is part of ensuring that our body is getting enough of what it requires to thrive. Each one of us requires a certain minimum amount of calories and nutrients for proper sustenance.

With regard to macro nutrients, there is a percentage ratio of fats, carbohydrates, sodium, and protein that our body requires for weight loss, weight gain or maintaining our body weight. If we don't get enough protein, our body can go into starvation mode and will begin to crave the nutrients, both macro and micro, that it is not getting.

Many people respond to this by eating processed or junk food which can provide calories, but not the nutrients. Some refer to this as "empty calories". This can then perpetuate overeating. When we eat, we must be mindful and aware of the balance of eating.

- If we have too much protein it can impair our liver and kidneys while also feeding the bugs within our body.
- If we have too much fats and carbohydrates, we begin to gain weight.
- If we have too much unhealthy carbs and glucose, we can increase our unhealthy fat levels in our abdominal area and develop glycation where the glucose binds with protein molecules and creates stickiness in the arteries leading to hypertension and cardiac issues.
- If we don't have enough nutrients, our bodies' ability to heal itself is minimized and compromised.

Learning how to eat sensibly and with mindfulness will help us create more harmony and efficiency within our bodies. In this day and age of technology, there is an app called **"My Fitness Pal"**, which is user friendly and helps users gain a greater awareness of the balance of calorie, nutrients, and macros with regards to eating.

In addition to the importance of what we eat is how it is prepared. If you are choosing to cook with oils, many experts including Andrei believe that the best oil to use include coconut oil and ghee. Other oils like canola and extra-virgin olive oils are better poured on salad versus heating up on the stove since it has low smoke point which creates toxic smoke. Heating these oils can create lipid peroxides which may be carcinogenic according to Andrei.

Due to these challenges, many plant-based people are not using oils at all. Here are five reasons for not cooking with olive oil:

1. Monounsaturated fats in olive oil are not heat stable.
2. Heart-healthy polyphenols in olive oil are easily damaged by heat.

3. Heating olive oil destroys omega fatty acids.
4. Low smoke point – breathing in toxic smoke.
5. Many olive oils are not real.

According to Katja Heino from Savory Lotus, many of the health benefits of olive oil, like its oleic acid, polyphenols, and omega fatty acids are damaged by heating it. She even says that many things labeled as olive oil are not even olive oil. A study by the UC Davis in 2011 found that 78% of the five bestselling imported brands of olive oil did not meet the international sensory standards for extra virgin olive set by European regulators. **(R 18)**

Mary Vance from MaryVancenc.com, suggests that the following olive oils are the purest and healthiest: **(R 19)**

- Kirkland Organic
- Corto Olive
- California Olive Ranch
- McEvoy Ranch Organic

Besides protein, fruits and vegetables and eating well, it is extremely important to drink well. What we drink will either support of sustain us in harmony or it could disrupt liver and kidney function. The most important thing to drink is purified water. It is the foundation to our health and well-being.

*To understand water is
to understand the cosmos,
the marvels of nature,
and life itself."*

~

Masaru Emoto

CHAPTER 3

WATER IS THE ESSENCE OF LIFE

Water is the essence of life. According to Dr. Masaru Emoto, "the average human body is 70 percent water. We start out life being 99 percent water, as fetuses. When we are born, we are 90 percent water, and by the time we reach adulthood we are down to 70 percent." (**R 20**)

Currently, due to choices made by humanity, the majority of our water supply from the reservoirs is contaminated. Many of our oceans are filled with plastics, sewage, mercury and radiation. Most of us are resorting to purchasing water from stores which are mostly kept in plastic containers which contain Bisphenol A (BPA). This chemical combined with plastic is carcinogenic, especially when exposed to the sunlight. Other options are filling reusable bottles with reverse osmosis at refill stations, getting a reverse osmosis or other water treatment system or at least the usage of some type of filter or filtration system in the house or business water systems.

In California, our water supply has fluoride added to it; a process called fluoridation. Other states, like Oregon, do not add it to their water supply. According to The International Academy of Oral Medicine and Toxicology (IAOMT), fluoride has been recognized as one of 12 industrial chemicals known to cause developmental neurotoxicity in human beings. Researchers have repeatedly challenged the alleged safety and effectiveness of fluoride.

According to Dr. Jon Dunn, Naturopathic Health Care, Inc., fluoride is an abundant mineral waste product of aluminum, phosphate, cement, steel and nuclear weapons manufacturing. **(R 21)**

It has also been linked with causing our pineal glands to calcify. As part of our body's Endocrine System, the pineal gland and pituitary gland functions are keys to communicating with our Divine Self or Godself. Calcification of these glands interferes with our spiritual awakening and evolution.

According to Global Healing Center, "the practice of water fluoridation has been rejected or banned in several countries including: China, Austria, Belgium, Finland, Germany, Denmark, Norway, Sweden, the Netherlands, Hungary, and Japan." **(R 22)**

Besides containing fluoride, tap water may also contain lead, copper and chlorine. According to Dr. Mercola, "most public water supplies are loaded with hazardous contaminants, such as disinfection byproducts (DBPs), fluoride, and pharmaceutical drugs." **(R 23)**

This growing awareness within people is why so many are purchasing filtration systems. **Lifetime Solutions and Kinetico** have great systems that remove toxins and hormones in our drinking water. **Kinetico** also has a special tank that removes the chlorine that goes through our shower head which may contribute to skin and other health issues when we get it on our skin or inhale the fumes.

Once the water is filtered through one of these systems, it is much safer to drink but it somewhat devoid of life force energy. One of the best waters to drink is Mount Shasta's Stewart Mineral Spring water. According to Dr. Masaru Emoto, it has a high amount of life force. Many people go to Mount Shasta Headwaters to collect the water that comes out of the underground aquifers of this sacred mountain. People love this water for its taste and what is believed to be its sacred and healing properties. The water travels for up to fifty years before emerging at the Mount Shasta City Park Headwaters having been filtered by the crystalline and volcanic rocks between the peaks of Mount Shasta which purifies all potential toxins.

However, unless you live at Mount Shasta, you and the rest of us are stuck with tap water. Actually, there are other wonderful fresh water aquifers coming to the surface at accessible springs. One source of finding them is https://www.findaspring.com **(R 24)**

Consciousness of Water

While we are learning how to return Earth's water back to its intended purity, there is another awareness that we can embrace. In his groundbreaking work, Dr. Masaru Emoto proved that due to water being alive and conscious we can change the energetic characteristic of the water molecules through our thoughts and intentions.

Dr. Emoto was able to show the world how writing certain words like love on a petri dish of water could change the molecular structure when the water was frozen. He discovered that words like love and gratitude would create beautiful and exquisite crystals; on the other hand, words with hate or anger would create distorted crystals. He also discovered how our thoughts and intentions could do the same. **(R 25)**

We can activate the energy of the water by writing positive and empowering words on the container of the water. I have done that as well as program the water with my intense concentration of pure love and healing energy and amplifying and intensifying that intention many folds through my Vogel Crystal wand. **(R 26)** I have also programmed the water with healing frequencies for an hour. When my mother was ill, I gave her this energized water to assist in healing her body. She found it quite nurturing and helpful.

Water and Body pH

Since our bodies are 70%+ water, the pH of water that we consume contributes greatly to maintaining our inner balanced pH. I like to also alkalinize my purified water with the **Wave Q.** I find that the water tastes lighter and better when it is more alkaline. Wave Q creates natural, mineral, alkaline, hexagonal-rich water with antioxidants. Drinking alkaline water helps the alkalinity of the body and hydrate the body with good absorption. **(R 27)**

In addition, I recently discovered an amazing machine that is conducive to harmony within the body. It is called the **Kangen 8.**

These devices filter your tap water, but they also produce ionized alkaline and acidic waters through electrolysis. These waters can be used for various purposes, including drinking, cooking, beauty and cleaning.

The nurse that told me about it stated it has helped to support the health of various family members who suffered from sciatica pain and cancer. My friend who is a homeopathic doctor stated that this is the primary system they use in Japan and is a system that she recommends.

Recently another friend of mine told me about a water machine that he has that creates ionized water. The machine is called **MMP-9090 Water Ionizer** and is made by **Tyent**. The machine creates an ionic charge in the water that passes through it which the company says helps to fight free radicals. The machine also creates various levels of alkaline and acidic water like the **K8** to be used for different purposes. It is also supposed to create hydrogen molecules in the water which are small enough to bring good hydration to all our cells. According to Steven Clarke, a Nano-Hydration Expert, the water from the machine could help with at least 170 different types of diseases or conditions. **(R 28)**

Tyent MMP-9090 TURBO Water Ionizer Features Snap Shot
- Automatic water outflow
- Voice announcement
- Touch screen with multi-color backlight
- Advanced water purification system
- Electrolytic antibacterial system
- Adjustable pH levels
- Automatic cleaning function

Although my household does not have one of these marvels, my friend who does have one stated to me that it has improved his energy and he no longer depends on coffee to give him energy. He also uses the water from the system to clean his fruits and vegetables and has noticed how there appears to be much more residue that was removed compared to using regular tap water.

Those of you who may want a more portable and basic hydrogen water infuser and ionizer may consider **Qlife.** (*It can be purchased online at https:// qlifetoday.com/*)

According to Dr. Mercola, the optimal pH of water we are designed to drink is between 6.5 and 8. If you are harvesting water from a natural spring it is smart to check its pH to determine if it requires adjusting. **(R 29)**

Tips for Purchasing Water

I usually bottle my own water to drink but when I am out on the road and want some good water to drink, a few of my favorites are Voss, Castle Rock Water from Mount Shasta, and Mountain Valley Spring Water. I like Fiji and Evian but they are sold in plastic bottles. According to Andrei, Fiji water contains a high degree of silicon and helps to rid the brain of aluminum.

I encourage everyone to always purchase waters that are in glass bottles to avoid BPA issues. Upon occasion I also enjoy carbonated mineral waters like Perrier and San Pellegrino. They both have a clean and refreshing taste.

I do not drink bottled water too often but, instead, I fill my **Hydroflask** with 4 - 6 glasses of water to drink from my **Kinetico** filtrated water system during the day when I am working. In addition, I drink a glass or two of water before and after work.

I usually add a high-grade Himalayan salt to each serving of water that I drink to get its many health benefits as well as make sure I am getting enough electrolytes and trace elements. The type that I take is a pink Himalayan salt called **The Original Himalayan Crystal Salt***. It is mined from caves instead of the open fields which may be contaminated. It is the best salt to add to our diet according to Dr. Barbara Hendel, author of *Water and Salt: The Essence of Life: The Healing Power of Nature*. **(R 30)** Andrei recommends about 1 1/2 teaspoon of this salt daily.

Another good salt is **Celtic Sea Salt**. Dr. David Brownstein is a well-known functional medical doctor and author of about 11 books favors this type of salt whereas Dr. Mercola likes the Himalayan.

When I am in the mood for something with more flavor and nutrients, I put one bag of **Spring Dragon Tea** and a handful of Goji Berries in with one of my containers of hot water. Once the tea and berries have steeped, I cool down the water and add organic raw local honey to taste. Spring Dragon Tea is touted as the healthiest tea in the world according to Ron Teeguarden, Taoist Master and father of Tonic Herbalism.

Many health-conscious people suggest adding a fruit to our water to bring life to our drinking water by the life force within the fruits. I concur.

In summary, drinking water that is infused with love, in an alkaline pH range, and filled with fresh organic fruit juice, antioxidant or the best quality Himalayan salt can do wonders for the body in bringing a greater degree of harmony and health.

Lemon Water in the Morning

Besides the above, I also drink warm water with a freshly squeezed lemon when I first wake up to clean my liver and jump start my digestive system. I do the same at night. It is important to swish and rinse your mouth after drinking the lemon juice to minimize the acidic harm on the enamel. Some people drink the lemon with a straw to bypass the teeth.

Another option is to do **coconut oil pulling** after you have lemon water. Due to its being anti-fungal in nature Coconut pulling helps to cleanse and heal your teeth and gums while also providing some protection to the teeth enamel. This is an ancient Ayurvedic technique that has been tested over the ages.

People used to use olive oil, but now coconut is the oil of choice due to its many blessings. Beyond cooking, some have noticed their gum and teeth getting stronger and healthier using it. **(R 31)** *Note:* it is best NOT to spit coconut oil in the sink, but rather into a can or something to keep from clogging up your drain!

Water as the Main Method of Hydration

All this leads to the awareness that drinking water is the main method of hydration. Conversely, drinks such as sodas, alcohol and coffee should be refrained from or minimized to promote greater health. As an example, a friend of mine stopped drinking coffee and did nothing else and all his aches and pain in his body left as well. Why you might ask?

- Coffee is a diuretic and can drain out many of our minerals and trace minerals which can have long term health consequences
- The caffeine is also quite taxing on the adrenal glands.
- It is also very acidic. If you are drinking a lot it can cause your pH to become so as well.
- Caffeine is also a vasoconstrictor.

Another friend, Dr. Mikaelah Cordeo, Ph.D., Spiritual author, healer, teacher, mystic and Messenger for the Ascended Hosts of Light, stopped drinking coffee and black tea as she was instructed by her guides and reported that it helped save her from a stroke. After three months of stopping it, she also noticed new circulation in her legs. She later read that caffeine was a vasoconstrictor.

However, if you must drink coffee, I recommend drinking only organic coffee like Bulletproof Coffee. Brands like Four Sigmatic Mushroom Coffee Mix with Cordyceps and Chaga may provide support in increasing energy and is a source of antioxidants. They also have one that contains Lion's Mane and Chaga for Cognitive Support. **(R 32)**

How Much Water?

How much water do we really require for optimum health? Most of have heard over and over again that we need eight (8 ounce) glasses of water daily. However, according to Kristen McCaffrey from Slender Kitchen, we can calculate what we need through our weight and activity level. She gives this formula to determine how much water to drink daily. (For example, if you weighed 175 pounds you would multiple that by 2/3 and learn you should be drinking about 117 ounces of water every day.)

Multiply your weight by 2/3 (or 67%)
Body Weight x .67= Basic water required in ounces

She also factors in our activity level as well by the following example. Add 12 ounces of water to your daily total for every 30 minutes that you work out. So, if you work out for 45 minutes daily, you would add 18 ounces of water to your daily intake. **(R 33)**

Example: (45/30) x 12=18oz
Body Weight x .67= Basic water required in ounces + 18oz

Despite the wonderful benefits of eating and drinking well, these things alone are not enough for us achieve radiant health. Much of our food chain has been contaminated for the most part. Many of the fruits, vegetables and herbs that we eat are grown in soil that is either contaminated or deficient of rich minerals. Fortunately, there is a way to navigate through all this and still get radiant health and harmony, but it will require modification, lifestyle changes and supplements. In the next chapter we will explore how we can break free from the toxic world we have co-created.

"Cleanliness is Next to Godliness"

~

Sir Francis Bacon

CHAPTER 4

DETOXIFYING AND SUPPLEMENT SUPPORT

I n a world full of toxins, millions if not billions of people are potentially suffering from a host of illnesses, autoimmune diseases, cancers, etc. It is likely that many will die or will suffer some type of chronic condition. Unless we make clear choices to reverse our direction, the incidence and prevalence of many illnesses and diseases will continue to escalate. The good news is that we can make new life choices that will assist us as individuals and uplift Earth and her kingdoms as well. By making better choices, we can clear the way for the Divine to create harmony, wellness and our inner Heavenly Kingdom or Universe.

Hard Reality

Due to the choices that humanity has made, we are currently surrounded by environmental toxins daily, and most of us are likely to have heavy metals tucked deep within us through our direct or indirect exposure to them.

Best-selling author, Anthony William (*Medical Medium*), believes that these metals can be genetically passed on from our ancestor's exposure. **(R 34)** However they arrive, once they are in our bodies, they stay unless we flush them out through some method of detoxification. If the metals remain over a prolonged time and the individual's immune system is down through severe stress, the body may develop an inflammatory response leading to pain, illness and disease.

Literally everything we use or are exposed to has some level of toxins. So, what should we do? It seems we should purchase a space suit or live in a plastic bubble. Fear not for there is a solution to our crisis. When we learn how to eat well, detoxify and take the supplements our bodies require for optimum health, we can begin releasing these trapped metals which adversely affect our entire nervous system and other body systems as well.

Also, according to Anthony William, heavy metals are a food of the Epstein Barr Virus (EBV) which wreaks havoc and inflammatory responses in our system through the fecal material that they produce and by the bodies of the deceased viruses. **(R 35)**

We may not be able to avoid the exposure to environmental toxins and metals but we can minimize it. Let us go over some of the common places in our day to day world that contain toxins and what we can possibly do about it:

Car Interior Toxins

People have been advised not to turn on the air conditioner when they first get in the car but, instead, open the windows to air out the car first to avoid the toxic benzene fumes emitted from the dashboard, air freshener and other plastic parts of the car. This is especially important on hot days. Benzene is carcinogenic.

Fluoride not only exists in the tap water in California, and other states, but it exists in many of our toothpaste. It has been linked with causing our pineal glands to calcify and adversely affecting the probiotics in our colon.

There are many toothpastes in health food stores that are free of fluoride. I use **Coral White** that I purchase from Valley Health Mill and alternate with Natural **Desert Essence's Natural Neem Toothpaste** that is also good for the gums which can be purchased from Whole Foods and online. Lately I have been using Auromere which is an Ayurvedic Herbal Toothpaste. It is readily available at Wholefoods and includes 23 Herbal Extracts including Neem and Peelu.

Amalgam tooth fillings contain mercury and have been associated with health-related issues including: anxiety, depression, irritability, memory problem, numbness, pathologic shyness and tremors. **(R 36)** It is also food for the Epstein Barr Virus. Many dentists are now trained to safely remove amalgams, which I highly recommend doing.

Removing them all at once can be harmful for your health since it can easily get into your blood stream during the dental work. Some feel that gradual removal is preferred. It is best to consult with a Holistic Dentist who understands the perils and complexities of the mercury issue.

Once amalgams are removed, it is equally important to chelate the mercury in a systematic way to ensure that it is out of our entire body systems. We will discuss more about this later in **Chapter 11, Detoxification and Purification.**

Bromine is another toxin that causes many health problems. According to the Dr. Edward Group from the Global Healing Center, bromine causes problems such as: disrupts thyroid function, increased Risk of Preterm Birth and Birth Defects, slows neural cognitive development, cognitive failure, contributes to mental illness, skin disorders, DNA damage, carcinogenic potential, toxic to kidneys and hearing loss. Among other places, bromine is found in soda, pasta, some vegetable oils, and flour and is used as a fire retardant in mattresses and baby products as well as cell phones and other daily used products. Consuming **iodine** can help detox the bromine in our bodies as it allows the body to release both bromine and aluminum. **(R 37, 38)**

Some of the plant-based foods **high in iodine (R 39)** include:

- Sea Vegetables including Nori, Arame Kelp, Kombu Kelp, Wakame Kelp and Hiziki
- Cape Cod Cranberries
- Organic lima beans
- Organic potatoes
- Prunes
- Himalayan Pink Salt
- Dark Chocolate high in Cacao

Aluminum - Unless naturally made, most of our **antiperspirants contain aluminum** which has been linked with health-related issues including dementia. There are some deodorants that do not contain it and offer some decent protection. My favorite is called **The Best Deodorant.** It has certified Organic Dynamic ingredients. It is a product from Benedetta Farm-Sourced® Holistic Skin Care. Another deodorant that I use from time to time is **Arm and Hammer Essential Deodorant.** It does not contain aluminum and parabens. An additional benefit is that it does not leave a stain on the shirt or blouse. I also like to use **Aubrey Men's Stock herbal pine deodorant.** It is aluminum free, vegan, gluten free, paraben free, phthalate free and cruelty free. It is also certified organic.

Formaldehyde - Our **floorings**, especially laminate and geo-engineered wood contain formaldehyde which has been associated with health problems. Chronic exposure to formaldehyde may also cause general damage to the central nervous system, such as increased prevalence of headache, mood changes, depression, insomnia, irritability, attention deficit, and impairment of dexterity, memory, and equilibrium, as noted on the website for the U.S. government's Agency for Toxic Substances and Disease Registry (ATSDR). **(R 40)** Hardwood floors may be safer than wood in comparison since they generally contain less VOC (volatile organic compound) that may be harmful for our health.

It behooves us to use products that have low or zero VOC to avoid our exposures to chemicals that do not agree with us. However, they are more expensive. A friend of mine owns a construction company and stated that linoleum is a flooring material that is quite safe since it is made from linseed oil and sawdust.

Makeup - Have you ever really read the ingredients of the makeup that you or your family members use? Many of the makeups that people use can contain harsh chemicals that are detrimental to the skin. It is best not to wear makeup but if you do, you might consider getting your makeups from a health conscientious company like **The Honest Company, Inc.** which was founded by Jessica Alba.

This is what she has to say about her company: "I founded The Honest Company because I wanted safe, effective products that perform. After all, you should not have to choose between what works and what is good for you." The Honest Company, Inc. is also certified cruelty- free by PETA's Beauty Without Bunnies Program.

A beautiful friend of mine, Tai-Monique, was an actress, model, dancer, entrepreneur and healer. She is now a lifestyle entrepreneur, coach, healer, educator and Reiki Master. She has been using makeup for many years and has been on a relentless search for a product that is both healthy for the skin and is Vegan. Her search led her to a company called **Arbonne**, based in Switzerland, and has been around for 40 years. They are Vegan and use natural plants and botanicals in their skin care products. They use pure, botanically based ingredients in scientifically tested products. Tai stated she sees and feels a difference with their products. She now feels that her skin is healthier and can breathe. Her skin, from what I can see, is smooth, healthy and radiant. Another good thing about this company, they also sell health and wellness products that detoxify the body to create beauty, health and harmony from the inside out.

Tai stated that Arbonne goes to all ends of the globe to extract the purest from plants to make the best formulations from science and nature. "Our philosophy is pure, safe and beneficial with a range of certifications that further aligns and meets our strict ingredient policy banning over 2,000 ingredients on our not allowed list. The European Union has banned 1,500. Their promise from the beginning is to set industry standards with the passionate intention to leave this planet better than they found it." She also stated that the company has a vast range of vegan skincare, beauty and holistic health and wellness products that help you feel and look good from the inside out that also offers a brilliant opportunity to create a life by design of extraordinary choice. To contact Tai Monique directly, visit: https://taimoniquekristjansen.arbonne.com.

Air Fresheners

Many of the **air fresheners** that we have contain toxic chemicals that are not good for those who have compromised respiratory status. **(R 41)**

The following are five chemicals that are often found in air fresheners:

1. **Volatile Organic Compounds** (VCO) - The most prevalent VOCs classified as toxic or hazardous in franced air fresheners

are acetone, ethanol, d-limonene, pinene and acetate, according to a 2015 study authored by Anne Steinemann and published in Air Quality, Atmosphere and Health 9(8), October 2016. (R 42) Depending on your exposure and sensitivity, toxic VOCs can produce a range of health effects, including eye, nose, and throat irritation, nausea and headaches, and even damage to liver, kidney and the central nervous system, says the EPA, which offers a complete list of symptoms.

2. **Formaldehyde** - "Formaldehyde is a known carcinogen." says Steinemann. "As for symptoms, you may experience eye, nose, and throat irritation, coughing, wheezing, bronchitis and dizziness." Reactions and reaction severity depend on your individual sensitivity", she explains.

3. **Phthalates** - One of the primary concern's health experts have about plug-in air fresheners is their wide-spread use of phthalates. According to a study conducted by the Natural Resources Defense Council (NRDC), 86% of air fresheners tested contained phthalates. Phthalates, which are also found in many plastics, aerosol sprays, paints, pesticides, cosmetics, and fragrances, are notoriously disruptive to the body. As the NRDC reported in their research, "Most phthalates are well known to interfere with production of the male hormone testosterone, and have been associated with reproductive abnormalities." Phthalates are on the State of California's list of toxic substances as "known to cause birth defects or reproductive harm". The NRDC also warns that airborne phthalates can cause allergic symptoms and asthma. Even trace amounts of phthalates can accumulate to cause these harmful side-effects.

4. **1,4 dichlorobenzene** - One of the primary ingredients in mothballs, room deodorizer, and urinal cakes, 1,4 dichlorobenzene (1,4 DCB) has been implicated in two serious health concerns: The compound may cause "modest reductions in lung function," according to NIH, and lifetime exposure has resulted in liver cancer in mice, according to the Centers for Disease Control and Prevention.

5. **Allergens** - If you have seasonal allergies, chronic asthma, COPD, or a common cold, use of an air freshener is a definite no-no, says

Dr. Janna Tuck, a practicing allergist in Cape Girardeau, Mo., and a spokesperson for the American College of Allergy, Asthma and Immunology. **(R 43)**

If you're worried about the health effects of VOCs, phthalates and other chemicals in home fragrance products, but you still want your home to smell like something, stick to natural sources, says Steinemann.

"If you really want an aroma, brew mint tea or grind up a fresh orange," she suggests. "Only natural, pure sources will be free of chemicals. Even essential oils emit similar chemicals to air fresheners."

We are becoming more and more aware of the **challenges of plastics.** Included in that list is that they contain flame retardants, bisphenols and phthalates, which are unhealthy for our bodies and are toxic for the Earth. Plastics came into use in the past 50 years. In that brief time, they have become a threat to our health, and Earth's ecosystems worldwide.

The good news is that the plastic habit is quite easy to replace with healthier and more sustainable options, like those we used before its invention. Here are a few easy to embrace suggestions:

- Use cloth reusable bags for groceries
- Purchase bulk foods rather than prepackaged. (Many people bring their own containers to put them in which assists even more)
- Purchase drinks in glass bottles rather than plastic
- Bring your own drink container to coffee shops, etc.
- Use glass storage containers in your home, rather than plastic

The health of our bodies and of Mother Earth requires that we all make conscious responsible choices.

Microwaves

Even our friendly **microwave** may emit radiation to our bodies that may lead to the disharmony of our well-being. One woman was complaining of headaches for a long time but after my friend told her to stop using it, her headaches went away.

In 1991, Swiss scientist, Hans Ulrich Hertel, did a study on the effects of microwaved nutrients on the blood and physiology of human beings. This small but well-controlled study pointed the firm finger at a degenerative force of microwave ovens and the food produced in them.

Atoms, molecules and cells hit by this hard-electromagnetic radiation are forced to reverse polarity 1 to 100 billion times a second. There are no atoms, molecules or cells of any organic system able to withstand such a violent, destructive power for any extended period of time, not even in the low energy range of milliwatts. **(R 44)**

To learn more about the study, I suggest you read the full article at the site at the link below. It is a hot topic but you should read the article and make your own educated decision. I highly recommend you read it. I myself do not use the microwave anymore. I intuitively and energetically feel that food heated in the microwave is unnatural, disharmonious and unhealthy for me and my loved ones. **(R 45)**

The more intense the heat to our foods and vegetables, the more the nutrients that are contained within them are compromised. In addition to avoiding microwaving of foods, many people are doing a raw food diet or do not cook their food at high temperature. Those of you who still like their food hot may consider using an air fryer instead of a microwave as a healthier alternative. In all fairness, I have to say that I have not met a person yet who has any issues related to long term usage of a microwave. Those of you who are more in tune with your body, like myself, may notice a difference. The best advice is to educate yourself and also see how it makes you feel.

Now that you are aware of many of the toxins and heavy metals around you, it is important to minimize your exposure to them, as well as learn how to detoxify it from your body to create greater harmony and wellness.

It is extremely important that we take action to detoxify on a regular basis to remove the toxins and metals that have been accumulating in our bodies for many generations.

Eating well, drinking well and detoxifying helps to reset our system and creates greater harmony and healing within us.

Techniques for Detoxifying

I hope by now you realize that most of us are more than likely filled with varying levels of metals or toxins within our body. If they are not removed, our bodies' ability to heal will be greatly hampered as we accumulate more and more toxins and metals. It is important that we employ methods to release them from our bodies. Below are some things I have done to help myself that you may find helpful. I have also included information that was shared with me from others who are concerned about their health. Keep in mind this is not a definitive list and that results vary depending on body types and different levels of overall health. The purpose of the information is to show you some of the possibilities out there that have been helpful to some people and may open your mind to a new way of thinking.

Water and Juice Detox

I usually do a **water and juice detox** regularly and eat fresh organic fruits and vegetables including cilantro, celery and parsley to help remove metals from my system. I drink hot warm water when I get up with freshly squeezed lemon in it and one glass before I sleep to help me detox and clean my liver. I sometime add raw honey in it as well.

Other Supplements for Detox

Besides that, I also take various supplements to cleanse myself further. They include **Green Barley Powder.** * I have been taking that for years and it helps me to feel a certain subtle feeling of well-being. A client of mine who introduced me to it stated that it helped with his prostate cancer. He noticed by taking it, his PSA levels had gone done.

A great movie to watch with regards to juicing and wellness is entitled *Fat, Sick and Nearly Dead.* **(R 46)** It is about a man who was morbidly obese and had an autoimmune disease. He came to America to regain his health by doing a 60-day detox program by juicing fruits and vegetables for every meal. He is closely supervised by a physician and makes an incredible transformation in his body, mind and emotions.

I have also taken **PectaClear Detox Formula*** on occasions. A customer taking this product has stated that many of the metals in their body have decreased after a follow up visit with their doctors to reexamine metal levels. According to the company, it removes heavy metal and supports superior cleansing and healthy detoxification.

I alternate with **Body Solution's*** detox solution. This is one that is based on a Native American Detox formula.

Iodine and Toxicity

Nascent Iodine* can help to detox the bromine, chlorine and fluoride in our bodies. It also rids the body of exposure to radiation. According to Janet Doerr, Intuitive Nutritionista and Energy Healer, iodine is a tricky one. We must be careful with how much we take to avoid overdose.

Iodine Toxicity may include the following symptoms:
More **Mild symptoms** of iodine poisoning include:
1. Diarrhea
2. Burning sensation in your mouth
3. Nausea
4. Vomiting

Severe symptoms of iodine poisoning include:
1. Swelling of your airways
2. Turning blue (cyanosis)
3. Weak pulse
4. Coma **(R 47)**

Consuming too much iodine can also lead to a condition called iodine-induced hyperthyroidism. This usually happens when people take iodine supplements to improve their thyroid function.

Symptoms of hyperthyroidism include:
1. Muscle weakness
2. Warm skin
3. Unexplained weight loss

Hyperthyroidism is particularly dangerous if you have an underlying heart condition, since it affects your heart rate. **(R 48)**

Consult with your local physician, health consultant or nutritionist on how much you should take or whether you need it at all. According to Janet Doerr, some people do a self-test by putting some iodine on their skin for 24 hours. If the stain goes away, it may indicate that the body needed the iodine. If the stain remains after 24 hours, it may mean that the body has enough iodine.

Nascent Iodine can be beneficial to the body but those with Hashimoto's syndrome (an auto immune disease of the thyroid) need to be careful taking iodine. According to Andrei, some of these Hashimoto patients will react negatively while others will actually benefit. He further stated that it is a blanket recommendation that when you have Hashimoto's, you avoid iodine until you bring the thyroid antibodies down which you can do with selenium alone.

Kelp, a natural form of Iodine, can be a good source of Iodine which is deficient in our diet. The iodized salt that we purchase loses most of its potency by the time it reaches our house. Good sources of iodine include seaweed but as we mentioned earlier, much of the ocean is quite toxic now. I have taken **I-53 Nascent** Iodine off and on. Iodine supports thyroid health, our immune system and metabolism. I swish it around my mouth to kill all bacteria in my mouth and I gargle with it if I have a sore throat.

According to Global Healing Center, it is good also for reducing the amount of radiation in the thyroid for those who exposed to it. It also supports breast health, ovarian health (cyst and reproductive ability), eye, skin and hair health, and neurological health. **(R 49)**

Chelation Therapy

Another method to remove the metals from your body is chelation therapy. According to WebMD, when metals like lead, mercury, iron, and arsenic build up in your body, they can be toxic. Chelation therapy is a treatment that uses medicine to remove these metals so they do not make you sick.

Chelation therapy uses special drugs that bind to metals in your blood. You get the chelating medicine through an intravenous (IV) tube in your arm. It is also available in pill form. Once the drug has attached to the metal, your body removes them both through your urine. **(R 50)**

Drinking Fulvic Mineral Water can help chelate heavy metals as well. Water, juice or other forms of fasting can help to detoxify our bodies.

Hatha Yoga and other similar yoga forms done in warm temperature can be helpful for releasing toxins from our bodies through our perspiration.

Superfoods to Help with Our Health and Detoxification

Spirulina and Chlorella

One of the most well-known of superfoods is Hawaiian Spirulina. It has been around for quite a while and has many great health benefits. Wellandgood.com is one of many references that document the many health benefits of spirulina. (R 51) In their words:

1. It is a powerhouse of nutrients including vitamins B1, B2, and B3, iron, magnesium, and potassium.
2. Assisting the body in flushing out toxins.
3. Boosts the immune system. Spirulina contains an antioxidant called phycocyanin that fights off anything that could damage your cells.
4. Lowers blood pressure.
5. Its ability to increase blood flow increases endurance for athletes.
6. Affects muscle strength due to its protein,
7. Fights cancer: Studies have linked spirulina to boosting the immune system enough to fight off cancerous cells—oral cancer in particular.

According to many health experts, Hawaiian Spirulina is the best.

It is important to note here that I have also heard and read about contaminated spirulina. One research team tested spirulina, AFA, and chlorella from all over the world and reported that the majority of them were contaminated with different types of metals such as arsenic, aluminum, mercury, or lead. The important thing is to make sure you get it from a reputable company and that it is organic, non-GMO and gluten free.

Chlorella is also good at detoxifying mercury and other heavy metals out of the body. It serves as a binder of heavy metals that have been chelated out of the body and into the blood stream.

A friend of my friend took **Chlorenergy*** for a while and when she went to see her doctor, he informed her that her mercury level in her body had improved significantly. That particular chlorella is made in Japan and it is touted as the best one in the world. I take it as well.

My friend was taking it religiously along with spirulina and eating lots of green leafy vegetables and found great benefits. When she took a saliva test for her alkalinity, the results revealed that her body was quite alkaline.

Some of the other benefits of chlorella **(R 52)** include the following:
1. Protein. It is 50-60% protein.
2. Some of the varieties of chlorella contain vitamin B12.
3. Iron and Vitamin C
4. Antioxidants.
5. Chlorella provides small amounts of magnesium, zinc, copper, potassium, calcium, folic acid and other B vitamins.
6. Fiber

Selenium is an important mineral that can be helpful for removing mercury from our bodies. Selenium acts as a mercury magnet with a very strong binding affinity for the toxic substance. This strong attraction allows selenium to mix and neutralize their reaction characteristics. This new Hg–Se substance that is produced is not absorbed by the body and gets flushed out of the system. **(R 53)**

Brazil nuts are by far the best source of selenium. Each Brazil nut is said to contain between 50-75 mcg of selenium. Taking a small handful, about four to six pieces, will supply most of the selenium you will need in the course of a day. However due to the variant amount of selenium in Brazil nuts it is best to eat less, rather than more to avoid toxicity.

In severe cases, acute selenium toxicity can lead to serious intestinal and neurological symptoms, heart attack, kidney failure and death. So, with power nutrients, less is generally better.

Signs of selenium toxicity include

- Hair loss
- Dizziness
- Nausea
- Vomiting
- Facial flushing
- Tremors
- Muscle soreness

However, toxicity is more likely to happen from taking supplements rather than from eating selenium-containing foods. **(R 54)**

Other good sources of selenium include many forms of fish, pasture-raised eggs, mushrooms, shellfish, and seeds. For adults it is best to consume between 200-400 micrograms of selenium daily. Too much selenium is toxic; however, the average American consumes just 60 mcg daily. While selenium toxicity is rare, it is important to stay close to the recommended amount of 55 mcg per day and never exceed the tolerable upper limit of 400 mcg per day. **(R 55)**

Chemtrails

Many of you may have heard about the Chemtrails that once seemed to fill our skies on a regular basis. Many place them in a category of a conspiracy theory but according to homeremedies1.com, Government admits to Chemtrails: The following video is an admission by Rosalind Peterson, President of the Agriculture Defense Coalition, who addresses the UN on the truth behind Chemtrails, geoengineering, and weather modification. The acknowledgement by the UN that our skies are being polluted with aluminum, barium, lead, arsenic, chromium, cadmium, selenium, and silver should give weight to the claims that Chemtrails cause a whole host of health problems in the general population.

Although it is going to take much legislative changes to halt the sprays completely, we can help ourselves to minimize the effects by taking supplements to release the heavy metals that we eat, drink and breathe in.

One of my friends who is very health conscientious told me about **ChlorOxygen** drops. They assist in the chelation of heavy metals.

Chelators and Binders

Chelators assist the body by pulling the metals out of the tissues. Foods that are **binders** escort the toxins out of the body via its elimination systems.

10 Foods to help eliminate heavy metals and toxins. (R 56)

1. Chlorella (binder)
2. Cilantro (chelator)

3. Cinnamon
4. Hemp
5. Flax seed
6. Magnesium
7. Saffron
8. Curcumin
9. Activating Charcoal
10. Diatomaceous Earth-
    (*Be sure to purchase food grade diatomaceous earth. Make sure to avoid breathing it! It can be harmful if inhaled.*)

Despite the benefits of removing the heavy metals, Andrew Hall Cutler, Ph.D., P.E., a chemical engineer and mercury chelation consultant, has frequently talked about the complexities of chelating mercury out of the body. He himself suffered health issues until he pinpointed it to the **mercury in his fillings**. He then went on a relentless search on how to rid his body of it and eventually developed a protocol on how to safely remove it from the body. He believes that the only way to remove or chelate mercury is through ALA (alpha lipoic acid) but due to its short half-life it had to be administered in a very specific protocol to ensure that it is released from the body otherwise it could be chelated and settle down in other organs in the body and wreak havoc and health issues.

Some of the illnesses that he believes are affected by mercury include: chronic fatigue, allergies, asthma, Parkinson's disease, multiple sclerosis, lupus, diabetes, depression and autism. His protocol came to be known as the Cutler Protocol. This is further explained in his book, ***Amalgam Illness.*(R 57)**

According to Kathryn Shanti Ariel, the Nature Whisperer, "in addition to food and herbs for detoxing heavy metals there are also homeopathic options. Having been diagnosed with arsenic toxicity when preparing to have her amalgams removed, Kathryn researched healing options which resulted in her using a combination of foods and homeopathy. The homeopathic remedies that she specifically uses are Arsenicum album for arsenic and Nat Mur for mercury."

Some believe that working with a highly qualified nutritionist, Functional Medicine Practitioner, or Naturopathic Physician to assess the body's needs before embarking on a heavy metal detox program is imperative. However, Andrei stated that the supplements that he sells at his store are quite mild and the effect of detox is cumulative and not aggressive like an alpha lipoic acid heavy metal detox program. He feels that his supplements do not have the Herxheimer Reactions that are more common in other more aggressive detox formulations that may cause symptoms like headaches, diarrhea or flu-like symptoms.

If you decide to engage in any heavy duty or aggressive heavy metal detox program, it behooves you to research further to and discuss it with someone who truly understands it like a Functional Medicine Practitioner or Naturopathic Physician with extensive experience with heavy metal detox especially with the complexities of mercury toxicity.

Supplements

Besides removing metals and toxins from our body, it may help us to take the supplements that give us the coverage and support that our food, fruits and vegetables may not be able to if they are grown in nutrient deficient soils.

In this day and age, we all need some degree of supplements in our diet. Some of us may need a multi-vitamin to give us a good coverage if we are not eating well or not getting enough nutrients from the food we eat. The brands I have tried include Super Nutrition Simple One Triple Power Multivitamin and Emerald Men's 45+ 1-Daily Multivitamin. I will note here that I believe we should only take what we need to create harmony and not more.

There are literally thousands of vitamins and supplements out there from thousands of different companies and sources. One thing I have learned is that not all vitamins and supplements are created equal. However, most people are not aware of this and will buy their nutritional supplements from either a wholesale discount warehouse or supermarket where this is no support or guidance. Savvy customers will purchase at a health food store or a Wholefoods store where there is some general support and guidance on what to get for their particular needs. It is best to consult with a health care provider like a holistic physician, naturopathic doctor, functional medical practitioner, chiropractor, nutritionist, etc. for what you need.

After my many years of my own research and years of consulting with very knowledgeable nutritionists, physicians, longevity experts and other holistic health care experts, I have discovered some of the best supplements on the market for improving harmony of body, mind and spirit. However, **before trying any supplements, it is very important to consult with your doctor** first due to our diverse bodies' needs.

Different illnesses respond differently to different drugs, supplements as well as herbs. Medications and supplements may have side effects and it is important that we know about it before taking it. Also, do your own research about the side effects of each supplement you take since it is most likely not listed on the bottle like it is in the pharmaceutical industry. Always consult with your doctor, nutritionist or health care provider about how much dosage to take for any medication or supplement you take. And always consult with your physician before taking a new medication or supplement recommended by another physician or health care professional.

Having said that, here is a list of some of most effective supplements I have found quite effective and has helped me or many others. I consult a lot with **Andrei Volhonttseff.** He is an extremely knowledgeable nutritionist that has helped thousands of people achieve radiant health. I owe much of my own health success stories because of him. Many people consult with him including medical doctors and nurses.

I will share what I have found very effective for me, my family and others who have used the products. I will also share what Andrei recommends for vitamins and supplements. I will not go over every vitamin and supplement, but those that are salient to me and appear to be quite effective. I will list various vitamins, supplements as well as conditions and what has helped people. Please realize that individual results may vary due to difference in genetics, blood types, and body chemistry and unique needs of our bodies.

We can save the lives of many people, including ourselves, and help end or minimize our sufferings by having the tools and knowledge to restore harmony within the body. The following list includes supplements that have made a big difference in my life as well as others and they include:

Fish oil- many people who are omnivore and health conscientious take fish oil for its reported health benefits. However, according to Professor Brian Peskin, BSEE-MIT, and founder of Life-Systems Engineering

Science, author of the **PEO (Parent Essential Oil) Solution,** fish oil does not offer true long-term health benefits to its users. He has written extensively about the fallacies of the benefits of fish oils and has discovered that the majority of the research that support that it is good are poorly done. The few other good references out there indicate there are no health benefits to using them. **(R 58)**

In his book, **PEO Solution**, written with Robert Jay Rowen, M.D., Professor Peskin gives ten - what he calls Inconvenient Truths - About Fish Oils but is quick to say there are even more. Dr. Rowen has spent five years analyzing Professor Peskins' research but came to the conclusion that his research was valid. Dr. Rowen is considered today's foremost pioneer of bold, innovative healing methods that are putting an end to our most common diseases. He is also a renowned international authority in oxidative medicine and is known as the Doctor's doctor.

He believes there are three major causes of chronic or degenerative illness/diseases: **improper nutrition, toxins** and **stress.** I am addressing all three in this book.

Professor Peskin advocates abandoning fish oil and start taking **PEO** (Parent Essential Oil). He refers to it as the only two, true, essential fatty acids - parent omega 6 and parent omega-3.

In addition, Professor Peskin has found that people who stopped taking the fish oil and started taking PEO had the greatest benefits. He has given us much information about the benefits of using PEO which include helping or supporting the following: the heart, appetite, diabetes, hormones/ endocrine, beauty, anti-inflammation, brain health and endurance.

Although I take the PEO oil myself, I know many people who don't. Instead, they take fish oil like most others and have had some benefits from fish oil. My friend who was experiencing chronic knee pain reported it feels better after he takes fish oil for a while. My optometrist recommends fish oils for her client if they have dry eyes. She stated that it seemed to help her clients. My dog takes fish oil (Grizzly Salmon Oil Omega-3 Fatty Acids) and it has helped her hair or fur to look healthy. A friend of mine did the same and had similar benefits from her dog.

Perhaps if others switched to PEO, their healing potential would be even more significant and more pronounced. The only place I have found the PEO oil* is at Valley Health Mills in Pleasanton, CA. Items can be ordered from the store and shipped to you. (*The* *throughout this book also indicates other supplements that are available at Valley Health Mills.*)

According to Andrei, one well known doctor, Dr. David Brownstein, changed his mind about fish oil after studying Professor Peskin's research. He now tells his patients and readers to not use fish oil but to choose the plant based PEO instead. He stated that Dr. Brownstein wrote an article about fish oil is ineffective and dangerous. He wrote that the anti-inflammatory effect experienced from people taking fish oil usually you experience it mostly during the first month while taking the fish oil but not so much after the first month. Andrei further states that fish oil can increase the oxidative stress damage to the body. One Study found that fish oil can increase the inflammation markers in the body in the long term.

Those who are vegetarian or vegans may also get their omega oils from plant-based foods such as seeds and plant-based oils. Examples of foods that contain Parent Essential Oils include the following:

- Pumpkin seed
- Flax seed
- Borage seed
- Evening Primrose seed
- Sunflower seed

Vitamin B12

According to Dr. Axe, a vitamin B12 deficiency is thought to be one of the leading nutrient deficiencies in the world. Vitamin B12 benefits your mood, energy level, memory, heart, skin, hair, digestion and more. Vitamin B12 is also an essential vitamin for addressing adrenal fatigue, multiple metabolic functions, including DNA synthesis, enzyme production, hormonal balance and maintaining healthy nervous and cardiovascular systems. **(R 59)**

Three brands I have tried include the following:

1. **NOW** brand **Methyl B-12** 1,000 mcg* and
2. **Isura's B12 Methylcobalamin***

Although both are chewable, placing a tablet under the tongue and letting it dissolve is the faster way of absorption into the blood stream. Methylcobalamin is the best form of vitamin B12 used by the body since it requires no conversion. I find Vitamin B12 quite helpful for increasing my energy level but it is recommended by some nutritionist to take it with a good vitamin B-complex to make it more effective.

3.   **Garden of Life mykind Organics B-12 Organic Spray is vegan and has Methylcobalamin.** This is my favorite versions of B12. I find it helpful in creating more energy

Vitamin E

Vitamin E may be helpful for the heart, blood vessels, hormones, Alzheimer's disease, liver, cancer, etc. It is also a great antioxidant but if used in conjunction with other antioxidants it can be recycled again according to some experts.

Vitamin E that contains **tocotrienols** can be quite effective in supporting the harmony in the body. Delta tocotrienol appear to be the best form to take according to research. **Kyani's** vitamin E contains tocotrienols which is purported to be the purest and most effective form of vitamin E. According to Dr. Norm Shealy, Kyani's vitamin E (tocotrienol) is by far the best form of vitamin E.

However, according to one vitamin E expert, Dr. Z, his alias a Vitamin E Expert, the best form of vitamin E is Delta Tocotrienol and should be kept cold due to its volatile nature. Keeping it refrigerated will maximize its potency. However, it is important to take it along with some healthy fatty food for better absorption.

Unique E* is a brand that Andrei likes. The company that makes it only specializes in vitamin E. It has d-alpha tocopherol, d-gamma tocopherol, d-delta tocopherol and d-beta tocopherol.

According to Dr. Z, Delta-Tocotrienol is also gifted with cardiovascular and cancer benefits.

•   It inhibits monocyte adherence to arterial endothelium in fatty streak formation - one of the first steps in plaque formation.

- It improves arterial health by preventing the artery walls from getting too narrow and forming blood clots.
- It inhibits liver cholesterol biosynthesis and decreases Total and LDL cholesterol and triglycerides.
- It fights cancer by targeting multiple cells signaling pathways and inhibiting cancer cell growth and metastasis.
- It induces apoptosis (programmed cell death) in cancer cells selectively and causes tumor regression by inhibiting cellular telomerase and promoting anti-angiogenesis (thereby starving the tumor) in cancer and macular degeneration.
- It also stimulates cytoprotective autophagy in certain cancers.

Vitamin E may also be helpful for someone exposed to radiation. **Radiation toxicity** is a real threat to our health and well-being.

Although most of us are aware of the Fukushima nuclear reactor meltdown and how the radiation has already spread across the ocean, most of us are oblivious to the radiation we are exposed on the daily basis. If we travel, fly, and just live with all the modern-day conveniences, we are exposed to radiation. **(R 60)**

We are also bombarded by invisible rays all the time, wherever we are. Known as radiation, these rays can come in the form of sunlight, microwaves, radio waves, electromagnetic waves from mobile phones and laptops, X-rays and gamma rays, among others. **(R 61)**

With high enough dosages, ionizing radiation can break and mutate our DNA, and disrupt cellular function, usually resulting in cancer.

According to *Hungry for Change*, there are 19 natural foods that can help with decreasing the radiation in our bodies and they include Spirulina, Chlorella, Seaweed, Kelp, Black/Green Tea, Garlic, Onions, Wheat Grass, Apples (and other fruits rich in pectin), Lemons, Parsley, Beets, Sauerkraut, Ginger, Avocado, Horseradish, Kale (and other leafy greens), Broccoli and coconut oil. **(R 62)**

Vitamin D-3

It is well accepted by many health experts that many people nowadays are vitamin D deficient. Our body makes that when we get enough sunlight exposure to our skin. One medical doctor said that our hands, face and head are like solar panels and absorb sun light into our body that helps us create vitamin D. The best time to be out in the sun is between 10:00 am to 2:00 pm. Vitamin D helps with our bones, immune system and aides our bodies to absorb calcium and phosphorus. However, we should avoid long exposures to direct sunlight due to UV ray damages to our skin and risk for skin cancers. According to **Dr. Sonia, Elite MD**, the Bay Area's Top Dermatologist, we can protect ourselves by applying a mineral based sun screen with zinc oxide or a chemical based one that contains titanium dioxide and reapply every two hours. She has a physician grade brand that she recommends called Vitamin C Sun Shield. It is Broad Spectrum SPF 40 and contains 7.0% Zinc Oxide and Vitamin C. She recommends using it indoors as well since UV rays can also enter the house. More information can be found at elitemdspa.com.

According to *Healthline*, other benefits of vitamin D include reducing your risk of multiple sclerosis, decreasing your chance of developing heart disease, and helping to reduce your likelihood of developing the flu. They indicate that it also helps with depression and aides with weight loss. **(R 63)**

However, Andrei, points out vitamin D is not actually a vitamin; it is a hormone. Calling it a vitamin is a misnomer. In fact, it is the oldest hormone and your body actually makes it.

A vitamin is something your body does not make that is essential for our body and vital for life. He says it does a lot of things in our body, but the primary function is to help calcium to be absorbed through the gut and get into our blood. It helps with increasing calcium absorption by about 70%. He goes on to discuss about the calcium paradox and how when people take calcium and vitamin D supplements for bone health, the calcium level in the blood rises and increases the possibilities of calcification of arteries and heart valves and people increase their risk for strokes, heart disease and kidney stones. Hence, he also recommends taking vitamin K2 as well to direct the calcium to the right place. This will be further explained in the following interview.

Magnesium is good for your immune system and stress. It also assists with directing vitamin D and calcium to our bones and is very important in supporting our heart and good health. According to Dr. Axe, it is involved in over 300 biochemical functions in the body, such as regulating

heartbeat rhythms and helping neurotransmitter functions. **(R 64, 65)**
Empower NUTRIENT'S Heart Healthy Magnesium* (Magnesium
Taurate) is what I take.

More insights from Andrei Volhonttseff

Andrei explained that there are nine (9) types of magnesium, and many
people are deficient of this mineral. It is either the second or third most
deficient mineral in our bodies. Some magnesium experts estimate about
80% of Americans are not getting enough magnesium in their diet. It helps
to make 300 - 350 enzymes in the body. He states that it is probably one
of the most important minerals for heart health to maintain normal heart
rhythm. He stated that there been cases where people were able to correct
their cardiac arrhythmia (irregular heart beat) using magnesium alone.

It is needed to energize the heart muscle cells as well as all the other
cells in the body because magnesium is needed by the mitochondria in the
cells to produce ATP (adenosine triphosphate). It is the chemical form of
energy that all cells use to do work. Deficiency in magnesium can cause
fatigue or lack of energy. Congestive Heart Failure patients have benefitted
from magnesium provided that it is absorbable. It can be very helpful
for preventing calcification of the arteries and heart valves. When there
is enough magnesium in the blood or serum, it prevents calcium from
precipitating out of solution and forming solids whether it's the arteries or
kidney stones. It is as important for the bones as calcium is, maybe more
important than calcium for many people.

He further stated that our bones are not just a collection of calcium
phosphate crystals. Bones are basically the main reservoir for minerals and
trace minerals in the body. There are at least a dozen minerals and trace
minerals that are very important for bone health in preventing osteopenia
and osteoporosis. One of the main one is magnesium which we need in
higher amounts as well as calcium; it is a macro mineral. Magnesium helps
to make the outer portion of the bones harder.

Magnesium as well as vitamin K2 helps direct calcium to the bones
where you want it and prevent it from being deposited in organs and soft
tissues where you do not want it.

Andrei points out the magnesium as a supplement is never just magnesium. It is always a type of magnesium compound and they differ and are not equal in terms of their absorption. At one end of the spectrum you have Magnesium Oxide (an inorganic magnesium used in most of the multi-vitamins and most of the calcium-magnesium combination products because it is very concentrated and inexpensive) is a poorly absorbed form of magnesium. A recent study found that it may only be absorbed at about 4%. Magnesium Citrate is better, Magnesium Malate is even better, but the best is amino acid chelated forms like Magnesium Glycinate or Magnesium Taurate.

Andrei's number one bestselling magnesium is Magnesium Taurate*. He likes the Taurate version because the amino acid taurine has more benefits throughout the body than glycine. He stated that Taurine is very good for **heart health, liver health, brain, kidneys and gallbladder** too. With the Magnesium Taurate compound you often get a double benefit. Both nutrients will help control blood pressure. It's the best form of magnesium for people **with high blood pressure.** Both nutrients support insulin sensitivity in the body which is blood sugar control. This is the best magnesium for **pre-diabetics and diabetics.** They are **also good for stress** because they have a **calming effect on the brain. (R 66)**

Gut Health and Wellness

Gut health starts from our mouth. What we put in our mouths, how much we eat and how fast we eat will affect how well the food is digested and how much work the stomach, small intestine and large intestine has to do. If we spend time chewing our food slowly and thoroughly, it gives time for our saliva to be produced in our mouth and begin the digestive process. This is a very important part of digestion that will minimize heart burns, stomach aches and improve your bodies absorption of nutrients.

According to the Tablet of Medicine by Bahá'u'lláh, "do not swallow until you have thoroughly masticated (your food)." Besides chewing your food well, it is important that we eat "real food" that include fruits (including the skin which is a good fiber and has good phytonutrients), vegetables, seafood, organic non-GMO tofu and foods with healthy oils and things that are not manmade). Your body knows exactly what to do with them for energy, body repair and gut, brain and heart health.

However, if our gut goes awry despite our healthy eating habits, the following information may be helpful with optimizing gut health further:

Discussion on Lectin

Dr. Steven Gundry, M.D., best-selling author, cardiologist, surgeon and the Director and Founder of the International Heart and Lung Institute as well as the Center for Restorative Medicine in Palm Springs and Santa Barbara, CA, has stated that much of the plant-based food that we eat contain a protein called **Lectin**. According to him, this can interfere with your digestion, energy, and overall health. **(R 67)**

Lectin Shield is a product endorsed by Dr. Gundry. He believes Lectin Shield could be helpful for supporting us with our digestive issues. So far, he has 80 five-star reviews which indicate that it is helping people. I have tried it and feel that it is definitely helping with my digestive system. My nephew took it and had great benefits.

Probiotics

Probiotics are the good bacteria that we need to properly absorb the nutrients from our food to support our energy, immune system, and overall health (physical and emotional well-being) and are essential for proper gut health and helping us achieve a healthy gut flora. Good gut health helps us to produce serotonin and dopamine. 80% of our immune system is from our gut. According to Global Healing Center, more than 90% of the body's serotonin is found in the gut. Serotonin is also one of the "feel-good" neurotransmitters and contributes to feelings of well-being and happiness. **(R 68, 69)**

If our gut is out of whack due to poor nutrition or due to taking antibiotics then we need to add them back in our system. Antibiotics are used commercially in our fish and meat. When we eat them, they get in our bodies and kill out the healthy bacteria in our gut.

"Most people are severely deficient in probiotics," says Dr. Josh Axe. "Why? Because these friendly bugs are killed off by antibiotics in medications, meat and poultry raised on factory farms, and hand sanitizers, as well as by pesticides in food, beverages, fluoride and chlorine in drinking water, and other toxins."

The best place to find probiotics is in fresh, living food like sprouts, alfalfa, broccoli, clover, fenugreek, lentil, mustard, sunflower, kale and other seeds like them.

Other sources of probiotics include the following nine foods: **(R 71)**
- Apple Cider Vinegar
- Dark Chocolate
- Microalgae- they comprise a mixture of plant including cyanobacteria, chlorella, spirulina, as well as brown, green, and red algae.
- Sauerkraut (Raw sauerkraut is an excellent source of friendly bacteria)
- Dill Pickles
- Olives Cured in Brine
- Kimchi
- Kombucha
- Beet Kvass

Other Supplements that May Aid Gut and Digestive Support

I have also found probiotic supplements that have been extremely helpful to me, my family and many others. They are as follows:

Just Thrive* is one of the best probiotics in the market in my opinion. Just Thrive contains three strains of bacteria (Bacillus Coagulans, Bacillus Clausii and Bacillus Subtilis HU58) plus a patented strain called Bacillus Indicus HU36®. This probiotic is one of the few that I know that can make it through the stomach acid and get to the gut. Many brands cannot. I have seen many good benefits from this blend especially with abdominal issues. My family takes this one regularly whenever they have any digestive or immune system issues. It contains 3 billion cells of bacteria per serving. **(R 72)**

ImmuProbio contain 50 billion living bacteria cultures. It is found in the refrigerated section of the store. I take this when I am feeling that my health is compromised and I need an extra boost.

Dr. Ohhira's Probiotics Original Formula* is another good brand that has been recommended to me that I use alternately.

My oversea relatives use **Ohhira Mountain Fruit Extract OMX** and have found it quite effective with their digestive issues and immune support. My relative found it very helpful in boosting his immune system when recovering from pneumonia. His wife stated that they purchase this type of probiotic directly from the probiotic rep who has been selling directly to physicians like the internal medicine doctors and immunologists for their cancer patients or those who have compromised immune system.

According to Andrei, it is important to alternate probiotic brands since different ones contain different strains of bacteria that our body needs. There are about 18 different strain of bacteria that our bodies need. He recommends rotating brands every two to three months.

Dr. Tobias GutMeister is a prebiotic and probiotic that seems to have much good reviews on Amazon. Some critics say that we can easily get prebiotic (food that supports the probiotics) in our flax seed, chia seeds or vegetables. However, I include it here as another alternative solution to check out further.

Garden of Life's **Dr. Formulated Probiotics*** has 14 types of probiotic strains. I have found this product helpful when I suffered mild food poisoning, stomachaches and diarrhea. The one I took had 50 billion guaranteed bacteria. They may be purchased also at Sprouts and Wholefoods. After I took three dosages of the probiotic, my stomachache and diarrhea had resolved. I felt some relief after the first dosage.

Puradyme.com has a good line of products and have their own powerful line of digestive support- **Liyfbiotic**-Multi-Strain Probiotics (L. Acidophilus DDS-1, L.Plantarum, B.,Bifidum, B. Longum, Bacillus Coagulum and Jerusalem Artichoke) and **Liyfzyme-Super digestive enzymes**. The combination may be very helpful with supporting your gut and digestive health. The product was formulated by Lou Corona, President and founder of Puradyme, who is known as "the healthiest man in the world."

I believe it is good to use probiotics only as needed with the guidance of a health care practitioner but when things are stabilized, we should try our best to get it from food and vegetables.

Gut health is extremely important in giving us overall good health and well-being. Anthony William has written extensively about it and how we can essentially reboot our digestive system and restore a good flora for vibrant and healing health. His book is called Medical Medium.

In addition to having probiotics for your gut health, it is important to have prebiotics as well. They are the food for the probiotic bacteria. There are different brands of prebiotic that can be purchased. However, they are more easily gotten from simple foods. Some of the common prebiotic in foods include:

1. Onion
2. Leeks
3. Scallion
4. Flaxseed
5. Cacao
6. Apples
7. Banana
8. Garlic
9. Asparagus
10. Almond
11. Chickpeas
12. Broccoli
13. Kale
14. Seaweed
15. Raw Honey
16. Berries

Discussion with Janet Doerr on Probiotics

Janet Doerr, the Intuitive Nutritionista, stated that probiotics are super important but it will be different for different people because all people have individual conditions in their guts to start with. A person may have a lot of fungus, they might have a lot of candida yeast, or they might have this or that, or they might have different parasites or they might have some other kind of unhappy bacteria and may be lacking certain good bacteria. So, everybody starts with something unique.

"One of the things we know is that if you take a probiotic with 50 billion live little guys in it and you put it in your stomach, the hydrochloric acid from the digestive processes is going to kill a huge number of those little guys before they even get past the stomach and go down the gut. But, some of them survive.

"So, is the probiotic helpful? Yes! Is it as helpful as the 50 billion on the label? No. What I ask people to claim is to say '**I choose that I have** the best gut microbiome on the planet.' Choose for that to be what they are creating, that I am going to have this super powered up, charged up, perfect microbiome. And then having claimed that, let their guidance system guide them step by step to whatever is perfect for them. When I said that, I heard that I should eat some kimchee (some sauerkraut stuff). And the answer is for a person to say 'OK, Universe, bring me exactly what it is that would be perfect for me.'

"I would encourage people to say yes to probiotics and yes to prebiotics. What are some of the prebiotics? **Organic raw fruits and vegetables, broccoli sprouts, sprouted organic sunflower sprouts.** Those things are loaded with yummy good bacteria...**fermented vegetables, sauerkraut, kimchee**...all those kinds of things...cultured food (i.e., yogurt, kefir). I generally encourage people to steer away from the dairy. They can have coconut milk yogurt, almond milk yogurt, goat's milk yogurt. Those are all lighter, higher frequency, cleaner, and healthier versions and still get all the good bacteria from the lactobacillus bacteria from a cultured food.

"So yes, the gut is super important - **Cultured foods, fermented foods, raw foods, probiotics and prebiotics.** All of the above! And which ones are best is very different for different people."

It is interesting to note how Janet makes her decision with which probiotic to take. She often asks her body what she should take then listens to its response in guiding her choices. It seems like it always guides her to what she needs. Learning a good muscle-testing technique for yes or no questions can be very helpful in this.

This practice of receiving inner guidance is very common with people who are intuitive and aware that their bodies are highly intelligent beings. The information also comes from the Body Elemental. Every human and animal have a Body Elemental overseeing them and providing guidance to those who will listen. These Divine Beings are part of the support for each and even human and animal embodied on Earth.

Interview with Alexis - Another Perspective

On the other hand, **Alexis,** her alias, a parapsychologist and a Medical Intuitive/Medium, is against taking probiotics supplements on a daily basis because she feels we all have different bacteria needs and the supplement may contain a bacteria strand that is not good for us. She has seen people taking certain bacteria that made them sicker. "A client of mine took a probiotic supplement and she and her daughter had a bad reaction to one brand of probiotic supplement and got quite sick. However," Alexis stated, "if you have been on an antibiotic and had some serious imbalance in your gut, I can see replacing certain bacteria for maybe a month but you also have to test which bacteria you do require.

She is also against just eating fermented food as a source of probiotic. She stated that the whole fermented thing is a rage now, and if you can't methylate certain fermented food, it is going to make you sicker. She further said, "We have a very delicate balance in our stomach, and so why would I ingest bacteria on a daily basis?" She pointed out to me that she is able to pinpoint which bacteria the individual needs.

With regards to the colon, she states that "all of the diseases start at the gut and that she sees a lot of magnesium deficiency in her patients." She usually recommends one of five different forms of magnesium to her patients. She sees so much deficiency because we burn them from stress and aluminum leaches magnesium. Most of us are aluminum toxic.

She states, "Although I believe that probiotics are very important for gut health, I do not believe in taking it daily for years. I take a probiotic supplement when I need it and usually it is for short term and have great benefits doing that as well as my family. I also will eat certain fermented foods only when my body craves certain ones like kimchi or sauerkraut, however, I always eat plenty of dark leafy vegetables and fruits as well."

I think both Janet and Alexis have valid points but both touch on something very important with our gut and health in general which is tuning into that Divine Presence within us to guide us on what we need for our body. I have always been guided to taking certain supplements or fermented food, when my body feels like I need it. Although it may sound like Alexis is against probiotics, she is more against jumping on the band wagon of taking something that may not be good for you.

Those of us who are in tune with themselves and the Divine Presence within may ask for guidance on what is best for you. Others may need the guidance of somewhat like Janet or Alexis who can tune in holographically to find out from your body what it needs. Others may feel more comfortable with expert advice from a Gut expert like Dr. Grace Liu, aka the Gut Goddess, Functional and Integration Medicine Practitioner.

Other supplements that may provide gut and digestive support include the following:

- **Slippery Elm*** is good for coating the digestive lining. Andrei and I have found it helpful for our digestive issues.
- **Colostrum LD*** is a touted as being very helpful with leaky gut syndrome and providing great support for our immune system. It helps with oral bacteria. According to **Sovereign Laboratories,** the natural antibodies in bovine colostrum take immediate action to destroy oral bacteria (the cause of gingivitis and a contributing factor to heart disease) and help shorten the healing process of cold sores. A little further down the G.I. tract, colostrum powder offers added healing for people with GERD and other stomach ailments. **(R 73)**

I highly recommend this product to help give your gut the help it deserves. It takes away the toxic material while bringing in the nutrients that our gut needs.

Colostrum 6 is a product a client of mine took with great health benefits. My client had been suffering with many digestive and gut issues for the past year and had poor health. Each time I would visit him, I noticed he had very low energy and had much pain. We would just sit and talk since he didn't feel well at all. The last time I saw him a year later, he was full of energy and stated he felt significantly better. He told me he had been taking Colostrum 6 for about a week and was surprised by the health benefits. He was actually quite happy and finally feeling good. **(R 74)**

I cannot verify all the claims but can verify that my client has improved significantly after trying the product for one week. It certainly appears to be doing a lot of good for my client in giving back his life. (*The products can be purchased from a local distributor or at the R 74 link above.*) For those who want to perfect their gut even further, you may want to check out Viome.com or Thegutinstitute.com. **(R 75)**

SIBO (Small Intestinal Bacterial Overgrowth)

Dr. Grace Liu is the founder of thegutinstitute.com and is known as the Gut Goddess. She is one of the top gut experts in the Bay Area. She has graciously shared 7 steps to stop SIBO.

1. She recommends **eating organic sauerkraut, kvass and kimchi**.
2. She recommends **boosting our gut flora by eating heirloom potatoes and other root vegetables, as well as ancient grains, legumes and lentils**. Always choose organic and opt for soaking and fermentation whenever possible.
3. If you're not severely immunocompromised, taking a soil based probiotic 1-2 times daily can be extremely helpful. Look for strands such as Bacillus subtilis, Clostridium butyricum, Bifidobacteria longum BB536, or Lactobacillus plantarum.
4. **Get plenty of fiber** - there are plants that provide bionic fiber to help heal the gut and keep it moving like inulin, psyllium, high - ORAC green powder and acacia gum can be beneficial. A tablespoon of each dissolved in 16 oz. of water is a great starting point.
5. **Work it out** - research shows that getting an hour a day of continuous low to moderate intensity exercise helps to keep your gut moving and overcomes broken myenteric -neuro junctions. Getting your 10K steps in is an ideal start!
6. **Avoid Allergenic Foods** (corn, soy, gluten/wheat, dairy, nuts and egg whites)
7. **Heal Your Hormones and Immunity** - SIBO calls for a selection of supplements that offer adrenal support, liver support and antioxidant for healing. Biocurcumin and berberine work well in combination with natural antimicrobials and antiparasitics.

You can get the full 7 steps at https://sibo.thegutinstitute.com. You can further improve your gut biome by getting a special kit at https://thegutinstitute.com/maximize.

Minerals

Besides gut health, it is important that we get enough minerals and trace minerals. Below are supplements that may help replenish our lost minerals and trace minerals. Minerals are important for our health and wellness. They are found in our fruits and vegetables. Although many of us try our best to get it from what we eat, our depleted soils results in fruits and vegetables that are similarly mineral deficient. If we are not getting enough minerals or trace minerals in our diets, we may need to take some form of supplementation.

Vital Earth Minerals Fulvic Mineral Complex* is a must have for anyone who exercises, sweats a lot or who wants to have good health.

Most people believe that athletes or those of fitness extraordinaire are healthy. Unfortunately, that might be further from the truth. According to Andrei, a couch potato can live longer than an athlete. Many athletes have a shorter life span due to their harsh training and the effects it has on their bodies. He stated that athletes who are fit are not necessarily healthy. In fact, he stated that many athletes have died at a very young age.

He believes that some athletes, including Olympians, train too hard and lose too much sweat. Most will drink some type of sweet beverage that only has some electrolytes like potassium and sodium chloride. However, what the athlete loses is a significant amount of minerals. According to Lydia from Divine Health, minerals are basically the spark plugs of life. Minerals are the catalyst that keep our 'battery' going and holding its 'charge.' **There are 103 known minerals at least 18 of these are necessary for good health. (R 76)**

Losing excessive minerals like magnesium and selenium over time can be detrimental to our heart. Andrei suspects some of the athletes may possibly be dying from heart problems due to the excessive sweating, lifestyle and other factors that lead them to losing minerals without replenishing them.

According to Lydia, many factors affect the minerals that are depleted from the body include: birth control pills, coffee, alcohol (speeds up the excretion of magnesium through the kidneys; it can also deplete, calcium, zinc, iron, manganese, potassium, and chromium), pregnancy, excess estrogen, hyperthyroidism, soda, sugar pharmaceutical drugs, cortisone, antacids and acid blockers, soil depletion, low stomach acid, excess insulin, stress (depletes magnesium), athletics/excessive exercising- taxes magnesium reserves), and The Standard American Diet (SAD diet). Suffice to say, we are all losing much crucial minerals in our bodies. It won't take much to empty our reserves of magnesium and selenium which will lead us to our premature demise. Fortunately, there is a solution.

Fulvic Mineral Complex is an excellent way to replace the minerals that may be flushed out of our bodies. It contains 70 minerals and trace minerals that will support our inner harmony and contribute to our radiant health.

Blk. is alkaline water that contains Fulvic Trace minerals- approximately 70 trace minerals and electrolytes. The bottle it comes in is BPA free. This is a great drink to get for hydration or dehydration which can be ordered online or purchased at Sprouts and Safeway.

The above is just to whet your appetite and pique your interest in being more proactive with your health. It is not a definitive list of all the important things that might help you but the purpose of my examples is to show you how there are myriad ways to help create harmony within your body, mind and spirit.

The important thing is to take only what you need after you consult with your physician or health care practitioner.

By now some of you might be overwhelmed by all the supplements that I feel were quite beneficial and important. There is an alternative approach that I have discovered that combines many nutrients, vitamins and minerals that is packaged for you to easily incorporate into your busy life. The company is called **Kyani**. They have three main products that include **Kyani Sunrise** (it contains the power of Wild Alaskan Blueberries plus 21 other super fruits which is also a good source of minerals and trace minerals), **Kyani Sunset** which contains the most potent form of vitamin E- tocotrienol (It is a great antioxidant and may support the heart, skin, immunity, diabetes and help to create greater harmony for those who have cancer.), Omega-3 fatty acids, Vitamin A (for immune support, vision, heart, lung and kidney support), Vitamin D3(immunity and bone support), Vitamin B1, B-2 and B-3 and Astaxanthin (one of the best antioxidants). It also has **Kyani Nitro** which is a good boost for energy and provides vascular and cardiac support.

I find this bundle quite comprehensive for someone who is on the go but want something good and effective to support their health and wellness. The Wild Alaskan Blueberry has five times the potency of a regular blueberry due to its ability to survive harsh weather patterns in Alaska.

(Those who are interested in this product can get this product at GoldenLotus.kyani.com).

Ocean Alive 2.0 Marine Phytoplankton is an excellent supplement is purported to contain all the nutrients we need at a cellular level.

Another product that seems to be getting a lot of attention and positive results and reviews is **Paradise Orac-Energy Greens.** It contains a lot of fruits, vegetables as well as herbs including Reishi and Cordyceps.

Besides what to take to support the chemical harmony within our bodies, it is extremely important we take actions to detoxify on a regular basis to remove the toxins and metals that have been accumulating in our bodies for many generations.

Eating well, drinking well and detoxifying helps to reset our system and creates greater harmony and healing within us.

It is one thing to take vitamin, minerals and supplements as a prophylaxis but let's explore some of the supplements, therapies and techniques that are popular for giving support with various conditions.

The following conditions have been listed along with some of the more effective supplements and treatments I have found for myself or clients who have used them. Remember, none of this replaces good medical care. They are only supplements to medical care, good eating and healthy living.

Boosting the Immune System

Having a strong and balanced immune system is at the foundation of optimal health for every living creature, including the Earth herself. 2020 is the year where having a strong immune system is imperative for our survival. Gratefully, there are many food and supplements that can support our immune systems while being in harmony with Earth and nature. We discussed extensively about the importance of probiotics and the gut health with regards to the immune system in the last section but the below will give your body further support once the immune system is compromised.

I have found the product **Sambucus Elderberry** with zinc*, and **Anti-V Formula Echinamide*** quite helpful when I have a touch of the cold or flu virus. It can help shorten the duration of the illness. (IS) Taking Zinc Gluconate at about 30-50 mg can be quite helpful. However, be careful to avoid taking too high of a dosage without consulting a health expert. Zinc is found in other supplements and multi-vitamins. Make sure to not take too much zinc as it can affect the needed copper in your body. However, some health experts say that we can even go up to 100 mg a day but only for a few days up to a week. Andrei stated that some health practitioners take somewhere between 25- 30 mg up to 60- 70 mg.

Andrea's favorite zinc is Zinc glycinate* because it is one of the best absorbed zinc. However, he stated that "zinc ions have a tough time getting across the cell membrane because of their electrical charge." Using a zinc ionophore can help it get into the cells much easier. "Once it gets into the cells and the concentration of the zinc ion within the cell gets high enough, it stops the enzyme that a virus depends on to replicate itself."

He further stated that there are two natural zinc ionophores (a compound that helps to move ions across the membrane)- quercetin and EGCg. The most effective quercetin is **Quercetin Photosome.** * His favorite is made by **Thorne.** He pointed out a study he once read that showed how by adding **EGCg** (can get from Green Tea and Matcha green tea extract) with the Quercetin Photosome, it can further enhance its effectiveness, absorption and potency.

NutriCology's Humic Acid* is touted as a powerful immune booster and support. One doctor wrote an article about how he no longer has a cold or flu for a year since taking this product. (IS)

If I have a sore throat, I will add three squirts of **Anti-V Formula Echinamide*** into a small amount of alkaline water. I mix it up and then gargle it for 30 seconds before swallowing it. I will do this a few times a day and it usually does the job for me. It contains Echinacea purpura, Lomatium, Astragalus, Licorice and Reishi mushroom. (IS)

I will use **Pathogen Assassin Immune Support*** if I want to bring out the big guns for putting the cold bug or virus in its place. It is purported to be anti-virus, anti-fungal, anti-bacterial and anti-parasitical. I once had food poisoning and took this product and found it was quite effective in helping me to get over the symptoms and recovering much more gracefully. One of its primary ingredients is Covalent Silver Ozone. (IS)

Others have found help with their immune system with **Colloidal Silver** (IS). However, very high concentrations can possibly turn your skin permanently blue. It is more volatile and needs to be kept in a dark glass container.

The reason the containers need to be dark is because silver particles are very sensitive to prolonged exposure to bright light, which, in turn, can cause your silver particles to oxidize and fall out of suspension. They will then coat the bottom of your storage bottle with what will look like a fine gray coating of silt. This, of course, will destroy the potency of your colloidal silver. So, colloidal silver always needs to be stored in a dark container that keeps bright light out. Doing so will vastly increase the length of time your colloidal silver remains fully potent in storage.

Andrei feels that the **Pathogen Assassin Immune Support** * gives better protection than colloidal silver but some people I know swear by colloidal silver.

It is good to note that what is well known is that different remedies work for different people. This is due in part to the difference in our body constitutions and the ecosystems in which we live.

When not feeling well, I take extra **vitamin D3** for about a week to enlist more support of the immune system. Regular usage is generally recommended to be started at 400-800 IU/day. This can also be achieved by about 15-30 minutes of sunlight per day. This can give you up to 20,000 IU of natural vitamin D. It is important to avoid vitamin D toxicity. 2000- 3000 IU is what is usually recommended to support the immune system. Some people take 5000 IU with no problems. There is a formula to calculate generally how much vitamin D you need – for every 25 pounds of weight you take up to 1000 IU. However, individual body needs will vary, when in doubt check your nutritionist or physician to do the necessary blood testing to determine your level of vitamin D to get an accurate baseline for how much vitamin D you will need for optimum health. This is the best way of determining how much you really lack and need.

It is also important to take it with vitamin K2, as we mentioned before, to help direct the calcium in your body to the right place and avoid excessive calcium buildup in the heart, arteries, or even affecting the brain, digestive system and the kidneys, so get medical advice on the right dosage here. Vitamin K helps with clotting of the blood, so if you are taking medications or have blood clotting issues, consult with your physician if it is ok for you to take it or not.

I also take **Immusupport Probiotic.** It will give me instant live bacteria to further boost the immune system of the gut. I alternate with **Thrive** Probiotic as well. These particular products ensure that enough of the probiotics survive the trip through the stomach and make it to the gut where they actually do the work. (IS)

Manuka honey is also a great support for the immune system. Manuka honey is from the New Zealand Manuka Tree and is a powerful part of nature's medicine cabinet. The higher the number on the bottle, the stronger it is. It is important to not add the honey to very high temperature water less it renders the enzyme in the honey useless. I usually allow the temperature to cool down a little before putting the Manuka or Raw honey into my cup of hot water.

Vitamin C is always a part of the healing process and I recommend it as well. One of the best forms of Vitamin C is **Empirical Labs Liposomal Vitamin C*.** It absorbs well in the body and taking higher therapeutic doses can be taken for a cold without causing diarrhea. Andrei takes 2000 mg / day just for preventative medicine but ups it when he feels his immune system is compromised. Dr. Thomas E. Levy, a board-certified cardiologist, feels it is the best form of vitamin C for the heart for support. (IS)

Intravenous Vitamin C can be quite effective for those who have a serious upper respiratory infection. This can be administered by a naturopathic doctor, holistic medicine practitioner or your physician. (IS)

Camu Camu Vitamin C*

I have also tried this more natural form of vitamin C which is a very high potency version that nature intended for us according to Andrei. I find is extremely effective when added with The Pathogen Assassin during a cold. It is utilized quite well in the body due to its co-factors. (IS)

A blend of Liposomal and Camu Camu may be a great way to go and the best of both worlds where you get great absorption, assimilation and utilization.

I have tried **Daily Wellness Immunity Support Blend** and have found it helpful to supporting my immune system. It contains apricot kernel oil, essential oils of frankincense, oregano, clove, spruce, rosewood and blue tansy. It is recommended that rolling the oil on the base of the foot is the best place for absorption of the product. *(It can be purchased at:* https://halfpintnaturals.com/collections/medicine-cabinet/products/daily-wellness-immunity-blend)

Coconut oil supports our immune system. Traditions Gold Label Virgin Coconut Oil* is Andrei's top pick Coconut oil. It is one of the healthy oils that our body needs that is made the old fashion way by hand. It is herbicide or glyphosate tested. It is farmed in the Philippines at Mt. Banahaw by a family. Coconut oil is believed to be good for our immune system and can provide metabolic support.

According to organicfacts.net, the following are some of its medicinal properties: It cures fatigue, has antioxidant, anti-aging and, antimicrobial properties, reduces hair loss; helps with candida, vermifuge, dandruff, and digestive disorders. **(R 77)**

It is also purported to have many health benefits including increasing our health cholesterol HDL and converting our LDL (bad cholesterol) into good cholesterol. There are many benefits including helping with weight loss and sex. According to Andrei, the saturated fat in this oil is healthy for us unlike what some of the bad press that it has received. Some of the bad press has come from so called health experts from an esteemed university.

According to Andrei, many of the contemporary experts based their knowledge on the old theory called the Lipid Hypothesis based on the research of Ancel Keys. He is known as the father of Lipid Hypothesis. He did studies on the diets of post-world war II populations in Europe. His research purportedly found that there was a link between heart disease, saturated fat and cholesterol in the diet. Over time that view was propagated and after initial challenges from the medical community, it eventually was accepted and also by the American Heart Association.

In recent years, they revisited the works of Ancel Keys and found that his work or research was fraudulent. He had data from many different populations throughout Europe and he had cherry-picked only those data that supported his theory. If he used all the data that were available to him from all the populations used in the study, there would have been no relationship between saturated fat and increase risk of heart disease. He has been discredited, but the dogma still remains. At the time, many other research scientists were appalled by Keys' shoddy research, but the media and top clients in the petrochemical industry embraced Keys' findings. **(R 78)**

Black Seed Oil - has been associated with benefits for blood pressure, digestive issues, diabetes respiratory illness and many other ailments. Research also seems to suggest benefits with viral infections. I how found it extremely effective with dealing with the early onset of a flu. A relative of mine was not feeling well and had a slight fever at 99 degrees. Due to the pandemic, the doctor was unable to see her. I had some black seed oil and gave her some. Two to three hours later, the fever was gone and she felt well again and was back to her baseline. I have taken it and feel that it is good at supporting the immune system. It is important to get 100% Pure Cold-Pressed Black Cumin Seed Oil.

There are many ways to improve the immune system but incorporating the **Wim Hof Method** into your life can be a free way of boosting your immune system. I have used it and have found that it was helpful when my immune system was weak. It helped me to negotiate through my cold much more gracefully. (IS)

Besides the above, if I sleep plenty (7-9 hours per night), hydrate well and meditate regularly, I can usually shake off the bug and virus. Keep stress by the wayside and these supplements and techniques can do wonders for many people. I write extensively about methods to deal with stress in my first book, *Dare to Imagine*. Incidentally, the **Wim Hof Method** is very helpful with helping us cope with stress as well. (More will be discussed on this method in the chapter on breathing).

Timing is everything. If you wait too late to intervene, the recovery period will be much more extended and the supplements become less effective. A layered approach with multiple methods worked best for me, but two helpful methods we can all do include: regular **exercise** which helps to boost the immune system and **Meditation** which improves the immune system by 40%. **Adequate sleep**, **eating well** and **minimizing your stress** will support your immune system as well.

Emotional Suffering

Depression

Millions of people all around the world suffer from some form of depression. Severe depression may be best treated initially with anti-depressants but with judicious use of it due to some of the adverse side effects. People suffering from less severe depression may find benefits with some of the more popular over the counter supplements out there like the **Jarrow Formula of SAMe 200** and **St. John's Wort. Vitamin E, Vitamin D3 and Niacin** are helpful as well. However, I find that a combined approach for this complex illness is the most effective. Getting rid of processed food, soda, sweets and coffee may be beneficial.

According to Carrie, alcohol and processed meat (hot dogs, sausage and other fried and fatty food) can also contribute to depression. Instead, get plenty of rest, water, organic food, organic fruits and vegetables will support and speed up the recovery process. **(R 79)** Carrie writes that the following foods can help with depression.

Plant based foods that are high in tryptophan include fruit including strawberries and bananas, oats, soy, nuts, legumes and some seeds including sesame, flax and pumpkin. Tryptophan is an amino acid which helps the brain produces a feel-good sensation by increasing the serotonin in the brain. (*The only recommendation I would make is to get organic products as much as possible to create greater inner harmony.*)

Carbohydrates (whole wheat bread or brown rice versus processed carbohydrates like white bread, sugar, candy or white rice) - I lean more towards getting it more from Mother Nature - like from fruits - instead. Also, eating more of what Dr. William Sears Calls the "right -carbs"- carbohydrates that have fiber, protein and some fat will help the body have a more sustained form of energy and feelings of wellness. They are found in fruits, vegetables and whole grain.

Salmon - If you are still eating fish, then salmon and other fatty fish containing Omega-3 fatty acids like salmon, tuna, lake trout, herring, mackerel, anchovies, and sardines can enhance your mood. It can be quite helpful with stress, brain imbalances and depression. It can help with repetitive thoughts and help brain produce more serotonin. It is a mineral of the brain that is quite lacking in our diet and taking it as a supplement can do wonders.

Having a healthy flora will definitely help with how you feel by producing opiates, serotonin and dopamine. Taking probiotics like **Thrive***, or other quality products, can be helpful for the short term in supporting a healthy gut which will allow us to experience greater peace, happiness and joy.

Camu Camu Vitamin C and essential oils can help with depression as well.

Anxiety or Stress

Taking **Rescue Remedy, essential oils,** drinking **Chamomile Tea or** using various essential oils like **lavender** can help one to feel less anxious and more relaxed. Yogic breathing techniques and meditation are very helpful.

In chapter 6, we will explore in the complexities of emotional turmoil in much greater depth.

Exercise can also help with anxiety, stress and depression by stimulating the body to release endorphins and dopamine to keep us happy.

Low Energy

Many times low energy is a result of the accumulation of toxins within our bodies. Once we release the metals through specific fruits, vegetables, vitamins, supplements, chelation therapy or other naturopathic methods that utilize intravenous chemicals to remove it, the result can bring much harmony to the body and result in more energy. Supplements that can support our energy include Magnesium Taurate, Tahitian Noni, NitroXtreme from Kyani, According to Dr. Norm Shealy, "NitroXtreme is the best product in the world for hypertension, overcoming fatigue and enhancing energy."

Vitamin B12 coupled with Vitamin B Complex, Ginseng Sublime and Qi Drops tonic elixirs from Dragonherbs.com can be quite helpful. I have found the Great Immortal tonic elixir from the Dragonherbs quite effective and it helps me to relax as well.

Astaxanthin 4mg with Phospholipids may provide DNA and cellular protection which allows the cell to work more efficiently and give us more energy.

According to Pyradyne.com, **Shou Wu Chih** is one of the most popular liquid tonic preparations for both men and women. It warms and invigorates the blood, nourishes the liver and kidneys and benefits the eyes. The prepared Shou Wu strengthens the bones and tendons. (**R 80**)

The Chinese consider it to be an herb tonic for longevity and sexuality; it replenishes Qi and the vital essence that is lost in sexual indulgence. It is a crucial herb to the blood, and research has shown that it decreases cholesterol levels and improves energy levels. It enhances the psychic network of the parasympathetic nervous system, allowing you to actually feel the inside workings of all the Pyradyne Systems and Nuclear Receptors.

It was one of the first herbal supplements that Ron Teeguarden tried that gave him an incredible amount of energy. It helped to spark his interest in eventually becoming a Master Herbalist.

I once visited a friend at Mount Shasta that I haven't seen in a long time. When I saw him, I could see he was being depleted of his Qi energy and was very weak. He was so weak he was using a cane. We later went to his house and within a short time, I began to sense a negative entity or entities at his residence. He apparently had been trying to leave Mount Shasta but somehow felt like he could not go and was trapped. Something bad would always happen if he would try to leave. I knew that his health would continue to deteriorate if he stayed so I gave him a heart to heart talk about leaving soon for the sake of his health. I truly believed that the entity was feeding off his energy. He eventually took my advice and moved out. I suggested drinking Shou Wu Chih and he did and he began feeling a lot better and with more energy. The last time I spoke with him he was doing very well.

I have found **Vibrant Health Green Vibrance** quite helpful for giving me more energy. It has 25 billion probiotics, vegetables, vitamins and many great nutrients for promoting optimal heath and energy. They sell this at Whole Foods. I take this daily. Maintaining gut health is the key to energy!

Niagen is a supplement that one of the great Yogis and spiritual masters at Mount Shasta takes to increase energy and well-being. It has a co-enzyme called NAD which is attributed to increase energy. He has noted an improvement within two weeks of taking it. According to Sean Johnson, author of F1000 Research, it is now clear that systemic NAD^+ decline is one of the fundamental molecular events that regulate the process of aging and possibly limit organismal life span. We are at an exciting point in time when we can effectively test the importance of NAD^+ for the prevention and treatment of aging and aging-related diseases in humans. **(R 81)**

Haritaki is often referred to as the King of Herbs. It (Terminalia chebula) is a tree native to southern Asia and India. The dried fruit of the tree has a long history of use in Ayurveda, the traditional medicine of India. Sometimes referred to as "chebulic myrobalan," haritaki is one of three dried fruits that make up the ayurvedic formula **Triphala.**

Available in powder or dietary supplement form, haritaki has a bitter taste. It is rich in vitamin C and substances found to have antioxidant and anti-inflammatory effects.

People use **haritaki** to promote healing from a number of conditions ranging from sore throat to allergies, as well as to improve digestive issues such as constipation and indigestion. In Ayurveda, haritaki is said to support the "Vata" dosha**. (R 82)**

Haritaki reputedly increases prana which is the super-fine essence of vata. Prana is the force that is present in every cell, in the subtle body, in the mind, and connected to our souls. It powers the body and keeps the mind supple and adaptable. It bestows creativity, enthusiasm, and strength. It is all this and more—and without prana, there is no life. This link to increasing prana could be behind the deep-rooted belief in India and Tibet that haritaki increases energy, intelligence, and awareness. **(R 83)**

Ashwagandha is an incredibly healthy medicinal herb. It's classified as an "adaptogen," meaning that it can help your body manage stress. Ashwagandha also provides all sorts of other benefits for your body and brain. For example, it can lower blood sugar levels, reduce cortisol, boost brain function and help fight symptoms of anxiety and depression. It is one of the most important herbs in Ayurveda, a form of alternative medicine based on Indian principles of natural healing. It has been used for over 3,000 years to relieve stress, increase energy levels and improve concentration. **(R 84)**

Triphala is an herbal concoction that's been used for thousands of years in Ayurveda. Traditionally used as a bowel tonic, it's often prescribed as a mild laxative. But while its laxative qualities are most widely known, the other benefits of this herb are perhaps even more noteworthy. Triphala means "the three fruits" and it's comprised of the Indian fruits amalaki, haritaki, and bibhitaki.

According to Kulreet Chaudhary, author of ***The Prime: Prepare and Repair Your Body for Spontaneous Weight Loss*** (Harmony Books, 2016), Triphala is one of the three Ayurvedic supplements that boost energy. **(R 85, 86)**

Chlorenergy* is touted as one of the best **Chlorella** in the market and can support increased energy and cellular health as well. Chlorella is a type of algae, which is a type of single-celled plant. There are countless types of algae, many of which are safe, although some can be very harmful to us. Chlorella is one of those that is not harmful, and it can even be very beneficial to us.

Chlorella is grown commercially and its popularity is growing, particularly in healthy-living circles. It is packed with nutrition and is low in calories, making it ideal for people that want healthy diets.

Chlorella also contains various compounds that can provide health benefits ranging from lowering blood sugar levels to giving athletes a performance boost.

Some of its many health benefits are as follows: **(R 87)**
- Binds heavy metals
- Boosts Immunity
- Lowers Blood Pressure
- Nutrition- it is a good source of nutrition and is a superfood
- High in Antioxidants
- Soothes Respiratory Conditions
- Boost Aerobic Performance
- Helps with Detox
- Good for Diabetics
- Improves Cholesterol Levels.
- Energy Boost

MCT Oil As the name suggests, medium-chain triglyceride (MCT) oil contains medium-length chains of fats called triglycerides. Due to their shorter length, MCTs are easily digested and many health benefits are linked to the way your body processes these fats. (R **88**)

MCT oil is most commonly extracted from coconut oil, as more than 50% of the fat in coconut oil comes from MCTs. MCT oil can provide sustained energy support. MCT oil is a supplement often added to smoothies, Bulletproof Coffee and some salad dressings.

MCT oil has also been dubbed a super fuel since your body absorbs MCTs more rapidly than long-chain triglycerides (LCTs). In the liver, the fats are broken down to be either used as fuel or stored as body fat. Since MCTs easily enter your cells without being broken down, they can be used as an immediate source of energy

When you are on a ketogenic diet, MCTs can also be converted into ketones in the liver. These ketones can pass through your blood-brain barrier, making them a convenient source of energy for your brain cells. **(R 89)**

Having good flora can lead to better mood as well as energy. When our gut is well, it absorbs the nutrients from our food to give us energy. If our gut and flora is out of whack and full of toxins and lack of the bacteria we need, our colon can't give us the proper nutrients that we need for our body for health, wellness, repair and energy.

A plant-based diet has been proven to improve the performance, endurance, strength and energy of many of our top cutting-edge athletes including football players, cyclist, runners, martial artist, weightlifters, body builders, etc. The film *Game Changer* will share with you who these great athletes are.

The **Stimulating Breath or Bellow's Breath** is a yogic breathing technique that can bring you instant energy or improve your Prana energy or life force. It also warms you up and wakes you up. It is a rapid breathing through the nose from 10 seconds to 1 minute. Dr. Andrew Weil has a simple and easy video you can watch to learn this effective and easy to learn technique.

Dragon Tail Meditation/Growing your Dragon Tail is a meditation or visualization technique originally taught by Grandmaster Mantak Chia. The meditator visualizes breathing in and out at the bones below the sacrum and opening it while extending or uncurling the meditator's dragon tail. He or she then imagines the tip of tail extending or growing it down to Mother Earth and into the center of the planet where there is this hot red lava and plenty of life force and Qi. The meditator then imagines hearing the pulsating heartbeat of Mother Earth. The meditator then visualizes or imagines the energy of the heart and Dantian pulsating as well and eventually becomes in sync with the pulsating heartbeat of Mother Earth.

The meditator visualizes and breathes while going down the tail and back down to the center of Mother Earth. The meditator then visualizes and breathes up the powerful Earth Qi spiraling up the tail until it reaches the sacrum, the Dantian and then to the heart lighting it all up with the pure Qi. Imagine and feel the pulsation of the three as one. Thereafter, breathe in and exhale the word ha and allow that heart fire to connect with all the other heart fires around the world. Do this a few times.

After I did this meditation, I felt rejuvenated even though I was tired prior to doing it. This is a modified version that was taught to me by Marian Brandenburg, a body healer, an intuitive massage therapist, Chi Nei Tsang Practitioner, and Ajna and Neuro Light Practitioner. She works during the winter at Grandmaster Mantak Chia's Tao Garden but is in San Rafael during the rest of the year.

Exercise is the best way to boost energy! Brisk walking, jumping jacks, trampoline exercise, jumping rope and dancing may be quite effective in increasing our energy levels.

Holistic Approaches for Common Ailments and Major Diseases Constipation

Those who are constipated are not eating enough fiber; this will render the gut being inefficient in getting the nutrients we need. According to *Everyday Health*, the national fiber recommendations are 30 to 38 grams a day for men and 25 grams a day for women between 18 and 50 years old, and 21 grams a day if a woman is 51 and older. Another general guideline is to get 14 grams of fiber for every 1,000 calories in your diet. According to Men's Fitness, the best sources of fiber include raspberry, avocado, chia seed, flaxseed meal, oatmeal, lentils, broccoli, cabbage, apples and Brussel sprouts. **(R 90)**

Besides eating fruits and vegetables that contain high fiber, we can get fiber supplements from **psyllium husk** or **NOW Organic Acacia Fiber Powder**. It is touted be a great pre-biotic and supports good flora.

Magnesium Citrate can also have a laxative effect and many of my clients have been prescribed **MiraLax** for those who have been constipated for days with great results.

Triphala can help with digestive health as well as with constipation as we have mentioned earlier along with many other benefits. It is often found in colon cleanse powders.

Yumiko Yoga, a Yoga Teacher, Reiki Teacher, Sound and Voice Healer, and Neo Healer in Tokyo, stated that many of her students have used a castor oil pack with amazing health benefits including improving menstruation and constipation due to its ability to improve blockages, circulation and elimination. She gets her castor oil packs at www.edgarcaycee.org.

Exercise also helps with improving digestion and elimination.

Hypertension

So many millions of people have high blood pressure. The causes of it may start with poor dietary habits, stress and too much sodium and sugar intake. Most people know that too much sodium causes increased blood pressure but few know that too much sugar or glucose can contribute to it. When we consume more glucose than we need, the excess will either be stored in the liver, become fat in our lower abdomen area and elsewhere or begin binding with protein molecules and begin to create a sticky material that leads to plaque formation and lead to hardening of the arteries in what is known as atherosclerosis.

If our blood pressure goes out of control it can lead to a heart attack, stroke or death. The majority of my clients have some degree of hypertension. Many are prescribed medications to control it. Besides medication, other methods that can help with hypertension include:

1. Juicing with celery first thing in the morning.
2. Decrease your intake of sodium with cooking and snacks.
3. Exercise at least 20-30 minutes a day a few days a week to stimulate greater release of nitric oxide levels in the arteries to increase

vasodilation, heal the arteries and dissolve the stickiness in our arteries that lead to plaque formation. Walk 10 steps if possible.
4. Qunol Mega CoQ10 Ubiquinol (available at Costco); it can be quite helpful.
5. Switch from table salt to Himalayan Salt
6. Kyani Nitro can be of assistance since it helps to increase the nitric oxide levels in the arteries.
7. Losing weight
8. Controlling stress through meditation, yogic breathing, yoga, Tai Chi, Qi Gong and exercise.

Andrei stated that what helps too is to eat more green leafy vegetables, non-starchy plants and fruits. He has found two products that are helpful:

1. Peptace Fish Peptides 500 mg
2. Life Extension Advanced Olive Leaf Vascular Support with Celery Seed Extract/

He also stated that it helps to increase our potassium level to about 2000 mg. According to the American Heart Association, the recommended amount is about 4,700 mg per day. However, always make sure you check with your physician on how much you can take due to the medications you may be taking or your unique medical conditions.

Cancer

So many people have cancer nowadays. Chances are that someone you know or love has cancer. I have seen people go into remission with conventional treatment while others have died. On the other hand, I have heard about people who had friends who have stabilized their cancer with the help of chemo, Brachy Therapy and various supplements, and lifestyle changes. Although I have not met any of these people who claimed to have a remission from their cancer, the information I got about them came from reliable sources.

Some of the supplements that have helped some people with cancer to restore more harmony in their body include **Kyani Products.** As mentioned before, they have a potent form of vitamin E that may be helpful to people suffering from cancer or other related illnesses or diseases. It contains Tocotrienol a very potent and pure form of vitamin E. Some studies seem to show how it could be helpful with cancer especially with Delta Tocotrienol **(R 91)** https://www.clinicaleducation.org/resources/reviews/the-next-generation-vitamin-e-how-tocotrienols-benefit-the-heart-brain-and-liver/

Kyani have many super fruits in their package giving good nourishment and support to the body to optimize the harmony within the body.

Curamed may be helpful as well since it contains a high amount of Curcumin. According to Cancer Research UK, a 2013 international laboratory study looked at the effects of a combined treatment with curcumin and chemotherapy on bowel cancer cells. The researchers concluded that the combined treatment might be better than chemotherapy alone.

A Medical Perspective

Dr. Donald Abrams, current Chief of Hematology and Oncology at San Francisco General Hospital and Director of Integrative Oncology Research at the University of California San Francisco's Osher Center for Integrative Medicine, noted a growing body of evidence linking vitamin D deficiency with breast cancer and suggests taking 1,000-2,000 IU preferably in gel cap form (to allow easier digestion), or with a meal containing some type of fat.

He and Dr. Melina Jampolis believe that nutrients are much better obtained from whole foods rather than vitamin and mineral supplements. He recommends following as much as possible an organic, plant-based, antioxidant rich, anti-inflammatory diet with particular emphasis on cruciferous (broccoli, cabbage), orange-yellow and leafy green vegetables and heavily pigmented, deeply colored fruits.

If you feel you must have animal protein, they recommend deep cold water fish (salmon, black cod, albacore tuna, herring, mackerel and sardines) and limiting or eliminating dairy, particularly non-organic, full fat dairy, since in epidemiologic studies they have been linked to higher levels of growth factors that may stimulate tumor growth. **(R 92)**

Sally Scroggs, MS RD LD, and Clare McKinley, RD LD, at the **University of Texas, M.D. Anderson Cancer Center** (one of the leading cancer hospitals in the world) explained that breast cancer risk could be decreased by up to 38% through lifestyle factors including maintaining a healthy weight, exercising regularly, and eating a healthy diet. In fact, less than 10% of breast cancer appears to have a genetic basis. **(R 93)**

According to the **American Institute for Cancer Research**, "no single food or food component can protect you against cancer by itself. But scientists believe that the combination of foods in a predominantly plant-based diet may. There is evidence that the minerals, vitamins and phytochemicals in plant foods could interact in ways that boost their individual anti-cancer effects." **(R 94) Lutetium 177** may be helpful with prostate cancer.

Alternative Approaches

According to another article, extensive research over the past several years has strongly indicated that **Tocotrienols** can efficiently prevent/inhibit the growth of different cancers such as cancer of the blood, brain, breast, cervical, colon, liver, lung, pancreas, skin, stomach, etc. **(R 95)**

Reishi and Cordyceps may help those suffering from cancer achieve greater harmony within. A friend of mine, Jocelyn Lew, has a special blend of the two made by Gano and has reported that some of her friends who suffered from cancer had some health benefits and felt better. In addition, these herbs have anti- aging qualities.

Another friend of mine, Silvia, her alias, gave me an old Chinese herbal recipe made with Reishi that has helped friends and family members suffering from cancer. Her aunt had nasopharyngeal cancer over 25 years ago and stomach cancer seven years ago. Her best friend's husband had thyroid cancer while her co-workers father had prostate cancer. They all drank the herbal soup regularly and their cancer appears to be in remission at this time. Keep in mind all these people were getting good medical care as well. The co-worker's father healed so well that his Stanford doctor wanted to follow him one day and study his lifestyle and assess what variables had helped him heal so miraculously. The amazing **Reishi aka Lingzhi herbal soup recipe** is as follows:

- Fill a pot with 8 cups of water.
- Add 5-7 dark colored Reishi mushroom pieces.
- Add 5-7 light colored Reishi mushroom pieces.
- Add 5 sweet dates.
- Add ½ of the dark of the big dark ball with seeds (Lo Han Go). Cut it in half.
- Bring this to a full boil for 10 minutes then let it simmer for 20 – 30 minutes. Drink warm and enjoy. Drink 1- 2 cups daily. You may eat the sweet dates.

Another friend of mine, Karen, her alias, had a friend whose mom had cancer in Korea and was told her prognosis was poor and that she would have to be fed through a gastrointestinal tube soon. The friend's mother decided to start juicing regularly and eat black garlic every day. She did this every day for a year and her cancer went into remission. She also changed her attitude about life and did everything possible to minimize stress which I believe had a huge impact on her cancer as well.

This is her recipe:

- Obtain some high-quality black garlic.
- Chop off the bottom stem/root.
- Put it in a rice cooker (fill up rice cooker about 80%).
- Press and keep warm for 2 weeks.
- After two weeks, put it in the refrigerator.

Turkey Tail mushrooms have been associated with benefits for many types of cancers including lung cancer. Back in 1976, a Japanese company had already patented certain extracts of Coriolus Versicolor under the name PSK and later PSP, which have since become recognized anti-cancer drugs in Japan. **(R 96)**

My friend who was a Homeopathic Doctor recommended **CBD oil, alkaline water and good nutrition** to support people who have cancer to achieve greater harmony.

She also said that healing sounds may be helpful as well especially when listening to the tone of **444 Hz.** It is believed that this sound frequency may make it hard for the cancer cells to flourish. The 444 Hz frequency is one of the "Solfeggio frequencies' capable of healing the body and mind.

She also recommended listening to the healing tones of **528 Hz** to heal the body further. **(R 97)** https://youtu.be/X1eFtSKABwg

According to Dr. Axe, there are twelve cancer fighting foods **(R 98)** https://draxe.com/cancer-fighting-foods which include:

1. Cruciferous vegetables (e.g. cabbage, broccoli, cauliflower, Brussels sprouts) and other vegetables like onions, zucchini, asparagus, artichokes, pepper, carrots, and beets.
2. Leafy green vegetables.
3. Berries (blueberries, raspberries, cherries, strawberries, goji berries, Camu Camu and black berries.
4. Brightly Orange-Colored Fruits and Veggies (citrus fruits,
5. Fresh Herbs and Spices (turmeric, cultured dairy products ginger, raw garlic, thyme, cayenne pepper, oregano, basil, and parsley
6. Organic Meats (beef, chicken and liver)
7. Cultured Dairy Products (raw milk, cheese). He also recommended about 6 ounces daily of probiotic yogurt, cottage cheese, goat milk kefir or amasai
8. Nuts and seeds (flax seeds, hemp seeds, sesame seeds, pumpkin seeds, sunflower seeds, walnuts, brazil nuts and almonds.
9. Healthy Unrefined Oils (coconut, flax, cod liver and extra virgin olive oil
10. Mushrooms (reishi, cordyceps, and maitake).
11. Traditional Tea (matcha green tea).
12. Wild Caught Fish (salmon, mackerel and sardines).

Ojibwa Tea

Another friend of mine, **Lisa White aka Meenakshi**, a healer, stated that a fibroid tumor in her uterus dissolved from drinking a special tea called **Ojibwa,** a Native American herbal tea.

Lisa White also recommended drinking a lot of carrot juice and eating habanero peppers and garlic. She stated that raw garlic seem to work best.

She gave me a recipe of healing called the **Kelley Eidem's Protocol(R 99)** and it is as follows:

- Grate one habanero pepper each day, putting it on bread. She recommends using the seeds.
- Grate two cloves of garlic each day, putting them on bread and covering it with butter.
- One Tablespoon of Emulsified cod liver once or twice a day. (She stated that TwinLabs makes some wonderfully flavored cod liver oils which can be taken before or after eating the sandwich with the same meal.
- Smother the grated garlic and habaneros peppers with real butter and eat it. Organic or raw butter is the best. No margarines of any type, including Smart Balance, etc.

Lisa stated that an alternative that she might use for habanero is ginger.

Laetrile

Some sources believe that **vitamin B-17, laetrile or amygdalin** can help people with cancer. It can be found in the pits of apricot, peaches, almonds and millets. However, this idea is controversial and the medical community feels that is not effective in helping with treating cancers. Furthermore, Laetrile was even banned in the 80s because it contained cyanide. Surprisingly enough it is still be used in some holistic clinics outside of the United States in clinics in Mexico like Hope4Cancer where they even do IV B-17 along with other modalities with some success.

Dr. Antonio Jimenez, M.D., N.D., C.N.C., Founder and Chief Medical Director of Hope4Cancer Institute, has been using laetrile since 1988 and has never had any toxic reactions. He stated that there are two main methods of taking amygdalin, B-17 (Laetrile) orally and through IV. He feels that the IV method is the best because you bypass the gut and it is absorbed into the body 100%. Dr. Jimenez is a strong proponent of Laetrile therapy. He rates the IV form as most effective. The second is oral and lastly, the actual kernel of an apricot, he considers best for prevention or early stages of cancer.

He states that every day, cancer becomes more complicated, and there are many variables to the cancer's progress and its healing. The doctor also points out that despite the benefits of Laetrile, it should be seen as an important part of an integrative and holistic cancer program instead of being seen and used as a magic bullet or as a sole treatment. **(R 100)**

Selenium

Many believe that selenium can be quite helpful to those who are suffering from cancer. Andrei feels that one of the best selenium is **LifeExtension Se-Methyl L-Selenocysteine.** Another natural source is Brazil nuts (one a day = full day's supply of selenium). **(R 101)** Although it is generally accepted that we should not be taking more than 400 micrograms, Dr. Gerhard N. Schrauzer (was the grand old man of selenium science) believed that 400 mcg was a good dosage as a prophylaxis against cancer.

Castor Oil Packs

Castor Oil Packs have been known for its health benefits for a variety of illnesses and is used externally. According to Yumiko, she has heard (in closed groups) about its effectiveness with cancer with many of its group members. She uses it in her own practice and finds it very effective. You can purchase the Castor Oil and learn more about how to make a Castor Oil pack at edgarcaycee.org.

Acupuncture

I had great opportunity in October 19th to meet with some of the top healers in the world as we dined together. According to one of the top acupuncture doctors in the world, **Dr. Steve Jackowicz, Mac, Lac, PhD**, certain cancers responded quite well with his treatment especially with those patients who had good compliance with his treatment regime. He stated that there are other great acupuncturists around the world who have successfully treated cancer to varying degrees depending on compliance with treatment regime. One lives in Massachusetts and has successful helped many clients with cancer (cervical uterine cancer, lung cancer, colon cancer, pancreatic cancer, prostate and breast cancer and oral squamous-cell carcinoma). He utilizes a holistic approach that incorporates the Best in Traditional Oriental Medicine, Acupuncture, Modern Medicine and natural yogic and holistic healing methods.

In my opinion, cancer has an emotional and spiritual component as well. I believe that anger turned inwards can settle in certain organs and manifest as cancer later in life especially when we are going through a lot of stress. Stress sustained over a long period produces cortisol which shuts down the immune system. Working with a therapist, a medical intuitive, healer or shaman on productively releasing those trapped emotions can be quite healing. Eating healthy and **drinking more alkaline water** can help create an internal environment that is not conducive to cancer. **Prayer and forgiveness** can also release some of the emotional toxic build up in our organs to promote healing. **Group prayers** are especially helpful with cancer patients. **Meditation and visualization** have its benefits with cancer as well.

The Gerson Therapy

The Gerson Therapy™ is a natural treatment that activates the body's extraordinary ability to heal itself through an organic, plant-based diet, raw juices, coffee enemas and natural supplements. **(R 102)** It seems like a viable method to help support people suffering from cancer and other diseases and illnesses.

You can get a plethora of cutting-edge information from **Ty Bollinger** about cancer at his various videos on YouTube. **(R 103)** In my educated view, treatments and techniques that employ holistic methods are the best. **Hope4Cancer** clinics approach to dealing with cancer is the ideal type of program that will best help an individual with cancer. It deals with the physical, emotional and spiritual component of healing. **(R 104)**

Vitamin D may be helpful as well to boost the immune system which is often weakened in a person with cancer. Some scientific studies indicate significant health benefits for those with various types of cancer.

HIFU, or High-Intensity Focused Ultrasound

Hifu, is a new, advanced treatment option for select patients with prostate cancer. This non-invasive procedure uses sound waves, instead of surgery or radiation, to image and destroy prostate cancers **(R 105).**

David Granovsky, Stem Cell advisor, blogger and author, recommends immunotherapy, cryotherapy (he is not talking about going to some liquid nitrogen that will increase the immune system as well but cryotherapy as an extremely targeted procedure) and HIFU in the treatment of cancer. This is huge in Asia and in Europe and in fact the Italian Institute of Urology considers it as the gold standard for treatment.

Keto Diet

Some feel that a Keto Diet can be helpful with cancer. I met a man once who had cancer and was in remission. He stated that it was his keto diet that helped him. He has regular meet ups with others who are doing the same and having similar benefits.

The keto diet is a low-carbohydrate diet. The diet's strict guidelines recommend eating more fat and protein while cutting most carbohydrates and sugars out of your diet.

No single food can cure cancer, but some research has shown a link between the keto diet and slowed growth of some types of tumors in mice. A few studies in humans with certain types of brain tumors have also shown promise. On the contrary, a very low-fat diet has been found to reduce risk of recurrence for certain types of breast cancer, **(R 106)**

Some of those who do the Keto Diet believe that the body gets into a state of ketosis and only the healthy cells survive while the cancer cell dies without the glucose.

A plant-based diet can be extremely helpful in supporting those who are recovering from cancer.

Diabetes

Diabetes is a Trojan horse of many illnesses and is a very serious disease that has destroyed the lives of millions of people. Healthy eating can usually steer one away from this disease especially when avoiding refined sugar, processed food and soda. Eating organic and real food decreases our likelihood of getting this disease.

There are supplements that seem to provide support for those with this disease. **Kyani** products appear to help improve the blood sugar level of some of its users (based on customer testimonials shared with me).

I actually had a client who had been taking it for a year prior to me meeting with him. He had suffered various illnesses and had diabetes. He was frequently hospitalized but after taking Kyani for a year with no other changes in his life, his health began to improve. He is no longer diabetic and has become more medically stable according to his family. However, it is important to mention that a healthy diet may have also been a contributing factor as well as lifestyle changes like exercise.

Professor Peskin was able to show how PEO* provides support for diabetic patients. Dr. Andrew Weil once talked about the **benefits of cinnamon with helping diabetic patients.** Although it is somewhat debatable with which type of cinnamon is better - Ceylon versus cassia? **(R 107)**

Eating a **well-balanced diet** and **exercise** is a must for a diabetic. Staying away from unhealthy high fats, sugar and processed food is also very important with diabetics.

A plant-based diet may be helpful in supporting those recovering from diabetes.

A Slovakian doctor has taken 91 of her type 2 diabetes patients off medication using an advanced plant-based protocol.

Under the guidance of Dr. Janka Lejavova, M.D., the patients followed the Natural Food Interaction (NFI) protocol, a whole food, plant-based approach that mixes and matches different plant foods in combination that are tailored to an individual.

The protocol, which was founded by David Hickman and Zuzana Plevora, has yielded impressive results in trials so far, with 96.5 percent type 2 diabetes remission rate in patients that have completed the protocol. **(R 108)**

Some have found help with the **Ketogenic Diet** while others have improved with an **intermittent fasting**. I had one client who was told to do intermittent fasting by his physician and is now no longer diabetic.

Magnesium Taurate* can help or be of support for those with diabetes as well.

Triphala has been used in India to help with high blood sugar and producing insulin from the pancreas.

Exercise and nutrition- Exercising regularly helps to stabilize insulin levels. Graze eating helps to also stabilize our insulin levels and helps our bodies to have more sustained energy. We should avoid all processed food, sodas and junk food. By doing that, we minimize our bodies being inundated with too much unhealthy forms of glucose which may convert to energy quickly but is short lived and contributes to the **inflammation, oxidation and glycation** in our bodies leading to pre-diabetes and type two diabetes and a host of other health related issues. Eating real food that our Creator provided to us is a healthier way that will lead to health and wellness. However, there is a balance and we must minimize on those fruits or foods that are high in glycemic index and calories.

Heart Disease

Heart Disease afflicts millions of people around the world. Many people have suffered a heart attack aka myocardial infarct. Many people must undergo a bypass surgery due to blockages on the heart artery or arteries. Others suffer from congestive heart failure. Changes in nutrition and lifestyle can reduce our risk of the above scenario. Supplements that may support healthy heart function may include **PEO and Kyani.**

According to Betternutrition.com, there are 9 Supplements for Heart Health. They are Coenzyme Q10, Pantethine, Omega 3's, Magnesium, Niacin, D-Ribose, L-Carnitine, Vitamin K, and Citrus Bergamot. **(R 109)**

I am one of many who think one of the most important things for the prevention of heart disease is **good oral care.** It is very important to brush and floss your teeth daily with both floss and an interdental floss brush. Using a tongue blade to remove bacteria on the tongue and rinsing your mouth for 30 seconds or more with a good oral care product can help diminish the bacteria in your mouth that might lead to gum disease or gingivitis. It can help to decrease plaque as well. I use **TheraBreath Periodontist Formulated Healthy Gums Oral Rinse.**

Co-Enzyme Q10 is essential to a healthy heart and body. According to Dr. Mercola, taking CoQ10 in combination with selenium may improve heart function and reduce cardiovascular mortality by nearly 50 percent among elderly people. It also helps decrease oxidative stress caused by damaging byproducts created by the mitochondria, minimize mitochondrial damage and promote production of new mitochondria. It has many good health benefits and important properties for wellness including being anti-inflammatory and an antioxidant. **(R 110)**

In an interview, Andrei describes **Ubiquinol*** as the best form of Co-Enzyme Q 10. There are many good brands, and his favorite one is sold through LifeExtension.

Andrei stated that vitamin C, vitamin E (mixed tocopherol; Unique Brand is his favorite), selenium, magnesium are all good for heart health.

Vital Earth Minerals Fulvic Mineral Complex* can be helpful to make sure we have all the minerals and trace minerals to support our vascular and heart health if we are deficient of minerals. According to Linus Pauling, an American chemist, biochemist, chemical engineer, peace activist, author, educator, and recipient of Nobel Peace Prize and Noble Prize in chemistry, he said that all ailments, illnesses and diseases can be traced to a mineral deficiency. Andrei further stated that if you want to boil nutrition down to a nut shell, it comes down to minerals. Andrei further stated that Worley Robbins, founder of the magnesium advocacy group on Facebook and the creator of the root cause protocol, likes to say there are no medical conditions and diseases but only metabolic dysfunction caused by mineral deficiencies.

As mentioned before, **Magnesium Taurate*** can support a healthy heart.

Liposomal Vitamin C is one of the best sources of vitamin C support for the heart according to a leading cardiologist, **Dr. Thomas Levy. (R 111)** With the liquid concentrated vitamin C, one can take highest dosage without the side effects of regular vitamin C supplements. However, Andrei has found that other natural sources of vitamin C like **Alive Wholefood Vitamin C from Nature's Way**, Camu Camu (are berries grown in the Amazon region of Peru and is the richest food source of Vitamin C in the whole world according to Andrei), Goji Berry, Kiwi Fruit and Acerola Cherry have the natural form of vitamin C that may be quite potent and only a smaller amount needed to be taken compared to other synthetic brands that contain ascorbic acid. Andrei said he once read a study that find that food derived vitamin C like the Acerola or Camu Camu is ten times stronger in antioxidant power than ascorbic acid, ascorbate and Liposomal C. Natural vitamin C is actually a package containing flavonoids, polyphenol and tannins, the C co-factors. A blend of Liposomal and Camu Camu may be a great way to go and the best of both worlds where you get great absorption, assimilation and utilization.

Stress Management, Meditation, Biofeedback, Yoga and Tai Chi may help improve heart health as well.

A good resource for heart health is a book written by **Dr. Dean Ornish**. It is called *Reversing Heart Disease* (**R 112**). Dr. Ornish teaches the reader how improve heart health and well-being through a holistic approach that embraces proper nutrition, exercise, life style changes, spirituality and mental and emotional well-being.

The **Ornish Diet** has been named the "#1 best diet for heart disease" by U.S. News and World Report for seven consecutive years! (**R 113**)

*****

A plant-based diet has been shown to decrease the risk of heart disease significantly over a course of time by decreasing plaque formation as well as improve vascular flow.

One of the best things you can do for your heart is exercise. In my practice, I see clients with pulmonary, orthopedic, neurological as well as cardiac issues. I see many clients who have congestive heart failure, have a pace maker or have undergone open heart surgery or a Coronary Artery Bypass Surgery. The most important thing for the heart is exercise. It stimulates the arteries to activate the endothelium to release nitric oxide. It helps to dilates and repairs the arteries and improve blood flow to the heart. It also dissolves the sticky things in our arteries that contribute to plaque and hardening of the artery. After heart surgery, the cardio vascular surgeon typically request for physical therapy to work with the patient on exercise and especially a program that works on walking. If you are unsure what to do, consult with your physician, physical or occupational therapist or health coach.

Pomegranate juice has been shown to help with glycation and by decreasing the sticky things in our arteries, our heart will pump more efficiently.

Watching your waist size is very important to your heart health. According to **Dr. William Sears** our waist size is a strong indicator of our health. Women's hip should be less than the hip and less than 35 inches. Men's waist should be 40 inches or less. The waist is measured at 2 inches above belly button and the hip is measured 7 inches below the waist.

If you are beyond your parameters research has shown that you are more likely to have diabetes, heart diseases, depression, cancer, dementia, inflammation in the body and you are more likely to suffer a heart attack or a stroke.

Dementia and Alzheimer's Disease

The incidence of **dementia** is on the rise. People are getting it even at younger ages. I suspect an environmental toxin exposure, poor nutrition and toxins may be partly to blame. Nonetheless, it is such a debilitating disease with at least 10 different types. I have dealt with many types of dementia and it is always a challenge especially at the later stages of the disease. There are about 7 stages and each getting worse until the person is no longer able to speak, walk and care for self.

Although it is currently believed that there is no cure for it, many doctors prescribe **Namenda** and **Aricept** to their clients in the early stages of the disease to slow it down. I have seen clients with some benefits and some with none at all. Besides medication, what else can be done? A psychiatrist once told me he gave his mother **Ginkgold** with some improvement. It helps to improve blood flow to the brain.

My mother suffered from dementia for 5-10 years prior to her transition. About five years ago, her dementia was obviously advancing quite rapidly. She began having behavioral problems, was hostile and was very uncooperative with her caregiver. She was volatile and her memory was deteriorating rapidly. She was on the verge of being placed in a nursing home or board and care. She was already on various medications to slow down the dementia as well as control her psychotic features but to no avail.

Since she was getting worse despite all the efforts from her physician, I began researching alternative holistic methods that might help. After trying **Mushroom Science's Lion's Mane Mushroom*** and other supplements **(Kyani Nitro, Kyani Sunrise, Kyani Sunset, SAMe, Curamed*** and **PEO*)** for a week or two, she became more docile and cooperative. Her memory and thought process began to show improvements. She lived at home, went shopping with her caregiver and was still able to manage to call me on the telephone and access her voicemail even until she was 90 years of age. She still remembered birthdays and was living a happy and fulfilling life to the end.

A friend sent me an article from the Dailymail.com about a mother who was suffering from Alzheimer's disease. Apparently, her son helped improved her memory by changing her diet. The mother ate a diet rich in walnuts, berries and brain-boosting foods.

Her son Mark discovered that Mediterranean countries had a lower rate of dementia and decided to put his mom on a Mediterranean style diet. He incorporated foods like broccoli, kale and spinach, sunflower seeds, green tea, oats, sweet potatoes and as a treat, dark chocolate with a high cocoa content into her diet. He also had his mom do cognitive exercises including jigsaws and cross word puzzles. As of this writing, she is now being held up by the Alzheimer's Society as an example of how the disease can be - if not completely beaten - arrested significantly.

A 2017 study by US scientists found that a Mediterranean-style diet gave participants a 30 to 35 per cent lower risk of cognitive impairment. **(R 114)**

According to Dr. Whitaker, there is no doubt that low-dose **lithium orotate** is exceptionally neuroprotective. It stimulates the release of brain-derived neurotropic factor (BDNF) and other growth factors that enhance the repair and growth of neurons. Scans of patients treated with higher lithium doses actually reveal increases in gray matter. **(R 115)**

In a study published in *JAMA Psychiatry* in 2017, Danish researchers examined patient registries of 800,000 people, aged 50–90, and found distinct relationships between diagnoses of dementia and exposure to lithium in drinking water. People living in areas with the highest lithium levels in their water were significantly less likely to have developed

Alzheimer's disease or vascular dementia, compared to those with the lowest levels. **(R 116)**

Doing **Super Brain Yoga** exercise can improve the amount of neural activity and improve bilateral integration and memory. Here is a link on how to do it. **(R 117)**

Some research on Alzheimer's patients has shown some improvement with the condition with patients who took **coconut oil.**

Ashwagandha - may be helpful with memory support and is also wonderful for the nervous system overall.

Curamed* - can be helpful as well with its anti-inflammatory properties and can be helpful with depression and memory issues. Curamed contains curcumin, the active ingredient of turmeric. Janet Doerr, Intuitive Nutritionista and Energy Healer, once had some brain fog due to aluminum getting into her brain. She began taking turmeric on a regular basis and found much benefit, she stated, "now, my memory is sharp as a tack again. So, I cleaned my brain back up. The turmeric helps to detox the body of aluminum."

She further stated, that "**blueberries** are good brain food and good for healing the brain after the aluminum or heavy is removed. They also increase stem cell production."

I have found that exercise, relevant music (music the individual thoroughly enjoyed prior the onset of dementia), comedy and dancing can improve the cognitive status of those suffering dementia.

Some research suggests that **intermittent fasting** can help with decreasing the risk of dementia. Professor Mark Mattson, professor of neuroscience, reports: "we're finding by putting electrodes in brains of animals during fasting their brain cells are more active." Professor Mattson studies have also found that fasting increases the ability of mice to remember and learn and it decreases their risk of dementia. With regards to humans, he states that people who overeat are at risk for Alzheimer's disease.

I found Dr. Frank Lipman's information for Alzheimer's dementia quite helpful. **(R 118)** He gives **10 recommendations for protecting the brain** against Alzheimer's and it includes the following:

1. Tame inflammation, round the clock.
2. More movement and a lot less couch-potato time.
3. Make quality sleep a top priority
4. What goes in your mouth matters to your brain. Dr. Lipman recommends organic leafy greens, colorful veggies, dark berries; nuts; healthy fats; and moderate amounts of organic; grass fed or pasture-raised animals. Drink oolong or green teas and ditch sugar, processed foods, and industrial oils.
5. Ditch sugar-and the Standard American Diet today.
6. Change your eating patterns (intermittent fasting-aka the 56:2 Diet or (8-Hour Window diet).
7. Take a brain-booster:
   a. Omega 3 fatty acids
   b. Methylated Folate and Vitamin B12
   c. Vitamin D
   d. Magnesium
   e. Nicotinamide Riboside
   f. Alpha Lipoic Acid
   g. Co-enzyme Q10
8. For those already suffering from cognitive decline, he recommended the following:
   a. acetyl-L-carnitine
   b. phosphatidylserine
   c. ginko biloba
9. Meditate, meditate, meditate!
10. Do not hibernate - circulate (and stated we should stay social and stay connected with friends, family, neighbors and community.

Other important resources I have found include:

1. A cutting-edge book on Alzheimer's Dementia written by Dale E. Bredesen, M.D. called *The End of Alzheimer's*. **(R 119)** and
2. *Learning to Speak Alzheimer's: A Groundbreaking Approach for Everyone with the Disease* by Joanne Koenig Coste (a great resource on how to communicate effectively and gracefully with those suffering with Alzheimer's). **(R 120)**

The **Neuro Light** may be helpful with improving memory and activating more parts of the brain to improve brain health, capacity, elasticity and shaping the brain in the way you want to improve according to Marian Brandenburg. It has two components: the brain gym (it helps to warm areas of the brain like the somatic or limbic area) and brain skills (you pick what skills you want to work on or improve on like peace, mood, cognition, dependency, etc.). It has helped even her stroke client to improve her memory, motor skills, ambulation and speech.

Research led by MIT has found strobe lights and a low pitched buzz can be used to recreate brain waves lost in the disease, which in turn remove plaque and improve cognitive function in mice engineered to display Alzheimer's-like behavior. **(R 121)**

"When we combine visual and auditory stimulation for a week, we see the engagement of the prefrontal cortex and a very dramatic reduction of amyloid," says Li-Huei Tsai, a researcher from MIT's Picower Institute for Learning and Memory. **(R 122)**

Several years ago, Tsai discovered light flickering at a frequency of about 40 flashes a second had similar benefits in mice engineered to build up amyloid in their brain's nerve cells.

"The result was so mind-boggling and so robust, it took a while for the idea to sink in, but we knew we needed to work out a way of trying out the same thing in humans," Tsai told Helen Thomson at *Nature* at the time.

On the spiritual side, I was recently taught the Sa Ta Na Ma Meditation by a friend, Felix Fojas, to balance the Air, Earth, Fire, and Water elements. He learned this from an Indian Yogi.

Sa Ta Na Ma Meditation is becoming scientifically recognized as a powerful tool for preventing or stopping Alzheimer's disease, increasing all aspects of cognitive function (perception, thinking, reasoning and remembering) and reducing stress levels while improving short term memory. There are three separate studies that have been published that the. Two studies were done at the University of Pennsylvania and continuing studying is being done at UCLA.

You can learn more about it at https://agelessartsyoga.com and even get a CD to support you with it. **(R 123)**

Activities that Provide Mental Fitness
1. Ma Jong
2. Sudoku
3. Crossword Puzzles
4. Solitaire
5. Read
6. Arts and Craft
7. Playing a musical instrument
8. Puzzles
9. Listen to music pertinent to times in life when you were well.
10. Exercise is good for the brain function.
    a. Exercise
    b. Dancing
    c. Ping Pong

Nutrients

Walnuts, blueberries and seafood especially wild salmon (it is high in omega 3 fatty acid) are very important for brain health and has been validated by scientific research.

Calcification of the Pineal Gland

Our **pineal gland** is the most important gland in our body for spirituality. However, it is being calcified by the fluoride in our toothpaste and water. In order to decalcify it, we need to activate it through meditation and spiritual practices. The following video link can help support it as well: **(R 124)**

Certain foods help support it like spirulina, blueberries, chlorella, iodine, parsley, oregano oil and the mineral boron. Foods high in Boron include: avocados, prunes, raisins, almonds, hazelnut, and dates, apple cider vinegar, beets, cacao, vitamin K, garlic, oregano oil and MSM.

Tonic Herbs include: chamomile, pine bark, lavender bud, wild indigo bark, violet, licorice and ginseng.

I also take Wild Purple Reishi and Tahitian Noni juice to support it. Drinking alkaline water, distilled water and sun gazing helps as well. The use of crystals over the third eye during meditation can help. Crystals like sodalite, lapis lazuli, quartz crystal, amethyst can help decalcify. Eating more greens and organic food is important for good pineal gland health. **(R 125)**

A spiritual friend of mine, Joanna Marie Fojas, uses Haritaki, Chaga, Spirulina, Chlorophyll and turmeric powder to support her pineal gland. She uses organic turmeric powder mixed in with apple cider vinegar or water and make it into a paste. She then puts it on her forehead and puts in on her third eye point. She does it for 21 days straight once a year. She also does Trakata meditation as well as sun gazing.

Janet Doerr mentioned that blueberries, especially wild blueberries, are good for the brain earlier but also mentioned it is good for the pineal gland.

One of the most effective method I have found to activate the pineal gland through modern technology is through the **Ajna Light**. Invented by Guy Harriman, it has been called a lazy man's meditation. I have used it on several occasions with incredible results ranging from mystical visions and receiving greater clarity and insight.

The machine can be set to create various levels of brain wave from delta waves, to theta waves, etc. A friend of mine tried it when she was very distraught and confused. After her session, she was able to see with greater clarity and her psychic ability began to be more pronounced.

When the machine is set to delta wave, it can help amp up the psychic ability of an individual according to Marian. The machine is supposed to be good at activating the pineal gland.

Besides the above, one can make **a decree and prayer** to clear the calcification of the pineal gland. One decree could be like the following: "I Am the presence of Saint Germain activating the violet consuming flame which burns and dissolves away the calcium in and around the pineal gland." It is important to visualize the activation of the violet flame onto the pineal gland. Usage of a crystal plus visualization can help dissolve the crystal as well.

Important Health Tips to Follow

At this point, you should be feeling a little more comfortable with how to achieve basic harmonious health and well-being. It is important to not jump on the bandwagon for the trendiest vitamin, supplement or medication but get what you need based on good science or get what is most harmonious with your body, mind and spirit. Most of the trendy things are not good quality and may even be laced with carcinogenic substances. I try to purchase those supplements that are recommended by good nutritionists.

Andrei likes to purchase the vitamins and supplements that are being sold to actual health practitioners. He wants to only sell things that are effective. Likewise, I only want to share information on things that are effective. Before you go crazy and start buying lots of vitamins and supplements, please follow the principles I share next:

- **Avoid doctoring yourself** to avoid creating medical issues that can cost you your life. I met a person who was taking niacin as a supplement at 500 mg/ day. He liked the effect of it so much that he began increasing his dosage until he was taking 9 pills a day. He eventually had to be admitted into the hospital due to declining health from vitamin B toxicity.
- **Always consult your physician, functional medical practitioner, naturopathic doctor, nutritionist, or other qualified health care professional** about what you are taking or what you want to take. It is very important the quantity you take, how you take it and when you take it. Some supplements are more effective at higher dosage and others are toxic. Certain vitamins such as Vitamin D, vitamin E, Vitamin K, and Vitamin A and Astaxanthin are best taken with fatty food. Some supplements are best taken on an empty stomach for better absorption.
- Most importantly, **listen to your body.** If what you take causes pain, strain, dizziness, brain fogging or other adverse side effects, you may need to contact your health care professional immediately to reevaluate the product or dosage. We all know that medicine has side effects but vitamins and supplements can as well.
- Remember **what works for one may not work for you** due to differences in body types, blood types and differences in body chemistry. Also, find out from your health practitioner what is the **best way to take the vitamin or supplement** for good absorption,

how much to take and **how long should you be taking it for**. Before you decide on taking anything new, be it medication, herbs, vitamins, minerals or supplements, **always check with your physician, pharmacist and qualified health care practitioner** as well as check online or book resources for any adverse side effects or contraindications to be more well informed. With medications, you can **purchase a *Physician's Desk Reference*** (that has all the possible side effects but might be too much for the lay person) or ***The Pill Book*** (15th Edition) which is a much more user-friendly alternative. **(R 126)**

- **Avoid following a fad** especially for a long time. Always check in with yourself and see if you are benefitting from the product or getting worse. If it is not helping you or you are getting worse, stop immediately or, if there are any withdrawal issues, taper it off slowly. Tune in to your I AM Presence and see if you should continue taking a product. Take things in moderation.

- Although I have shared a lot of good information in this book, you **should always do you own research** to verify for yourself if what I say is true. You should do research on anything with which you are unfamiliar.

- When trying something new, always **search online about adverse effects of the product or contraindications.** That will minimize any potential problems in your health.

- I'd like to also share some wisdom from Bruce Lee that will come in handy when using this book: 1. Research your own experiences; 2. Absorb what is useful; 3. Reject what is useless; 4. Add what is specifically your own.

- **Realize that nothing is set in stone.** The field of Health and Nutrition is ever changing. We learn more and more about how the body works. You must continue to update your knowledge as new and cutting-edge information is shared.

- **Search** for the supplement you want to use at the **website of a credible source** and see what the experts have to say.

- **Regularly check all your supplements, multivitamins, minerals, and fruits and vegetables to make sure you are not overdosing.** For instance, if you are taking a selenium supplement at 200 mcg, take a multivitamin (which may have 25 mcg of selenium) and have some Brazilian nuts (each is 50-75 mcg of selenium), your selenium level could easily be at a toxic level if it reaches over 400 mcg.

• **Always listen to your body on what it wants and needs.**

There is a plethora of information about herbs, supplements and minerals online and in many resource books out there. So, go and start getting yourself more educated and empowered about health and wellness. Not all herbs and supplements are helpful in every circumstance. For instance, some supplements like **Gingko Biloba, Turmeric and St. John's Wort should not be taken with blood thinners.** Anti-inflammatory supplements may be helpful for many with pain but after surgery, your doctor may not want you to take it **to allow the body to heal better without it.**

With regards to vitamin and minerals, it is always best to get it from natural sources (fruits and vegetables) if possible, for the best form for absorption and utilization from the body.

By now many of you are asking how many supplements can you take and have them still be healthful rather than a hindrance? That is something that many nutritionists cannot answer. However, there are many out there including health practitioners and nutritionist who take many supplements and are having great benefits. Andrei takes about 25 supplements himself. Another scholarly nutritionist takes over 20 as well. Andrei stated that a well-known author and educator takes about one hundred supplements and appears to be doing well. Another famous author takes about 200 supplements.

In my first book, I wrote about some of the supplements I took and then was told by a nutritionist that I was taking too much. However, in retrospect, I was probably taking just enough but my supplements needed to be tweaked a little to higher quality supplements. I have come to realize that many nutritionists do not know much about supplements and prefer to avoid commenting on it and rather focus on healthy eating. However, as we have learned earlier, that is not enough to help us achieve optimal health and harmony.

For supplements, how much or how many to take really depends on what you are taking. My rule of thumb is that you should only take what your body needs to create harmony and supports the free flow of energy within your body for radiant health. Taking high quality supplements recommended by a qualified nutritionist or health care practitioner can make a difference on how much supplements you can take.

One important thing with supplements, vitamins and medications is to avoid increasing the dosage without the blessings and approval of your physician, nutritionist or health care practitioner.

Andrei sees his physician and gets a blood workup annually, and it is always normal. I highly recommend everyone do the same both to see if you are missing nutrients or are too high in anything which can be picked up through the liver enzymes level. When the liver enzymes are too high, it may be indicative of us taking too much supplements and/or vitamins.

With the intention of keeping my liver in harmony, I show the list of supplements and vitamins to my nutritionist and physician and they review it to see if anything needs to be tweaked or discontinued. I also get as many of my nutrients as possible directly from my food.

In achieving radiant health and harmony, it helps to look at the various needs that we have in the context of the problem or issue. The more we approach an issue or disharmony in the context of physical, mental, emotional and spiritual bodies, the more effectively we can clear the way for the Divine Presence to reestablish harmony again. It is important to make sure we address the five elements (water, earth, air, fire and metal) when doing a comprehensive holistic program.

Besides healthy eating and drinking and taking the vitamin, supplements and minerals you need, practice the following to support your mental, emotional, and spiritual needs to optimize your well-being and internal harmony:

- Meditation or U.U.M.M. Meditation
- Wim Hof Method (the exercises, cold showers or ice bath, exercise and the focus within to activate the energies and awareness).
- Exercise regularly (Yoga, Qi Gong, Tai Chi, aerobics, brisk walking, Second Brain Activation or any exercise that activates the digestive system, etc.).

- Fill your heart and mind with positive thoughts of love, compassion, kindness, mercy, forgiveness and gratitude daily and throughout the day.
- Devotion and Prayer.
- Love yourself and surround yourself with people who love you. Meditate and feel God's love fill your entire being.
- Fasting, detoxifying heavy metals from the body and ensuring that you are getting a sufficient amount of minerals and trace minerals for optimal health.

By doing the above seven categories, you will be addressing the five elements that will support your body systems to allow greater harmony and healing. The Divine Presence within will optimize and support your recovery and return to health.

Those of you who want to take nutrition or wellness to an even higher level may want to learn more about our APOE gene. Depending on which APOE gene you have, there are certain foods that you eat that will either activate or turn off a disease process like dementia, heart diseases, etc. Pamela McDonald, NP, Integrative- Medicine Nurse Practitioner, has written a book about this subject which Dr. Wayne Dyer supported and endorsed. It is called the *Perfect Gene Diet.* (R 127)

It is good that we could eat and drink well for optimum health and harmony but there are some of you who are suffering with so much pain you can't even think about anything else other than just making it through the hour or day. I have seen thousands of people suffering from pain and have seen what works and what does not work. People in pain cannot progress with achieving harmony until they can get a handle on their pain. This next chapter is for all those who have been suffering for many years. Your cries have been heard and may the next chapter bring you some relief, insight and hope.

*"Health is the greatest gift,
Contentment the greatest wealth,
Faithfulness the best relationship."*

~

Buddha

CHAPTER 5

END SUFFERING AND EXPERIENCE RADIANT HEALTH

Chronic and Severe Pain

During my lifetime, I have seen so many people suffering from pain – from as young as a seven year old youth with juvenile arthritis to many elders who are crippled by their pain due various reasons including osteoarthritis, spinal stenosis, rheumatoid arthritis, bursitis, rotator cuff injuries, edema, low back pain, cellulitis, neuropathy, etc. There are also millions of people who suffer from some form of autoimmune disease that has given them debilitating pain from Chronic Pain Syndrome, Fibromyalgia, Hashimoto's Disease, Multiple Sclerosis, etc.

According to Healthline.com, in 2019 more than 30 percent of adults in the U.S. are living with chronic or severe pain. **(R 128)**

Many of my clients have been helped by medication but others have found no relief. Some medications help with the pain but have bad side effects like severe constipation. Other pain medications that contain opiates can be quite addictive and going through the withdrawal can be extremely uncomfortable and very disturbing. One client was trying to wean away from her medication that contained opiates and went through extreme withdrawal symptoms. She felt so anxious and wanted to just pull off all her skin.

Some of the withdrawal symptoms occur as early as within 24 hours after stopping the drugs and include: muscle aches, restlessness, anxiety, tears and runny nose.

Later symptoms, which can be more intense, begin after the first day or so. They include: diarrhea, abdominal cramping, goose bumps on the skin, nausea and vomiting, dilated pupils and possibly blurry vision, rapid heartbeat, and high blood pressure.

Although opiates and opioids can be effective with pain management, even when used responsibly, they can lead to addiction and I personally would only use it as a last resort, and only for a very limited period of time.

For those who are interested, information about weaning off opioids is available at the Mayo Clinic's link at: **(R 129)**

At the time of this writing (2020), the National Institute on Drug Abuse, states approximately 2.1 million people in the United States and between 26.4 and 36 million people worldwide abuse opioids. **(R 130)**

It is really an epidemic at this time and will continue to be that way until people embrace better and non-addictive solutions.

I have been able to help myself, my family and many others manage and often get rid of their pain altogether by utilizing a more holistic and integrative approach to pain management. Sometimes it is the marriage of western and holistic medicine that brings relief.

It has been my experience that much of the pain is some type of inflammatory response. Pain can sometimes go hand and hand with mental or other emotional distress. Some people never seem to get healthy because of what they may see as benefits, such as attention, sympathy and help from friends and family.

We can easily detect this by checking the blood pressure and pulse rate of a person suffering from pain. If they are truly in a high amount of pain (mental, emotional and physical), then their blood pressure and heart rate will be elevated significantly. If not, it is probably in their head or they are trying to get some secondary gain out of the pain. Many times, this can be happening at even a subconscious level and even the person with the pain may be oblivious to the secondary gains. Such an individual may need psychological help and respond better with a behavioral modification approach including hypnosis.

For those who truly desire to live a harmonious and radiant life, this chapter is for you. Fortunately, there are many things you can do to help decrease or get rid of your pain. I think that starting to eat better and drinking better as we talked about in earlier chapters would help the body heal itself and remove some of the causes if not all of pain. However, sometimes things like severe osteoarthritis in a joint are so painful that it is essentially bone against bone. In such a case, an individual may need to have a shoulder, hip or knee replacement to end the pain. Choosing a good surgeon and physical therapist is going to make a difference in your recovery and they are not all the same. So do your homework.

If you are eating and drinking well and do not have any type of orthopedic issues that requires surgical intervention then the following sections may be helpful to you. Incidentally, there are times when exercise, yoga and proper physical or occupational therapy can help the individual avoid even having surgery. I have helped many clients avoid surgery despite having a rotator cuff injury just by doing occupational therapy and exercises.

Pain Management and Reduction

Pain is a hot topic and how to manage it is quite complex but I will go over how we can begin to gain relief from it and help our bodies heal from the causes. Heal the cause and the pain will be gone. It is that simple.

Pain has many components including physical, spiritual, mental, emotional components. Pain is somewhat complex and interwoven with the various components making it sometimes difficult to treat.

There are many methods to helping a person who is suffering physical pain. They include herbs, occupational therapy, physical therapy and various modalities. We will explore each in more detail.

Body Work (may also help with emotional and mental pain). It helps to improve blood flow, release endorphins into the body, decreases swelling and supports the immune system.

There are many types of massages out there that can provide much relief to pain if done correctly. They include: Swedish massage, Thai massage, Acupressure massage (Shiatsu massage, Tui Na Sports massage, Seifukujitsu massage, Jin Shin Jyutsu˚ and Jin Shin Do), Balinese massage, foot reflexology, etc. I have tried various types and one of my favorites is Balinese massage. I tried that when I went to Bali, Indonesia. I found it to be the most relaxing and it was good in releasing my body aches from many days of travels. However, after having a massage session with Marian Brandenburg, I have come to have great respect for her ability to heal the body and understand body wellness. She has studied much about healing with Grandmaster Mantak Chia.

She is an outstanding massage therapist and healer. She can actually pick up on stored emotions in the muscles and organs during her session since she is also an intuitive. She stated that pain is a messenger. She also is the only person I know of in the Bay Area who would know how to do **Chi Nei Tsang**, a cutting-edge massage technique that works directly on the liver, spleen, gut, and intestines to improve those organs health resulting in Qi and blood flow for wellness. This technique was taught by Grandmaster Mantak Chia.

I also like Acupressure Massage because I find it relaxing, holistic and targets important acupressure points for health and wellness. Although I am not fan of foot reflexology, it can be quite therapeutic for the entire body through its network of connections to all the organs of the body. Not one style will be good for all people. Find the one the suits your needs.

Those who need deep tissue massage may like a Swedish massage. Choose the style that best resonates to your mental, emotional and physical needs. Doing regular massages can help reduce the buildup of emotional tension and stress that leads to pain in the neck, shoulder and lower back. Preventative medicine is the best medicine.

Other types of body work that can help with pain include:

- **Myofascial Release** This is a method that can be done by a chiropractor, physical therapist, an occupational therapist or massage therapist to release tightness of the myofascial tissues. These tissues are connected to muscles throughout the body and provide support. Treatment is done through stretches, massages and stimulating certain trigger points to provide release of tight tissues or sheaths.
- **Feldenkrais Method** - The Feldenkrais Method uses a process of organic learning, movement, and sensing to free you from

habitual patterns and allow for new patterns of thinking, moving and feeling to emerge. **(R 131)**

- **Rolfing** - According to Jenny Rock, Certified Advanced Rolfer, Rolfing is a systematic and holistic method of manipulating the muscle and fascia to help the body return to structural balance in movement and gravity. **(R 132)** Once this happens, Rock says the body's natural mechanisms take over and finish the job of correcting these imbalances.

Alternative Medicine and Therapies

Many alternative medicine and therapeutic approaches can be quite effective because of utilizing a more holistic approach to dealing with the pain. This includes and is not limited to Chiropractic Medicine, Cranial Sacral Therapy, Acupuncture, Moxa Cupping (The use of **Moxa Cupping** has been popularized by Michael Phelps and many in Hollywood as a great method for pain relief. It removes the toxins in our body, reliefs pain and improves blood flow), Oriental or Traditional Chinese Medicine, Ayurvedic Medicine, etc. I have found Moxa Cupping extremely helpful with reducing the amount of pain on my arm through its ability to improve circulation and clear adhesions.

Cryotherapy could also be an effective method for helping to decrease pain and inflammation. It helps to increase endorphins and produce norepinephrine in the body to combat pain and inflammation. However, you should check with your physician first if you have any medical conditions. It behooves you to study the **Wim Hof** method of breathing prior to doing your cryotherapy session. It will help you tolerate the cold better. It also alkalizes the body and shuts off the pain signals. I also add **Bellows Breathing** to warm my body further. Through the two methods, I have been able to stay in very cold water up to my head for about 18 minutes and felt so rejuvenated after that cold-water therapy. However, if you are not properly supervised or trained, you might suffer hypothermia.

A great way to decrease the pain and inflammation in your body is to do **Earthing.** Spend 20-30 minutes a day walking barefooted in nature. Our bodies will accumulate electrons that help to heal our bodies. If you are unable to easily walk, then standing or sitting on the earth with bare feet can also be very helpful.

Earthing Mats are an alternative to outdoor Earthing. If you live where walking outside barefoot is really not practical or even possible, then the use of an Earthing Mat can provide you with some similar benefits. They are not as good as the real thing but hold a strong second place and can be used at home or in the workplace if you are sitting at a desk all day. **(R 133)**

Reiki is a very well-known energetic healing method that can be helpful with accelerating the healing process and releasing some of our pain. The practitioner uses universal energy to bring balance in the body and to release toxic and painful energetic patterns that are trapped in our bodies and organs. It is usually done with a practitioner working directly over a person's body through the practitioner's hands. Many times, the practitioner will use crystals as a tool for healing as well.

My Reiki instructor was involved in an accident and it was through Reiki that she was able to manage her pain. Her recovery through Reiki led her to study it and become a Reiki Master.

I have used a form of Reiki to help my family decrease or release their pain which in turn allows the body to heal. I used it to facilitate the pain release and then healing of an imbalance in one of my dog's hips. She limped until I gave her a healing session. The full story is in **Beyond Imagination**.

Practicing the Wim Hof method is a good method to help us decrease our pain by helping us to be happy, healthy and strong. It also alkalizes our bodies and helps the body to produce endorphins. Alkalizing the body helps to turn off the pain signal according to Wim Hof. The endorphins further help our ability to manage pain.

In this busy life of ours, it is sometimes hard for to find time to seek an alternative practitioner. Those who have the time may not have the financial resources to see the much needed practitioner due to insurance coverage issues. For some, the over the counter approach may help for less serious and complex pain.

Over the Counter Relief

There are many over the counter pain reliever out there. I only share about the ones my family, clients, friends and I have found helpful.

Electric Medicated Balm External Analgesic can be helpful in minimizing some of the agonizing pain. My mother found it quite helpful for many years. Although she tried many pain relief gels, this is what she found that helped her the most. Friends of ours have used it with good benefits. They sell this in many stores in Chinatown, San Francisco.

DMSO* (Dimethylsulfoxide) has been used by some to effectively help manage their pain. This can be purchased from Valley Health Mill in Pleasanton, California. Dr. Hector Oksenendler reports that some of his clients who used this found it helpful.

Many people, including my mother, have found benefit with **Curamed***. It is a highly concentrated curcumin (the active component of turmeric). It has provided many people relief from pain. My mother's pain was controlled by this supplement which has great anti-inflammatory properties. **Curamin** is quite effective for more acute pain whereas Curamed is more for chronic pain and disease symptoms according to Andrei. However, those who have gall bladder problems or gallstones may want to avoid turmeric as well since it might make the condition worse.

I have tried both and have found Curamed at 750 mg more effective in pain control than Curamin with my acute pain. Andrei points out how some people find it even more effective to pair Curamed with **BosMed 500***. They seem to have a better result with pain management. It contains a high potency of Boswellia. I have tried them together and have noticed an improvement with pain. **(R 134)**

According to Terry Lemerond, author and educator, **Boswellia** can stop the leading causes of most disease: inflammation and oxidation. Its most important benefit is its ability to modulate a particular inflammation pathway called the 5-LOX (5-lipoxygenase) pathway. The 5-lipoxygenase enzyme activates inflammatory leukotrienes, compounds that contract smooth muscle tissues in the body. **(R 135)**

However, if you just had surgery, your physician may not want you to take an anti-inflammatory in the beginning during the early healing phases since some inflammation is part of a normal healing process.

Consult with your physician when it is appropriate for you to take the anti-inflammatory supplements or medicine. Turmeric also has blood thinning properties and may be contraindicated with those individuals who are on blood thinners or have bleeding ulcers. Those who have gall bladder problems or gallstones may want to avoid turmeric as well since it might make the condition worse.

Homeopathy Remedies

According my friend Flenje, a registered physical therapist who is also a doctoral candidate in Physical Therapy, homeopathy can offer great health benefits as well. She shared with me four **homeopathic remedies for pain relief:**

- Bryonia 6c- good for acute and severe pain
- Dulcamara 6c- it helps with pain associated with the elements, especially when the air is cold or damp. During this time the joints may be stiff and painful.
- Hypericum perforatum 30c- great for nerve pain which are burning, sharp and radiating.
- Rhus toxicodendron 6c- can help with muscles and joint pains due to lack of movement.

Topical Creams, Patches or Gels

Biofreeze is an analgesic gel that helps with curtailing the pain and may last one to three hours. It has a cooling effect. Many therapists, chiropractors, and massage therapist have this in their office and use it with their clients. Even my acupuncturist has it in his office. I have recommended it to many clients with good results as well as used it myself on many occasions. It can be purchased online or at stores such as Target, Walmart and Bed Bath and Beyond.

Salonpa sprays or patches have been used by many people to give relief of pain including some professional ballet dancers I have met. Some of my clients have tried **Salonpas Lidocaine Plus Pain Relieving Liquid** and found that they were able to have pain relief for at least a few hours.

Others prefer more heat and use **Sombra gel or cream**. It warms up when it is absorbed in the skin. Some people have added heated grated ginger to further help with minimizing the inflammation, swelling and pain which can be purchased at this link: **(R 136)**

Some have found good lasting relief with **lidocaine patches prescribed by a physician.**

Arnicare Gel has been helpful with some of my clients for pain control. One of its primary ingredients is arnica which in homeopathic form is commonly used for pain, bruising, swelling and even to reverse shock. "However, the strength required to reduce or reverse hypovolemic shock is in tablet form of 30c to 200c dilution," according to Kathryn Shanti Ariel.

Many of my clients have been prescribed **Voltaren Gel** to help sooth pain that may be more intense and have found some relief. That needs to be prescribed by a physician.

I had one client who could not find any relief from any medications nor any of the common over the counter pain control ointment or gel but did find some relief with **Penetrex.** It contains arnica, vitamin B6 and MSM. It has 4.5-star reviews from Amazon.

Herbal Supplements and Holistic Methods

The herbal supplement, Boswellia, comes from the same tree as Frankincense incense. Studies show that boswellia may reduce inflammation and may also be useful in treating the following conditions.

- Osteoarthritis (OA)
- Rheumatoid arthritis (RA)
- Asthma
- Inflammatory bowel disease (IBD)

According to Dr. Mercola, **wild lettuce** can be helpful with pain. He stated, "If you've suffered anxiety, headaches, or muscle or joint pain, you might already be familiar with wild lettuce." It's also effective at calming restlessness and reducing anxiety, and may even quell restless legs syndrome. When using a wild-lettuce supplement, take 30 to 120 milligrams before bed. **(R 137)**

MSM

According to a book called ***The Miracles of MSM,*** MSM can relieve a variety of pain including back pain, headaches, muscle pain, arthritis, athletic injuries, etc. In addition, Health Line shares this information: Methyl-sulfonylmethane, more commonly known as MSM, is a popular dietary supplement used to treat a wide array of symptoms and conditions. It's a sulfur-containing compound found naturally in plants, animals and humans. It can also be produced in a lab to create dietary supplements in powder or capsule form.

MSM is widely used in the alternative medicine field and by people looking for a natural way to relieve joint pain, reduce inflammation and boost immunity. Studies have shown that MSM significantly reduces inflammation in your body. It also inhibits the breakdown of cartilage, a flexible tissue that protects the ends of your bones in joints. **(R 138**

Janet Doerr stated that MSM (organic sulfur) is very helpful for reducing pain especially when it is a joint kind of issue. She noticed that when they got her dog on glucosamine because of severe joint pain *and* if it had MSM in it, suddenly her dog is running about all happy.

Other things that may help include **Kyani NitroFx. It improves the nitric oxide level in our bodies** and the flow of the arteries that may lead to the painful area. It may also help to decrease the inflammatory response and bring in nutrients for healing and recovery.

Kyani NitroFx is a proprietary blend of noni concentrate that has been proven to increase the production of Nitric Oxide (NO). Also known as "The Molecule of Life," Nitric Oxide repairs, defends, and maintains every cell of the body. Benefits of Nitric Oxide also include increasing energy, supporting healthy circulation, and encouraging the body's natural inflammatory response. Helping your body produce Nitric Oxide, Kyani Nitro ensures adequate nutrient delivery for optimal wellness. It helps to improve the flow within the arteries that may lead to the painful area. It may to help decrease the inflammatory response and bring in nutrients for healing and recovery. **(R 139)**

CBD Oil

Sometimes when the individual is not getting any relief from their pain, **CBD - Cannabis Oil** may be of great assistance. Many people have found great relief from their pain when using the oil including myself, my mom and my friends. The brand that I tried is called **Papa and Barkley** which I ordered from Elemental Wellness Center in San Jose.

I have recently discovered a brand of CBD oil which helped me considerably. It is called **Can Be Done Topical Salve. (R 140)** It contains Cannabinol 500 mg, arnica herbal infusion or oil and Copaiba essential oil. I found it helpful with some of my muscle pain. You can purchase it at **Good Common Sense** Naturals Store.

According to Wendy Schulte, owner of the store and Cosmetic Formulator of the pain salve products, their pain relief salve is made from organic CBD and as the finest ingredients and essential oils. It is 100% THC free and has non-GMO essential oils. It does not contain synthetic ingredients or glycerin.

They have three versions of the salve. One for mild pain with 250 mg of CBD with lasting effects of 1-2 hours, the second one is for moderate pain with 500 mg of CBD with lasting effects of a few hours and a third one for severe or chronic pain with 750 mg of CBD which lasts 6-8 hours.

Wendy points out that what makes their product better than many out there is that her CBD oil is made from CBD isolates. Many other companies out there use what is called full spectrum that contains THC and hemp oil. These are 20-30% weaker than the more concentrated isolates type that Wendy uses in her product. You can order it by sending her an email at _sales@goodcommonsense.com._ She has been quite successful with helping many through her products and has been in business for 10 years.

A friend of mine had been suffering from severe pain (a solid 8/10 pain) which kept her awake at night despite her trying other traditional or conventional methods for pain management; she was only getting a couple hours of sleep due to her post-surgical hip pain and arthritic pain of lower back and non-operated hip.

She accidentally found a CBD oil at a local farmer's market and decided to give it a try after hearing many good things about cannabis. She bought both the cream and oil. She tried the cream and had immediate relief. After she tried some oil, she was able to finally sleep eight hours, something she hasn't been able to do for eight months. In fact, the pain went all the way down to 2/10 now, and she is just overjoyed.

Another friend of mine had some spinal problem (degenerative disc disease) and had a bad injury that caused her to be in severe pain. She ended up on a wheelchair. She took CBD oil for three weeks at the request of her doctor and was able to be weaned off all her pain meds. She can now walk again. The brand that she took and swears by is called **TruHemp.** She stated that their oil is non-GMO, organic, full spectrum and 3rd party tested and has zero THC in it.

Some doctors prefer some THC in it to help those in severe pain like one of my former clients.

Janet Doerr stated that **CBD oil** is fabulous for many people. She even has her dog (who is 14 and has a lot of arthritis) on pure CBD oil.

I discovered a blend of CBD oil at **Resonant Botanicals,** in Seattle. It was developed by biochemist, Michael Yocco. I like that it is organic and blended differently than many of the CBD oils I have seen or tried. They are blended with botanicals and include natural terpenes, MSM, magnesium and essential oils.

They also have a special blend that is specific to the neuropathy pain plus they have a blend that helps you during the day and when you sleep. I tried some on my sore muscle and found it helpful. **(R 141)**

Acupuncture

Acupuncture is one of the best methods for treatment issues of body pain, says Dr. Alex Feng, Ph.D., O.M.D. L.Ac. (He is also a spiritual leader, master of healing, Qi Gong Master and Daoist Master. A former director of Integrative Medicine at Highland Hospital, he is now on staff at Alta Bates Summit Medical Center.) *San Francisco Magazine* named Dr. Alex Feng one of the ten best acupuncturists in the Bay Area.

I have tried acupuncture and found it quite effective in providing me pain relief and healing of my injured arm. After receiving one acupuncture session on my painful limb, my pain had decreased moderately. My fingers which were stiff were much more flexible after one treatment. The next day I found that the improvement in pain relief carried over and I did not have to use any CBD cream for relief.

Acupuncture improves blood flow to the injured area and aides with the healing and recovery. It is a great method for helping the body to heal from pain but has also been known to help with sleep, digestive issues, respiratory issues, mental, emotional issues and many other issues that affect our well-being including cancer, chronic fatigue syndrome, diabetes, stroke, etc.

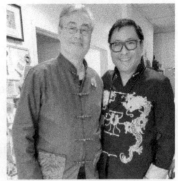

Dr. Alex Feng and Blake Sinclair

Medical Intervention

I once had a client who suffered from a great deal of pain (body and nerve). She took pain medications but found little relief. She even sought help with a chiropractor and acupuncturist and found some relief. However, what she found was the most helpful solution for getting rid of her nerve pain was a procedure called **Radio Frequency Ablation**. It can be done anywhere in the body where there is pain including the back and head according to my former client.

With Radio Frequency Ablation, a needle is inserted in the area of the nerve pain and a radio frequency is sent to the area and adjusted until a pulse is felt. Once it is felt, the frequency is set to that range and left on for about eight minutes. After the session, the pain goes away and can last for one month up to six months. There are also implants that can be put in the body that automatically sends a Radio Frequency to dissipate the pain signal.

Sometimes it is necessary and may be beneficial to get physical or occupational therapy to help with the healing process for certain conditions like shoulder, neck, and lower back pain.

Physical and Occupational Therapies

Many people suffer some type of shoulder and lower back pain due to stress, poor body mechanics and or injury. They might have tried over the counter approaches or pain medication but have not found adequate relief. Sometimes it helps to see a professional like a physical or an occupational therapist.

Many of us carry the stress on our shoulders and necks for many months until the muscles get so tight and inflamed. The result is severe pain. Lack of activity, poor posture and poor body mechanics can make it worse.

If you are repeatedly getting pain on the shoulder, neck, wrist and lower back while at work, you may benefit from an **occupational therapist** to evaluate your work and your workstation to assess your body mechanics during work and your ergonomics while sitting at the computer or desk during work. Many times, a lesson on proper body mechanics, exercises and instructions on how to rearrange or modify your office and workshop will help to improve the body mechanics of the shoulder, elbow, or hands which may lead to a decrease in body aches. It can also help reduce the incidence of carpal tunnel syndrome and cervical and lower back pain. They can also use different modalities to help alleviate pain like using a Ten's Unit, Ultrasound, Paraffin Wax, cupping or other cutting-edge technology.

A Physical Therapist can be effective with helping you to reduce your pain through exercises, soft tissue mobilization, trigger points, stretching, as well as using cutting-edge technology to improve circulation and help the body to heal faster with some form or Low-Level Laser Therapy, Ten's Unit, Ultrasound, etc.

It may seem that the two different therapies are the same, but occupational therapy helps issues that affect the functional ability of an individual with regards to their body mechanics during various activities of daily living task or skills. Since function is tied in with the upper body function, their focus tends to be more related to the upper body. Whereas the physical therapist focuses more on general strength, mechanical and mobility issues; hence, their focus is more on the legs. In reality the two therapies overlap quite a bit.

A Physical Therapist is more likely to use some form of modality to treat your pain; however, more and more occupational therapists are becoming skilled with doing it as well. Whether you get an occupational therapist or physical therapist to assist you is not as important as having a therapist who is well-versed with your issue.

I have found a myofascial release tool called an **Uno Roller with Surface Skin technology** that has been quite effective in decreasing the pain and tight muscles while improving the blood flow to the painful area. It was designed by a physical therapist and can be purchased at Fleet Feet in Pleasanton, California. **(R 142)**

Hot and Cold Modalities

The judicious and prudent use of a **heating pad** can be helpful for body aches, pain and muscle tightness. The heat helps the muscle to relax and release the tension. It also opens the arteries - vasodilation - to allow better flow to the painful area and allow nutrients of healing to come in. Clients with diabetes should not use a heating pad unless under the supervision of a professional.

I have also found much success with the **Heat-Wave Synergy stones.** You heat the stone(s) in a microwave for a minute or so and use it to provide deep tissue pressure or massage. It is made of ceramic and is a good conductor of heat that penetrates deeply beyond just the skin layers. I have used it on my family members and myself with good success with clearing tight muscles.

In one instance, I had much pain after a severe cramp episode during my stay in Seattle.

I woke up with a severe cramp of my calf muscle but I stopped the cramp within 3 seconds using acupressure. However, the next morning I had moderate residual pain in the calf. I was able to decrease the pain by 30-40% with visualization and massages but some pain remained when I would walk a certain way. I limped during the day because my calf was tight. I found this product in Seattle and the salesperson tried it on me for a few minutes and I felt instantly better. The products are **Heat-Wave Synergy Stones** of which I purchase two at that time.

I used them on myself I found that they released most of the remaining tightness and pain on my calf. I found them quite effective, gaining greater understanding by watching an instructional video on how to use it.

I used it on a client who had 10/10 pain on her lower back in a therapeutic way to activate the parasympathetic nervous system and improving blood flow in the back. I also did soft tissue massage and some gentle Tui Na Sports massage and the pain in the lower back went away after my session.

It is a great tool for a physical, occupational and massage therapist but anyone can learn how to use it if they watch the many instructional videos they have. **(R 143)**

If you wish to use this product note that care must be used in using it with the elderly who have thin skin or compromised health. It should not be used with people who have compromised sensory perception or diabetes. It is important to check the temperature prior to applying it to the skin especially with the elderly. Sometimes a cloth barrier may be needed when using it on sensitive skin or when it is hot. When in doubt contact the company on how to use it properly or discuss it with your local physical or occupational therapist.

Warning: Diabetics sometimes have a hard time perceiving pressure and heat properly due to neuropathy or poor circulation. Placing the heating pad on the affected area for 15-20 minutes at medium temperature is a good start. (High temperature should never be used unless supervised by a professional therapist). Slowly increase the time as tolerated. This is best for chronic pain.

If the pain is acute, the use of an ice pack to decrease the edema and numb the pain may be very helpful. (Make sure there is a barrier to the skin if dealing with a diabetic). Fifteen minutes a few times a day can help. Sometimes an alternating approach of heat and cold is good as well. If in doubt, ask your doctor to send you to an outpatient clinic for physical or occupational therapy.

Here's a trick I once learn from a conference. Some therapists fill a small paper cup with water and freeze it. After it is frozen, they trim part of the top of the cup and use it like a roll on to ice painful parts.

Happy Feet Happy Body

Having a good pair of running or walking shoes can be extremely helpful with creating the proper base of support for realigning the ankle, knee and hip for proper positioning. Improper fitting shoes can put a strain or torque on the knee and hip and cause more pain than necessary. I like to shop at stores like **Fleet Feet** in Pleasanton, California where they analyze your gait pattern, take a 360-degree picture of your foot and help you choose the proper shoes and semi-custom arches based on your gait, foot arch and anatomy of your foot. By getting proper shoes, the pain on my hip resolved. If your issues are more complicated then you can consult with a physical therapist and orthopedist to fabricate custom shoes and or arches.

Those individuals who have special orthopedic needs may need to be evaluated by a physical therapist and orthopedist for custom orthotics to further improve their gait and base of support to alleviate pain on the ankle, knee and hip.

High Tech Tools for Healing

The Bioflex Laser therapy appears to be a very effective method for managing an assortment of musculoskeletal (spinal pathologies, soft tissues and sport injuries, arthritis, etc.) pain. It was developed by Dr. Fred Kahn, MD. FDA approved units may be purchased at https://bioflexlaser.com / products/ **(R 144)**

Laser Technology combines super luminous and laser diodes to irradiate diseased or traumatized tissue with photons. These particles of energy are selectively absorbed by the cell membrane and intracellular molecules, resulting in the initiation of a cascade of complex physiological reactions, leading to the restoration of normal cell structure and function. It also helps with wound healing, dermatological disorders and neurological disorders.

My client's granddaughter had a concussion and received this type of therapy and found that it was quite helpful in her recovery in dealing with the pain from the head injury.

Some people find relief with the **Ten's Unit** to block the pain signal. There are many OTC ten's units you can purchase at the stores. It is best to be trained initially by a licensed physical or qualified licensed occupational therapist.

Meanwhile, some find relief with **ultrasound.** Ultrasound therapy is a treatment modality used by physical or occupational therapists to treat pain conditions and to promote tissue healing. While ultrasound therapy is not effective for all chronic pain conditions, it may help reduce your pain if you have any of the following: **(R 145)**

- Osteoarthritis
- Myofascial pain
- Bursitis
- Carpal tunnel syndrome
- Pain caused by scar tissue

Cold Laser Therapy or Low-Level Laser Therapy (LLLT) can be quite effective in helping with pain, swelling and inflammation.

It is a treatment that utilizes specific wavelengths of light to interact with tissue and is thought to help accelerate the healing process. **(R 146)**

Low Level Laser Therapy has been used by Physical Therapists with excellent results. I have witnessed extraordinary improvements with clients who used it.

One client had severe pain and after one treatment had a 90-100% reduction in pain. It was night and day with this client who had a treatment.

Some people including athletes have used **Silk'n Relief** to successfully treat their pain. It has Bipolar RF and IR heat energy, infrared, and low-level light therapy. This machine may be used at home and is FDA approved; it may be purchased online. **(R 147)** It may be helpful to have initial instruction from a qualified occupational or physical therapist trained in physical modalities.

The HiDow XPDS 18 Modes Tens Units can be helpful for pain management and aids in the healing of the injured area. It has 18 modes of varying degrees of massage which can be very relaxing on tight or tense muscles. When tight muscles are released so is the pain associated with the tension, thus breaking the pain cycle and allowing the area to more easily heal. It helps with acute and chronic pain. The unit has been sold to physical therapists and chiropractors but is available for consumer usage. Again, getting initially trained by a physical therapist or occupational therapist is a good idea.

LED LightStim may help with pain management as well. LightStim is a handheld LED device that delivers low intensity light energy similar to a process called plant photosynthesis whereby plants absorb light energy from the sun. How does LightStim work? LightStim emits UV-free rays that convert sunlight into cellular building blocks that stimulate the body's natural process to build new proteins and regenerate cells. **(R 148)**

One of my clients had a unit and she had used it in the past when she had shoulder pain and found it quite helpful. When I first met her, she was in much pain on her right shoulder due to a fall. There was no acute fracture but I suspected a mild rotator cuff injury. She had started using the unit over her shoulder and found that after a few minutes it was feeling better. LightStim patented LED Light Therapy is a natural way to ease pain. LightStim for Pain emits warm and soothing light energy proven to temporarily relieve minor muscle and joint pain and stiffness, minor arthritic pain or muscle spasms through the temporary increase in local blood circulation, and the temporary relaxation of muscles.

Dr. Tennant has invented the **Biomodulator Plus and Pro** which helps with pain issues and helps the body to grow new cells for healing. **(R 149)**

VITAFON-T- is a vibroacoustic apparatus made in Russia. **(R150)** It is recommended for use by Commission of the Russian Health Ministry. Its recommended usage includes over 38 conditions. Some of the conditions that it is recommended for include but is not limited to the following:

- Fractures
- Spinal Traumas
- Insomnia
- Arthritis
- Flaccid Paralysis
- Alleviating Fatigue
- Prevention of colds
- Constipation
- Gastritis

This type of treatment utilizes a range of frequencies and amplitude of vibration, analogues to that of a living organism. It helps to decrease inflammation and improve blood flow. Instructions are given from the manual on specifically where to place the vibraphones for treatment. Zones are identified throughout the body for easy identification.

Chakra Sweep PEMF (Pulsed Electromagnetic Field) - According to Norman Shealy, M.D., Ph.D., PEMF has been used for 25 years and has been shown to

- Increase ATP production in the mitochondria
- Enhance the sodium-potassium pump
- Increase cellular pH to make the cells and body more alkaline
- Improve oxygen uptake and assimilation into the cells
- Lower blood viscosity and improve circulation and microcirculation
- Create a healthy level of electroporation (openings in the cells for improved nutrient transport and waste elimination)
- Reduce Pain

Dr. Shealy further wrote that clinical benefits of the Chakra Sweep are greatest in reducing pain and in improving depression, anxiety and sleep. He has also been found it to reduce blood pressure, improve oxygen saturation in COPD, and assist opioid addicts in relieving craving. **(R 151)**

Dr. Norman Shealy is one of the world's leading experts in pain and depression management. He was the first physician to specialize in the resolution of chronic pain. He is an author, inventor (has 14 patents in Energy Medicine), editor, President of Shealy-Sorin Wellness and Holos Energy Medicine Education and Winner of the first Harold G. Wolff award for excellence in pain research. (the Shealy-Sorin Gamma PEMF. *is available at https://normshealy.com/.)*

Management of Common Pains

I feel that it is important to **always consult with your physician** to assess any underlying illness, disease or pathology before you begin any home remedies or treatment. You may have a pinched nerve, torn ligament, bone fractures, compressed disc, etc. which may be better treated by surgical intervention. Equally important is to make sure your physician is aware of any exercise regime you are contemplating.

Despite the many pains that exist out there, there are some remedies that may help some of our common pains and they include the following:

Low back pain

Low back pain is very common and most of the time can improve with yoga, physical therapy, Pilates and exercise. Two great resources for back support include *Treat Your Own Back* by Robin A. Mckenzie **(R 152).** I have used some of exercise tips with great relief. The other book is *The Back Pain Help Book* by various health professionals. **(R 153).**

A friend of mine Yumiko Yoga, a Yoga Teacher, Reiki Teacher, Sound and Voice Healer, and Neo Healer in Tokyo, recommended using a product called Egyptian Oil for alleviating stiffness especially in the back. She recommends massaging it on the spine and that the product helps with pain as well since it promotes circulation. You can get the product at https://heritagestore.com//

Dr. Hector Oksenendler, RPT, DC, feels that **chiropractic adjustments** along with proper exercises is the most effective way to treat lower back pain. He talked about how we must be cautious about how to do many of the in-vogue back exercises out there. For instance, he stated that it is important to maintain the lordosis curvature of the spine when doing any lower back exercise to protect the back. He believes that Pilates is one of the best forms of exercise an individual can do to help the back as it strengthens the body's core or trunk muscles providing overall support of the vertebrae and spinal column. I concur with Dr. Oksenendler. I have studied Pilates and have found it helpful for strengthening my core, spine and lower back issues. Make sure you tell your Pilates instructor if you have any injuries, limitations or pain so that he or she could modify the exercise for you so you could do it in a way without hurting yourself or aggravating the pain.

However, check with your doctor if Pilates will work best for you. The workouts can be quite intense for an elderly person or one who has health issues. Otherwise, it is a great workout program for the core. (There are Pilates instructors who are more skilled and trained to work with the physically challenged and the elderly). In addition, Dr. Oksenendler stated that snorkeling or swimming for about an hour can do wonders for the back, if you are able. He also finds suspension exercises very effective for improving back problems.

It is important to sit and sleep on proper density chairs or bed to minimize the strain on the spine with worn out furniture.

Neck Pain

Prior to any therapy on the neck, the individual should see an orthopedic doctor to rule out any herniated disc, spinal stenosis, cervical fractures or any nerve compression or impingement disorders. Once you are clear to get treated on your neck, physical or occupational therapy can be helpful with your recovery.

I find that **acupressure** can be quite helpful with stress induced tensions. If there are no contraindications from your physician, having **gentle traction and massage** on the head and neck from a qualified occupational or physical therapist can be helpful but a good chiropractor can do wonders since the spine is their expertise.

General Shoulder Pain

I have helped many clients significantly reduce shoulder and neck pain, or get rid of it all together by natural methods. The client usually has a dramatic improvement with active and passive range of motion on the shoulder joint after the pain is minimized or resolved.

Our bodies require touch, compassion and love. Getting a good shoulder and neck release from a caring and nurturing physical therapist or occupational therapist, chiropractor, or massage therapist can be so healing.

I see many clients with shoulder disorders ranging from rotator cuff injury, shoulder replacements, arthritis and just stress-induced tension. Many of those clients will have tight shoulder muscles and manifest moderate weakness. I have seen many thousands of clients with shoulder issues and have been extremely successful with restoring function to most if not all of my clients who are motivated or have a good support system. Orthopedic doctors are always amazed at the level of success I have achieved with my clients.

I have found the following to be the most effective way to treat the shoulder: usage of ice during the acute phases, judicious use of heat on the affected limb after the acute phase, soft tissue massage, self-range of motion or stretching, acupressure exercises, pendulum exercises, wall glide exercises and dowel exercises in supine position during the initial phase and doing it seated when the muscle pain has subsided significantly while the muscle strength has improved moderately.

Theraband exercises can also be quite helpful with improving the strength and decreasing the pain. It must be done only when the muscle has healed enough and is ready for it. If it has not healed well enough, it is possible to strain the muscle from the Theraband. It is best to be evaluated by your physician, physical and/or occupational therapist on your readiness for the exercise and how to use it to exercise correctly.

Shoulder shrugs and rotation forwards and backwards can release some of the tension of the shoulder and decrease pain and tightness.

Using an overhead pulley (which are nominally priced and readily available on Amazon) can be quite helpful for those who have excessive shoulder tightness. They are a basic pulley system that has at least 3- 4 parts including: 1. a rope 2. a pulley; 3. Two handles and 4. A bracket or tab that secures between the door and door frame. Using such an exercise device can be helpful for maintaining flexibility of the shoulder muscles and accelerate the healing process. It must be done lightly and gently to avoid straining oneself. It is best to get a consultation from an occupational therapist on how to set up a good exercise program with incorporating this device into the treatment regime.

The above are all part of a good occupational therapy or physical therapy program. The expertise of the clinician depends on his or her experience with treating the shoulder issues or disorders.

I have recently discovered an amazing tool that is great for releasing tight shoulder muscles and be done by yourself. It is called a **Muscle Hook** and is so versatile and effective. It can be purchased at Target and comes with instructions on how to use it. It is also great for releasing tightness with impingement of the shoulder.

Impingement of the Shoulder

This type of impingement may be due to poor body posture, repetitive movements, imbalance of muscles and poor alignment of tendons or bursa in the shoulder bones. The rotator cuff tendons and the bursa are commonly affected. Stretching exercises can help improve the humeral alignment to decrease pain. Ice can help if there is inflammation of the bursa. Heat can help to relax the tight muscles. The judicious usage of a pillow between the legs and arms at night can provide relief when you sleep.

In order to get complete healing, you will most likely need to see an Occupational Therapist who is also a hand therapist or an outpatient Physical Therapist well-versed with shoulder impingement. You will need manual therapy, stretching, trigger points and specific exercises to strengthen the supportive muscles around the shoulder like the rotator cuff muscles, the trapezius, pectoralis minor and others. Cupping and ultrasound are also quite helpful. If the condition doesn't improve within 8 sessions, you may need to get a cortisone shot to stop the inflammation or seek alternative healing methods.

Carpal Tunnel Syndrome

This occurs when the median nerve and tendons that go through the carpal tunnel (a narrow passageway or tunnel made of bones and ligaments on the palm side of the hand at the wrist) and is compressed and inflamed due to repetitive movements and poor positioning or mechanics of the wrist. The nerve innervates the palmar surface of the thumb, index, middle and part of the ring finger. Symptoms may include numbness, tingling, pain, muscle atrophy at the base of the thumb and weakness of the hand, wrist, forearm, and may go even as far as the shoulder.

Treatment may include anti-inflammatory supplements like Curamed, Boswellia or medications prescribed by your physician. Biofreeze and icing are good in decreasing the pain as well. Therapy aimed at stretching the wrist and strengthening it is important.

It has been known that magnet therapy has helped many with pain relief, especially with high gauss magnets. My friend Mikaelah Cordeo reported finding great relief of pain and symptoms using a magnetic necklace that she wrapped around her wrist and thumb for a number of weeks.

It is important to wear a night time carpal tunnel or wrist brace to allow the wrist to be positioned in a neutral position to help decrease compression on the median nerve to promote healing as well. It is sometimes necessary to wear it during the day as well depending on the nature of your work and whether you use your hands a lot or not. You can easily find a prefabricated one from Target, CVS Pharmacy, Walmart or your local medical supply store. However, if you find that it is not as comfortable as you would like you can have a custom-made splint made from orthoplast from an occupational therapist who is a hand therapist or who has experience making splints.

With regards to exercises, there are many YouTube videos on great exercises for your carpal tunnel. Here are a few of my favorites:

1. Extend your arm out in front of you with palm extended and facing down. Next, slightly extend your wrist and moderately flex your fingers as if you were placing your hand comfortably on a tabletop. Hold it for 5-10 seconds.

2. Extend fingers straight and keep wrist in the neutral position for 5-10 seconds.

3. Turn your palm facing up and gently grab hold of you thumb with your other hand from the palm side and slowly stretch and extend the wrist downwards for 5- 10 seconds.

4. Hold your hand in prayer position for 10-30 seconds; slowly turn your wrist down so you have upside down prayer position for 10-30 seconds. Lift or adjust elbow as needed.

5. Put your thumb in your palm – same hand – and close your fingers over the thumb. Position your forearm in a neutral position where palm is neither facing up or down. Flex downwards and back to neutral position 10 reps.

It is equally important to have your workstation ergonomically set up to allow the wrist to be comfortably positioned in a way to avoid excessive wrist extension or flexion when you are doing much typing, such as a readily-available, computer keyboard, wrist support pad. Either repetitive movement or poor positioning of the wrist can lead to tightness around the carpal tunnel leading to pain, numbness and weakness. It is not conducive for your wrist to hold it in a bad posture over an extended amount of time. Learn to take breaks frequently and just shake your hands out for a few minutes or do wrist rotation exercises. An occupational therapist who specializes or has experience can easily evaluate your work station for proper ergonomics.

General Muscle Pain (from sports injury or from sprain)

R.I.C.E. is especially effective during acute injury or sprain. It stands for Rest, Ice, Compression and Elevation.

Kinesio Taping can help reduce pain, provide support, and improve healing. After injuring my arm, my son offered to Kinesio Tape my arm. I had injured my rotator cuff muscles (especially the subscapularis, teres minor, infraspinatus and including my deltoids). My son had learned how to do it from school while pursuing his doctorate in Occupational Therapy; he also learned some on his own through self-study.

After he strategically taped the injured areas, I immediately felt like my arm had more support and had less pain during movements. I highly recommend using Kinesio Taping after an injury to help improve function, support and recovery time. It can be done by an occupational therapist, physical therapist, sports doctor, athletic trainer, etc. It is important to also include a P.R.E. (progressive resistive exercise) program to strengthen the weakened muscle.

I began a light exercise program on my arm after it began to feel better with the Kinesio Taping which helped to further decrease my pain. I believe that the stronger our muscles get the less pain we experience. I have observed this also in many of my clients. The trick is to exercise the muscle within the pain free range and slowly increase the resistance or weight as tolerated.

Neuropathy Pain

Terry Naturally's Healthy Feet & Nerves is a popular hit for many years at Valley Health Mill. Many customers have found some benefits with their neuropathy pain. Others have taken Benfotiamine (fat soluble Vitamin B1) and have had benefits with their neuropathy pain. It is believed that vitamin B1 helps support the myelin sheath around the nerve to improve nerve conduction.

If the body is recovering from nerve damage, Kathryn Shanti Ariel recommends homeopathic Hypericum, which assists with the actual healing and reconstruction of nerves. **(R 154)** Using this along with vitamin therapy such as Vitamins E and C, along with Coenzyme Q10 can be of great assistance in the healing process.

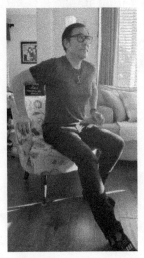

Resonant Botanicals' Neuro-Soothe was developed over the past couple years to create lasting, effective relief from symptoms associated with Neuropathy, Fibromyalgia and Dystonia. **(R 155)**

Some clients have found benefit from neurological medications prescribed by their physician. Two medications that many of my clients take are Gabapentin and Neurontin. Physical Therapy treatment targeted towards increasing the blood flow to the feet can be helpful with the treatment of neuropathy as well.

One exercise I learned from a neuropathy conference is sitting on a chair with arms on it. Place both hands on the chair arms (if possible) and have one knee flexed and the foot is below the knee. Extend the opposite knee about 30-45 degrees with the foot in front of it.

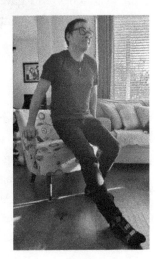

The individual pushes on the arms of the chair until the buttocks are off the chair by about 4-6 inches. Thereafter, the individual slowly lowers him or herself back down to the chair.

This can be done 10 – 15 times or more as tolerated. If the individual is in ill health or weak, this can be done with the supervision of a friend, therapist or family member.

Once one side is completed, do the same on the opposite side. The knee that is flexed is getting a load on it and causes blood flow towards it. The physical therapist who did the lecture found that many of his clients with neuropathy had improved with these types of muscle loading techniques. Essentially it improves the blood supply to the nerves so they can work properly.

Migraine Headaches

MigraSoothe, Vitamin B2, Magnesium, Feverfew and Butterbur have helped people with the migraine headaches. Saje's Halo essential oil can provide some relief as well. My friend Yumiko uses peppermint (essential oil) for her migraines and has received good relief from it. She gets her oils from www.youngliving,com/ which has a special way of blending the essential oil and it is pure and organic. According to Betty, her alias, Young Living Oil is far superior than other essential oils for the following reasons:

1. They have a seed to seal promise from the Young farms.
2. They have a million-dollar laboratory built to test the quality of their products to the highest level of plant constituents (ie. Terpenes, limonenes, etc).
3. The essential oils are created by the father (Gary Young) of modern-day essential oils.

She had the great pleasure of meeting with the Young founding family and discovered how they had such high integrity.

I have tried Solaray's MigraGard with some success. Pyradome is a technology device I have used on occasions and has helped to alleviate light headaches and gave me more clarity. **(R 156)** Meditation, stress management and biofeedback training are also helpful.

Gout in the Big Toe

Gout brings severe pain and inflammation that occurs when there is too much uric acid in the body. The pain can be quite severe and debilitating. I once had it and was unable to walk for a few days. Icing it can keep the swelling down but taking Tart Cherry can produce quite fast relief. I took it and the next day my pain had diminished significantly and I was able to walk again. Purium's Apothe Cherry has been reported to very effective with the pain as well.

Abdominal Pain

Leaky Gut Syndrome

Besides **Colostrum LD*** that we mentioned earlier, a friend of mine who is extremely health conscientious resolved her Leaky Gut by taking **collagen powder, probiotics, and L-Glutamine Powder*** to strengthen the wall of her gut and was able to successfully resolve her Leaky Gut issue. However, care must be taken when using glutamine.

DO NOT take glutamine if you are diabetic or have seizures, suffer from bouts of mania, severe liver disease with difficulty thinking or confusion, or if you are sensitive to monosodium glutamate (MSG). **(R 157)**

Crohn's Disease can benefit from the above as well. Cat's Claw may also be beneficial to those who suffer this debilitating digestive issue.

Cat's claw is used as a dietary supplement for a variety of health conditions including viral infections (such as herpes and HIV), Alzheimer's disease, cancer, arthritis, diverticulitis, peptic ulcers, colitis, gastritis, hemorrhoids, parasites, and leaky bowel syndrome. **(R 158)**

Cat's claw (Uncaria tomentosa) 250 mg per day may help fight inflammation. However, Cat's claw may make leukemia, as well as autoimmune disorders, worse, and may worsen low blood pressure. So, it must be used carefully. **(R 159)**

A friend of mine, Patti Gee, a massage therapist and Holistic Health Practitioner, recommended **Enerex Digest Best** to provide good digestive support and it contains L-glutamine which is a big plus. **(R 160)**

Other herbs that may help include:
- **Boswellia**
- **Tumeric**
- **Green Tea**
- **Marsh Mallow**- An herb that comes from the Althaea officinalis plant has been identified as useful in treating Crohn's Disease.
- **N-Acetylglucosamine**-N-acetylglucosamine supplements used in one study were found to reduce colon inflammation in children with Crohn's with no negative side effects. **(R 161)**

- **Vitamin D-** Chronic vitamin D deficiencies are common in people with Crohn's. Some researchers have found that chronic vitamin D deficiencies can lead to inflammation in the stomach and colon.

By adding vitamin D back into the diet, people with Crohn's might help minimize symptoms and increase immune system health. Since Crohn's is caused by a malfunction in your autoimmune system, providing a boost to your body's immune system can be a bonus. **(R 162)**

- **Vitamin B12-** It also protects nerve cells and helps make red blood cells. **(R 163)** It can be difficult to assimilate for some people. Check with your physician for optimal) absorption.

There may possibly be an emotional component with Crohn's Disease or other digestive disorder and inner child work or work towards healing emotional trauma can be helpful with the recovery of this illness.

Abdominal pain from food poisoning may find some relief from probiotics and or **Pathogen Assassin Immune Support liquid.**

Many people take antibiotics for some type of bacterial infection but fail to follow up taking probiotics. Consequently, many develop some type of digestive issue because the antibiotics have killed off not only the bad bacteria but also the good ones in our gut. It is important to take probiotics anytime any antibiotics are use. Most brands are not compatible with antibiotics with the exception with **Thrive.** It can be taken simultaneously with it.

However, Alexis is not a proponent of long-term usage of probiotics. Getting some after an antibiotic treatment is acceptable for her but she frowns upon those who use it on a daily basis and prefers to look deeper into her client's colon and complete system to see what else may be causing the colon issue like low magnesium or too much heavy metals or toxins there. Others have found additional benefits by adding Slippery Elm Powder to their health regime. It helps to coat the digestive lining and provide relief as well.

Joint Pain

Ultimate Joint Support KollaGen II-xs™ can be helpful for those who have joint issues. I have taken it initially when I had knee pain. After taking it for a few months, my pain subsided significantly and now I do not have any knee pain.

Biofreeze Gel can provide some temporary relief for those who are suffering from osteoarthritis and is readily available at Walgreens, Target and Walmart. Many physical therapy clinics, chiropractor's office, rehabilitation facilities have this product to provide instant relief to their clients. It is used by many athletes and even dancers.

Heat- judicious use of a heating pad can provide great relief as well. Avoid high temperatures especially for a prolonged period especially with the elderly and those with diabetes. Heat improves circulation and relaxes tight muscles. The improved circulation accelerates the healing process and many times helps reduce pain, especially chronic pain, dramatically.

Post-Surgical Pain

Patti Gee also recommended **Enerex Serrapeptase for postsurgical pain as well as arthritis.** Serrapeptase is a naturally occurring enzyme that was originally isolated from silk worm larvae. The enzyme is produced by bacteria in the gut of silk worms, and is responsible for helping the silk worm digest the mulberry leaf (its natural food) and the cocoon when it emerges as the moth. Serrapeptase is an anti-inflammatory that has been used to treat conditions like arthritis and even to unblock coronary arteries. **(R 164)**

Serrapeptase is a natural enzyme that effectively reduces pain, inflammation, as well as mucous build-up. Whether symptoms stem from injury, surgery or disease such as arthritis or sinusitis, its action disrupts pain pathways and restores your body's persistent inflammatory response to reduce swelling and improve circulation. This productive and efficient "miracle" enzyme can easily bring comfort and relief for better health.**(R 165)**

However, many orthopedic doctors prefer their patients not take any anti-inflammatory in the early phases of healing to allow the body to go through its necessary healing first. Always consult with your physician first before trying anything new.

Garden of Life Vitamin Code Raw Calcium may be helpful for those who are healing from a fracture. It contains magnesium, vitamin K, vitamin D and other vitamins. The combination of the three may help speed up the healing of the bone.

If the pain in a joint is severe, it is sometimes necessary and helpful to have a **cortisone injection.** However, frequent injections are highly contraindicated. According to the Mayo Clinic, complications of cortisone shots can include: Joint infection, Nerve damage, Thinning of skin and soft tissue around the injection site, Temporary flare-up of pain and inflammation in the joint, tendon weakening or rupture, thinning of nearby bone (osteoporosis), whitening or lightening of the skin around the injection site, death of nearby bone (osteonecrosis), or temporary increase in blood sugar. **(R 166)**

Tendon and Ligament Issues and Support

Neocell's Super Collagen* can be helpful for supporting tendon and ligament injury. A friend of mine had injured his ACL and has been in pain for several years. He tried this product and found great relief in a matter of weeks. He will continue to take it until he is ready to have his ACL ligaments repaired.

My nephew is a fitness buff, body builder and works out a lot with heavy weights and hence gets some joint pain. He has found that **Extreme Joint Care** has been quite effective for him in alleviating much of his joint related pain.

Biosil is an excellent supplement that supports skin, bones, nails and joints. It is made with a special molecular blend of silicon that is highly absorbable. This product has been promoted by Christie Brinkley and she takes this product as well. I also take this and find it helpful for my joints and skin.

Words of Wisdom from Various Healers about Pain

Interview with Lisa De Witt aka Meenakshi, Healer and Reiki practitioner. Lisa has been a healer for many years and has had much success in her practice. We are fortunate to have her share some of her secrets and knowledge of how to deal with pain. This is what she has to say about pain: "Pain is a very broad concept since there can be so many causes for pain. Like anything else I am seeking the cause of the pain. Is it due to trauma, infection, inflammation, or?

"For physical trauma, I would probably do a spiritual healing and then suggest **homeopathic Arnica** or **Bellis Perennis. Rescue Remedy** (a flower essence remedy) is a natural remedy for emotional trauma and I also suggest it for people who are trying to quit smoking. I've seen a lot of people with previous **bone fractures** who are still having pain many years later and it's usually because their body needs **more calcium, magnesium and vitamin D** to help the bone heal. Once they do that, the pain gets better. It's hard for them to believe that all their doctor needed to do was tell them to increase their bone building vitamins!

For people with arthritis I usually suggest they try **Epsom salt baths** and look into increasing their iodine.

"In all cases I recommend people do some kind of **cleansing diet** and drink water to **rehydrate.** Divide the body weight in half and that is how many ounces of water a person should drink per day. I recommend people get their vitamin levels up before they do any kind of fasting because so many people have vitamin deficiencies even if they are overweight. Many women tend to be low on iron and many people are just not getting enough minerals or protein. Many people have undiagnosed parasites which need to be addressed.

"**Food grade diatomaceous earth** alone with other herbs such as **Kroger's Wormwood Combination, ginger chews, pumpkin seeds** and **cayenne pepper** will eliminate many **parasites**. Many Chronic illnesses will clear up after a person eliminates parasites which weaken the immune system and allow fungus, bacteria and viruses to come in. People are dying because some doctors are refusing to acknowledge that so many are infested with parasites. These people look worn out and wonder why they feel so tired all the time. They pretty much always have digestive issues. The tests aren't sensitive enough and unless a person literally has worms crawling out of his body, most doctors will not listen."

Words of Wisdom from Various Healers about Pain

Janet Doerr, the Intuitive Nutritionista, recommends other things for pain management, including **arnica cream and arnica homeopathy** which helps with bruises and swelling. It is very helpful if it is a muscle issue. She also has found benefits with essential oils like **Frankincense oil.** It is very good at reducing inflammation. She stated, if a person has a sore knee, it can be rubbed on; it can be diluted. She had a cousin who diluted the oil and put it on her dog's joints that were inflamed. After it was put on, the dog was very comfortable. **Boswellic acids** can be bought in capsules and is very helpful for reducing inflammation and discomfort.

She also talks about pain from energy approaches. She stated that if there is pain, the energy is not flowing through the meridian from say the foot to the hand - all the way through the body - through the energy pathways called the energy meridians. Many people get great relief from **acupuncture** after a car accident or an injury. Also, when their work includes a lot of stresses and strains on their body, especially repetitive motions, acupuncture can be great. Janet feels that **Reiki** is another great form of energy healing that is helpful for pain management.

Janet recorded an MP3 called **Energetic Pain Pill** and made two versions, one spoken and one where she did not speak. During the speaking one, Janet would invoke the Ascended Masters and angels and she stated she would call forth from the plant kingdom, Redwood trees and healing herbs like turmeric and boswellic acid.

She would speak with the intention of love, compassion and with the greatest respect and compassion for the person having a pain experience to help them relax and work their way through it. When she is speaking, she is also intending Light Codes for healing.

She stated she also taped some energy when she was in a Redwood grove in California and used that as a silent under layer in the MP3. Then she made a second one, and she read her script in her head and thought about bringing all the same energy in but made no noise and did not speak out loud. In both versions she still intended that all the energy, love and compassion would be in the MP3s. One day when she had much pain in her ribs and could not find relief, despite trying various healing methods, she listened to the silent version, found relief and was able to fall sleep.

Janet also points out the pain and issues of the body may also have emotional energies embedded in it, especially in our various organs. Sometimes, the energies that are causing the pain have ancestral origins and are patterns that we energetically inherited so to speak. When there is an emotional trauma in the past of our ancestral lineage that is not resolved, it may work its way within our body and organs and cause much suffering. These are many times the core of many of our sufferings. We will discuss more about this in the chapter about emotional suffering.

Besides dealing with pain through herbs, supplements, MP3s, and energetic healing, Janet has also talked about healing yourself through your intention, visualization, energetic healings and meditation. She once had a left hip that had severe arthritis. The doctor said she needed surgery but she decided not to have one so she worked hard on healing herself. To make a long story short, she was able to heal her left hip joint, avoid surgery and now can do anything she wants with her legs.

Alexis, her alias, is a **Medical Intuitive** and **Parapsychologist.** She would ask why are we in pain? "We're toxic, we're inflamed… yeah there are few of us who are involved in horrible accidents, had a broken bone but we are a culture that is so empty. Everybody is on some drug, or something, or they smoke something or they regulate their mood on drugs, on alcohol, food or sugar, caffeine and pain pills because people are not comfortable with their bodies anymore."

She stated that **CBD oil** can help with pain **and inflammation**. She is a fan of CBD oil and even uses it with her cat. However, she also points out that a lot of times pain is **biochemistry**. For instance, one of her relative had a limp and she had him analyzed with her dousing devices like a pendulum and put them on various modes and determine that his hip pain was in metabolic mode. Thereafter, she went to assess further from her charts and found that he had a vitamin D deficiency. She put him on 5000 IU of vitamin D3 for three days, and then his pain went away completely. She said that if the body gets what it needs, it heals. She said, "I have many miracles…I could probably cite 20 miracles."

With regards to supplements, she states that "there are many supplements we can also use for pain but before she recommends it, she ask does the body need this, can it use it; you would be surprised at how many things we need but cannot use. There are a lot of things we cannot use, cannot break down, cannot metabolize it properly; we're missing co-factors due to a glitch in our matrix. This is my protocol when I recommend a supplement:

- Does the body need it?
- Can the body use it?
- If it can, what form does it need it?
- What's the dose needed?
- How often is the dose needed?
- What is the initial building dose?
- What is the maintenance dose?"

Her approach is logical and easy for her clients to understand and follow.

Regarding pain and inflammation, she stated, "You have to ask yourself why you are having inflammation. I want to find out why you are having inflammation. To me supplements for inflammation are just suppressing the issue. Otherwise you could be under curcumin for the rest of your life."

She prefers to go to the root cause of the pain. She stated, "I heal the system so the symptoms go away. I heal the system that is causing your specific inflammation and then the inflammation goes away."

Millions of people suffer from some form of **autoimmune disease.** According to Anthony William, many of these individuals have Epstein-Barr Virus. According to Anthony, the Epstein-Barr virus (EBV) has created a secret epidemic. Out of the roughly 320 million people in the U.S., over 225 million Americans have some form of EBV. **(R 167)**

It feeds on the metals that are tucked within our organs like our liver, spleen, thyroid and brain. The viruses' excrement as well as deceased bodies causes inflammation which can result in pain throughout the body. Anthony William has written extensively on how to use fruits, vegetables and various supplements to help us recover from the virus and to release the metals from our bodies. Many of us may have Epstein Barr Virus but it may be dormant most of our lives until we experience great or sudden stress in our lives. The stress is a trigger for the virus to awaken and begin wreaking havoc to our organs, brain and nerves causing severe pain from the inflammatory response of the body trying to get rid of the excrement and remains of the virus.

Stem cell research is a new frontier of science that has opened a new window of hope for millions around the world. David Granovsky, a stem cell expert, advocate, advisor, and author, stated that stem cells can help with pain management by addressing issues of inflammation in the body and through its ability to regenerate new cells in the body for healing. I will elaborate more about what he says about stem cell technology in Chapter 15.

Good stress management, healthy eating and drinking and detoxing regularly can help us minimize getting ill from the virus. **Pharma Gaba** has been clinically proven to decrease cortisol production which is the stress hormone. **Curamed** may help with the inflammatory response of the body and reduce pain. **Kyani's Sunrise** (super fruits) **and Kyani NitroFx** may help with the inflammation and healing as well.

Additionally, Anthony William has excellent information on how to systematically treat and improve many of our common autoimmune diseases. I highly recommend reading his book, *Medical Medium,* and his other two books as well.

Cheryl, her alias, is a Seifukujitsu Healer or Restoration Therapist and instructor and Licensed Massage Therapist. She recommends Seifukujitsu (the healing division of Danzan Ryu Jujitsu) and suggests that it can be quite effective in treating various ailments including the following: inflamed eye muscles (red eyes or strain), nasal illness, toothache, tonsil tightness, vocal cord constriction, asthma, headaches, stomach and intestinal issues, abscess in nose, coughing and bronchitis, noises in ear (tinnitus), stomach ulcers, sciatica, insomnia, high blood pressure, spinal disorders, constipation, congested spinal muscles, sore spine and bone bruises.

Cheryl also stated it can help patients with stroke, including those who are anxious, depressed, suicidal or have arthritis, contractures, scar tissues, frozen shoulder, epicondylitis, etc. Anything that can be restored or balanced may be helped. Many of the therapists are quite mechanical and some are not. They do not manipulate or adjust but massage and create more balance for the body and system. She tried this on my sore muscle and within a few minutes my pain subsided significantly by 90%. (*You can get more information by exploring* https://AJJF.org.)

I believe that proper hydration with alkaline and hydrogen infused water can be very helpful with pain management.

Another extremely important factor with pain management is following a plant-based diet. It helps to improve vascular flow and decrease the amount of inflammation in the body.

In summary, it is important to do one thing at a time. Putting too many different ointments, gels, supplements and medication together can have an adverse and dangerous reaction in your body. Also avoid applying ointments and using heating or cooling elements simultaneously.

Before getting a product, do your own research and read available reviews. Read the labels and see if there is anything that you are allergic to. Find out through your web searches or books to find if there are any contraindications with using the product with your unique problem, illness or disease. If you cannot find it, you can try contacting the manufacturer of the product. You can also consult a professional when in doubt but most importantly listen to your body and that Divine Presence within you with what you need.

If you have many unique and complex issues, consulting with your physician can be quite helpful. Then when you try something, pay attention to how your body is reacting to it. Is it helping your problem or creating new ones? Products that are good for you will support your body in healing itself and improve how you feel, move and function. The important thing to realize is that you have many options in life and that there is hope for you.

So, the good news is that we can also affect the amount of pain we have by exercising regularly and eating healthy (eating lots of fruits, vegetables and food with healthy fats). At one point in my life, I had much pain in my arm, but the pain subsided as I cut out processed food, sugar and greasy food from my diet and started exercising. I later learned from Dr. William Sears, a Harvard-trained physician and health expert that exercise stimulates the endothelium (the inner lining of the blood vessels) to release Nitric Oxide. This improves circulation, dilates and repairs the arteries and removes the sticky stuff in our arteries. All this led to the healing of my pain. Incidentally, Dr. Sears considered a healthy endothelium to be the '**fountain of youth**'.

There was a dramatic improvement with pain relief in my arm. Perhaps exercise and eating healthy food is a good start for any pain management program.

Besides the physical pain that we have, many of us suffer some form of inner emotional pain or turmoil that can be quite crippling. Let us explore further in the next chapter on how we can be free from this type of insidious emotional pain.

"The more we ignore or suppress certain emotions, the more we are controlled by them."

~

Geri Scazzero

CHAPTER 6

HEALING THE EMOTIONAL BODY

E motional imbalances and pain can be just as or even more debilitating than those of the physical body. Part of this is that they are often misunderstood, resulting in their being misdiagnosed or ignored all together.

Currently, emotional pain and suffering afflicts millions of people all around the world. Some of the common emotional imbalances include guilt, anger, depression, anxiety, poor self-worth, and PTSD (posttraumatic stress disorder). The causes of these emotional imbalances and resulting pain are many, some from direct experiences of abuse or neglect, while others can be the result of a person being highly sensitive or empathic, especially if they are not aware of this gift.

Being an empath means that a person is highly sensitive to the energies of other people, animals or other life forms. I will discuss this in more detail later in this chapter.

Sometimes the emotional pain is so overwhelming that people are pushed to the edge where they see no way out and succumb to committing suicide.

Suicide occurs throughout the world, affecting individuals of all nations, cultures, religions, genders and classes. In fact, statistics show that the countries with the highest suicide rates in the world are incredibly diverse. For example in 2019, among the top five are the eastern European country of **Lithuania** (31.9 suicides per 100k), the eastern European country of **Russia** (31 suicides per 100k), the south American country of **Guyana** (29.2 suicides per 100k), and the Asian country of **South Korea** (26.9 suicides per 100k). **(R 168)**

It happens worldwide and includes the United States of America where there were 47,173 people who committed suicide and died in 2017. **(R 169)**

Other times the pain is so great, it leads some to take their anger and depression out towards others in the form of mass shootings.

It is obvious that emotional pain is a real problem that requires great compassion and a holistic approach to healing in order to remedy it at the cause. At the root of these challenges is the duality-based way of living that we have created and sustained, and that many are now choosing to leave behind. Due to its nature, duality is conducive for creating and contributing to mental and emotional suffering in ourselves as well as towards others.

Understanding Emotional Pain and Its Effects

There are two main ways that people express emotions and emotional pain: 1. Through external expression and 2. By internalizing or hiding our emotions

Many of us who internalize our emotional pain do so to avoid dealing with it at a conscious level as part of our coping mechanism. Although we can hide it from our conscious awareness, the pain will hide in our bodies in different places depending on the type of emotional pain we are experiencing.

According to *Higher Perspective* **(R 170),** there are nine types of pain that are directly linked to emotional states. Each type of pain has a different type of issue:

4. Pain in the head – can be caused by day to day stress.
5. Pain in the neck – our own issues with forgiveness of self or others.
3. Pain in the shoulders – may relate to carrying an emotional burden.
4. Pain in your upper back – may relate to feeling you do not have enough emotional support.

5. Pain the lower back – may be related to money issues.
6. Pain in the elbows – speaks to inflexibility with changes in your life.
7. Pain in the hands – lack of willingness to reach out to others.
8. Pain in the hips – fear of moving.
9. Pain in the knees – can be a sign that your ego is a little too big and that you are thinking of yourself a little too highly.

Emotions Buried Alive

Emotional issues which are not dealt with will many times, bury themselves in our various organs and will manifest as aches, pains or diseases later on in life. By releasing the emotions or addressing them in a constructive and loving way will allow the energy to shift and healing to occur.

Another great reference is Louise Hay's book *You Can Heal Your Life* (**R 171**) which goes into considerable detail of how and where emotional energies reside in the body, what their affects can be and how to release and balance them. Louise has written extensively about how our emotions and behavioral issues hide throughout our body. She writes about how to analyze what problems we are having at different parts of the body and what our body is attempting to tell us.

For instance, if we constantly have joint and knee problems, Louise feels that the possible cause could be with our stubborn ego, pride; and our inability to bend. Issues of liver may be related to core issues of anger and primitive emotions. She offers great insight to the possible root causes of our problems which many times are mentally or emotionally based. She gives us great affirmations to help integrate or resolve the mental, psychological or emotional issues.

Another wonderful reference of this type is *Feelings Buried Alive Never Die* by Karol Truman. (**R 172**) Truman provides a comprehensive and enlightening resource for getting in touch with unresolved feelings which, she explains, can distort not only happiness but also health and well-being. Leaving no emotion unnamed, and in fact listing around 750 labels for feelings, Truman helps identify problem areas, and offers a "script" to help process the feelings, replacing the negative feeling with a new, positive outlook.

Chinese Medicine Perspective

The understanding within Chinese medicine is that our feelings of anger, jealousy and contempt are stored in our liver. If they are not released and replaced with peace and harmony, they will over time cause the liver to malfunction leading to illnesses and diseases of the liver.

According to Grandmaster Mantak Chia, sadness, depression, and grief are stored in our lung area while the spleen stores our worry, anxiety and mistrust. Hence, learning how to be more aware of our pain can be quite insightful on how to heal it. **(R 173)**

Face Reading as a Diagnostic Tool

Rebecca-Danbi Kim is a **Feng Shui Practitioner** who also does **Face Readings** and **Personal and Home Energy Clearing.** She is a friend of mine who recently gave me a Face Reading. Face reading first appeared in China in the 6th century B.C. Doctors in China have used the ancient science of face reading since the time of Confucius as an aid to diagnosis and help their patients. Close observation of the face provided deep knowledge of the personality of their patients as well as insight into the state of their health and impact of their unique experiences on their journey in their life. **(R 174)**

When I had my first Face Reading, I was amazed by its accuracy. A thorough reading was done on my entire face including analysis of my ears, ear lobes, eyes, forehead, hairline, lips, etc. Depending on the size, prominent features, wrinkles or bumps on certain places on the ear, certain information could be ascertained about some emotional event than may have transpired during a certain time frame. I found the whole reading extremely fascinating and I learned a lot from my session. What amazed me most is the fact that our face is another place where important emotional and ancestral data and life events are stored.

By analyzing the ears, we can tell the amount of vital energy or Jing Qi that the individual was endowed with. The ears can also indicate wisdom, psychic faculties and gifts. By analyzing it further, the practitioner can tell when in close time frame something important happened to an individual and whether the individual received many ancestral gifts or not. One ear represents the experience from birth to six years old while the opposite ear represents age seven to thirteen. The ears represent our kidneys as well and our kidneys represent our connections with our ancestors. Our ear lobes can indicate our financial style.

By analyzing my ears, Rebecca could tell at age two to three I had some emotional trauma and was indeed correct. I remember clearly at that age I saw my parents fight right in front of me.

The forehead reflects the times in our twenties while the eyes and eyebrows reflect the time in our thirties according to Rebecca. According to John Stan, the nose is the forties, the mouth is the fifties, the chin is the sixties and the jaw is the seventies. Then the face starts marking up the sides of the face until the age of 100. **(R 175)**

The Face Reading can reveal three meanings or components:
1. The emotional meaning (for instance, our eyes) tells us how we communicate.
2. The physical health component.
3. A Timing component.

Rebecca mentioned that our face is a map of our inner and outer journey and energetic patterns within and without us. She further mentioned that any physical change to our face will respond to a corresponding change within us and our life path. A lot of times when people do plastic surgery on their face, they are also altering their lives and destinies as well. And usually, it is not in a good way. We are born with the features we were meant to have and have a specific meaning and purpose and design for our life path.

They have a specific meaning and purpose. It can cause energetic shifts that the system does not know how to deal with and that can cause a lot of problems as well. Lips can reveal how satisfied we are in relationships. By enlarging them, it has caused some people to have issues with their relationships from stories she has heard from other Face Reading experts. However, she also mentioned that whenever there is an internal energetic change, we can also see it in the external side of our face too. Sometimes wrinkles can even disappear or a groove might look less prominent or even go away. It depends on whether it is something that can be worked through and how much of that inner change happens.

Rebecca then talked about how the forehead can indicate the level of creativity especially if it is rounded. It relates to intuition as well as ancestor's skills, talents and karma or challenges passed down from the ancestor. Meanwhile the sides of our forehead (where the hairline is) indicate whether we have a mind that makes intuitive leaps in thinking, and decision making may be assisted by intuitive flashes or have a great inner sense of knowing.

She talked about the underside of the eyes which is connected to the kidneys. Puffiness below the eyes can be quite normal for someone who is intuitive but it can also represent hidden tears. It happens when there are some emotions that have not been processed.

There is so much more I want to share but the important thing I wanted to share with you is how beautiful we were designed by our Creator. He or she made us in a way to record our journey once we incarnated into this planet.

By consulting with someone like Rebecca, she can help guide us on understanding our own roadmap of our life journey. We can then learn so much about ourselves and realize what our strengths and weaknesses are and what we need to do to grow further. **(R 176)**

There is also a Face Reading that is done in Chinese Medicine to determine the presence of illnesses and organ and Qi flow and wellness.

The Whole-Body Perspective

According to **Janet Doerr,** the Intuitive Nutritionista, gall bladder issues may reflect bitterness. **(R 177)** She observes that the energy in the prostate can be different for different people. "Sometimes I have found it is anger towards other men. Deep anger at what other men (beings in male bodies) have done from a lower ego-based consciousness, causing harm to the Earth, to women and children, or through war, greed and suppression of other people. Lung problems may be related to grief issues."

Regarding the colon, Janet explains it may represent some emotion that is horrible or disgusting. About the pancreas, she states it is about blood sugar management. People may not be allowing themselves the sweet things in life.

- Do you have somebody to cuddle with?
- Do you allow yourself to go listen to music?
- Do you allow enjoy expressing yourself in art or has all of that been suppressed?
- If it has been suppressed, it wouldn't surprise me that we are going to see a relationship between people who have Type 2 diabetes and how many of them would report that they go to a job they hate and they do not allow themselves to do anything in their life that they enjoy.

Another thing that Janet Doerr offers is **Ancestral healing.** When there is an emotional trauma from our ancestor, the energy is often carried over from one generation to the next in our DNA, cellular memory, and in the energy field of the ancestors. Sometimes we may have a problem that does not seem to go away despite the best medicines, herbs and supplements due to these ancestral patterns and energies that need to be addressed. They are energetic remembrance of the energy of a prior ancestor. Sometimes these patterns can give rise to many different diseases and illnesses in our various organs.

By addressing the emotional issues attached to the organ, joint or body part, the body begins to release the illness, disease and disharmony associated with the trauma and begins to heal. Often the healing incorporates taking vitamins, minerals or supplements to further assist in the healing process. It also helps to guide the individual to see the origins of the emotional issue or trauma that is at the root cause of the pain, illness or disease.

Janet guides the individual to see the trauma in a higher perspective or neutral viewpoint to transcend any guilt or shame associated with it and help shift the energy to more of a neutral energy. The emotional trauma is seen as just a neutral experience, neither good nor bad. As she guides the individual to look back into a situation, she guides the individual to see the trauma from a neutral viewpoint (that the issue was just an experience which is neither right nor wrong), learn from it and helps the individual to now love themself.

As we look back in the experience of life, instead of saying they were wrong, this was good, or this was bad. All of this creates a polarized field of energy; instead if we can get to a neutrality point where we say let it be. She helps her clients shift the energy to a neutral view of that experience. She then shows the client how they did the best they could and to just let it be.

She uses decrees and light codes which help the person see from a multidimensional view. She also works with different rays of Light, (Violet Flame which helps to transmute all which no longer serves us and releasing anything that is not love). She calls in great beings of Light from other realms to assist to help clear some of the negative beliefs the individual has been clinging onto to help them step into their own sovereignty without the energetic entanglement. These teams of Light are often those who overlight Janet and the individual who she is assisting. However, at times additional Beings may join in to aide in specific situations.

She describes her processes as follows: "I start with the current health issue someone is experiencing and look at the underlying energy, and sometimes I ask well what happened right before it started and other times I go..., 'Well, this has been going on for quite some time. Let's talk about the energy. There's this heavy energy in your body.' Then I lead them through a process of dialoguing to find out if the energy is even there, could it be from the ancestors, could it be from the mother or father. And very often there is a taking in of energy and belief system from a parent earlier in life, because as a child we want our parents to be happy. If they are not happy, we might think (sub-consciously), gee, maybe I can take some of this energy into my body to help. Now, they are wearing their parent's energy and later in life, it can manifest as a health issue."

This is an example of how working with a counselor, life coach, marriage family therapist, Taoist Master or healer, who is aware of these multibody (holistic) relationships may be helpful in assisting us to see more clearly what type of issues we may be storing in different parts of our body. Seeing them, and understanding how to return the whole body back to balance and harmony is a vital component to our overall health and well-being.

Restoring Emotional Balance

The good news is that most of these illnesses can improve with the proper mental and emotional help, support and resources. More importantly is the understanding that it is only through returning to our True Divine Nature that we can end the emotional suffering completely, replacing it with balance, harmony and joy.

My first two books *Dare to Imagine* and *Beyond Imagination* (R 178) go into more detail on how to discover our true nature in following a path to enlightenment and God-Realization. If you have not already read them, I encourage you to do so to receive the wisdom they contain and partner it with what you are receiving in this book.

As we learned earlier, all the toxic foods and drinks we eat and drink and toxins we are exposed to can lead to disharmony of the body and its biochemistry which in turn leads to illnesses, diseases and physical pain. In addition, they often contribute to our mental and emotional suffering as well. The important thing is to stay away from artificial sugars, processed food, food coloring, preservatives, GMO, soy products, dairy products and other harmful chemicals.

Due to the effects that our food and water quality have on our overall health, eating organic fruits and vegetables and drinking healthy water will abate some, if not all, of the emotional suffering. However, some emotional pain is so great that it immobilizes the individual's ability to function in society. In such a case, the individual may need to get medical care to stabilize. The important thing is to seek help at a crisis center or call the suicidal hotline. Talking to a caring person can help de-escalate an emotional meltdown.

Those of you who have exhausted all of your resources on the things that can be done to help with depression may consider one last method - **Ketamine;** it is categorized as a dissociative anesthetic. It has helped some people but does come with some degree of risk due to its possible adverse effects on blood pressure and heart rate. It can be addictive and cause hallucination too. However, if it is used prudently and judiciously with the appropriate client, the benefits can be huge in curtailing an individual's suicidal ideation and the effects can possibly last for a year. This may be just enough time for an individual to get more help and tools to learn how to better cope and deal with depression. Ketamine treatments are administered by a doctor and through a series of IV infusion.

In 2014, researchers found that a ketamine infusion significantly reduced symptoms of post-traumatic stress disorder (PTSD) in 41 patients who had undergone a range of traumas. **(R 179)**

However, it is not FDA approved yet and is still quite controversial and great caution must be exercised before even contemplating this type of approach. I only share this here because a friend of my friend was severely depressed and was quite suicidal and desperate. By utilizing this treatment, he was able to navigate out of his depression and suicidal ideation. He had tried anti-depressants (SSRI- Selective Serotonin Reuptake Inhibitors) as well as Benzodiazepines for depression and anxiety respectively with some success for a few years but after a while, it was losing its effect on him and he suffered adverse withdrawals symptoms from the latter which caused him to go to the hospital. Some of the symptoms included spasms and the body going into shock.

A friend of mine sought ketamine therapy as a last resort after trying medications as well as many holistic supplements but not achieving the emotional results he was looking for. He went through a series of 5 IV infusion sessions of ketamine. He felt immediate relief after the first session. His attitude and outlook had changed and he felt much better despite the many lingering issues in his life including compromised housing, health and financial situations. After he was done with his treatment, he continued to take a ketamine nasal spray three times per day to help him in maintaining the gains he had made. It has truly made a difference in his life and has helped him live in more harmony and seeing himself more empowered and less as a victim.

Note: This may not be for everyone but it has definitely changed the life of my friend and has its place in the treatment of depression and anxiety. Yet, my friend's experience indicates that it may be helpful for some who have moderate to severe depression.

When the individual is stabilized, going to a holistic medical care facility like the ones owned and run by Dr. Daniel Amen can be extremely helpful. They have a very comprehensive program and use a **SPECT Scan** to analyze the brain with regards to any contributing factors to the emotional pain. Such factors may include environment toxin exposure, drugs, and even tumors. They may prescribe medications or herbal supplements to better help the individual to stabilize their emotional disharmony. **(R 180)**

Besides holistic psychiatric care, healthy eating and drinking choices, using supplements as required, and meditating, there are other alternative methods which can be quite effective with helping to restore our emotional harmony. One method is the studying and practicing of Buddhism which when done with sincerity can help to end much of the suffering we create from our minds like depression, anger, anxiety and stress.

Often when we are depressed, angry, anxious or stressed out in other ways, we are either brooding over past issues, worried about what tomorrow or what the future may bring and missing out living in the moment – being in the Now.

Both spiritual and scientific understandings are showing us that it is from the Now that we create our lives.

Living in the past or future often creates stress which shuts down the immune system if it happens over a prolonged period.

Buddhism focuses on mindfulness and being present in all that we do. Being present is the only true reality since the past is indeed the past, and the future does not yet exist. Dwelling on the past or worrying about the future leads us into living in an illusion which is easily influenced by subjective memories and emotions. This keeps us in a state of illusion and suffering. Learning the meditation technique from Buddhism can lead to greater mindfulness and increase ability be present. Once we learn to be present, we can focus our energy in truly living more fully.

Buddhism also teaches about detachment to allow us to be more in touch with our True Divine Nature. When we learn how to be detached from our negative emotions, thoughts and desires, we can begin experiencing more of our true self or true nature, which is Divine Love. When we learn to detach from material things, fame, fortune and the excessive material comforts of life, we will gain more freedom to experience the fullness of life and the Divine nature of thing.

One of the most powerful tools within the Buddhist practice which support health and inner unity and mindfulness is meditation. It utilizes much breath work which is quite helpful for relaxing us and dissociating from stressful thoughts and emotions. It is also known that in the silence of the moment granted to us through meditation is where we truly connect with God. It is also in that space that our multi-body systems are allowed to receive the great prana (Divine Love and Light) of Creation which is the core of all true healing.

In addition, practicing important concepts of Buddhism such as compassion, kindness, mercy, forgiveness and service heals the heart, mind and soul and makes the world a better place. They indeed help to create Heaven within ourselves as well as around us.

The Breath and Emotional Health

Just being mindful of our breath can be so healing. It gives the mind and emotions a break, allowing them to relax, heal and recharge, so to speak. When we learn to still our minds, soon the negative emotions and thoughts no longer hold us hostages but float by like clouds in the sky of our inner Universe. Hence, meditation can be extremely helpful with anger management, depression and anxiety. In the past I suffered all three of these imbalances but found relief from doing daily meditation.

Breathing is essential for our survival and health. Breathing properly can lead to improved meditation which leads to greater health, wellness and harmony. Breathing improperly can lead to stress, illness and even death of the body.

Breath is one of our primary body activities that connects us to our Divine Self. Our core breath is a silent mantra of I AM that I AM. It also helps to activate the parasympathetic nervous system to put us at ease and relax us. The Buddhist Masters from all around the world have all discovered the powers and wonders in controlling our breaths for greater spiritual practices and mastery. However, many Indian Yogis have also found various types of breathing to help the body in different ways to promote wellness, harmony and health.

Yogic breathing exercises like **4-7-8 breathing** can bring great calmness, helps with cravings and with sleeping. **(R 181)** Meanwhile **Alternate Nostril Breathing Technique or Nadi Shodhan Pranayama** can be quite balancing and soothing when one is anxious. It helps to restore the mental and emotional imbalances of the brain. **(R 182)**

The **Wim Hof Method** can be quite helpful with anxiety, stress and depression according to what I learned from the Wim Hof Method workshop in San Francisco in 2018.

Bach Rescue Remedy, FES Five Flower Remedy and **CBD Hemp Oil** can help us feel more relaxed and less anxious.

Rescue Remedy is a homeopathic (flower essence) method of healing. This mix was created by Dr. Bach to deal with emergencies and crises – the moments when there is no time to make a proper individual selection of remedies. It can be used to help us get through any stressful situations, from a last-minute exam or interview nerves, to the aftermath of an accident or bad news. **Rescue Remedy** helps us relax, get focused and get the needed calmness. It is a blend of five different **Bach Flower Remedies**: Impatiens, Star of Bethlehem, Cherry Plum, Rock Rose, and Clematis.

More importantly, Rescue Remedy or FES Five Flower Remedy can reverse shock, both hypovolemic and anaphylactic, by bringing the body systems back into balance. Flower essences act first on the emotional and mental bodies which then assist in balancing the physical body. **(R 183, 184)**

Rescue Remedy and Five Flower Remedy are examples of flower essences or remedies. Kathryn Shanti Ariel explains that "flower remedies are the energy of certain flowers captured in a water base through sunlight infusion, and which is then stabilized with a small amount of alcohol. Flower remedies directly address an animal or human's emotional state in order to help facilitate both psychological and physiological well-being."

By balancing negative feelings and stress, flower remedies can effectively remove the emotional barriers to health and recovery. "Behind all disease lie our fears, our anxieties, our greed, our likes and dislikes," wrote English physician Edward Bach in the early 1930's. Dr. Bach based his revolutionary belief upon his personal observations of patients whose physical illnesses seemed to be predisposed by negative psychological or emotional states such as fear, insecurity, jealousy, shyness, poor self-image, anger, and resentment. Today, numerous studies conducted at major universities and medical centers have verified Dr. Bach's early conviction, revealing a definite connection between negative emotional states and a reduction of the body's natural resistance to disease.

A friend of mine found great benefits with **Highland's Nerve Tonic** and with **Rescue Remedy** for her mother who suffers dementia. She uses it when she gets very anxious and agitated.

Animals also suffer from PTSD. Kathryn Shanti Ariel talks about this in detail in her book *Holistic Emergency Care and Trauma Recovery for Animals,* which also covers extensive information on Flower Essences, Healing Herbs, Homeopathic remedies, and Energy Healing tools. **(R 185)**

I personally have used Rescue Remedy for years as a backup support in some trying situations and have found great relief. I also used 'Return to Joy' - an **Anaflora Flower Remedy** to help heal my dog's PTSD after he was savagely attacked by two large dogs. Although the veterinarian stated that my dog Max would never be the same, eventually he returned to his mental and emotional well-being through the help of flower essence, our love and energetic healing. I ordered the flower essence from Anaflora. **(R 186)**

A more recent healing option, **CBD oil,** has helped many of my friends, some relatives and clients to feel more relaxed and less stressed out. Some have reported that their depression and anxiety seemed to be helped by it. Free of THC, CBD oil contains focused energy that assists the body to release emotional and physical pain and allow healing to occur.

Recently a friend of mine told me more about **Lithium Orotate**. According to **John Gray**, (a relationship counselor, lecturer, and author), lithium is a most important mineral. He stated it is the number one missing mineral in our brain which allows our brain to make an adequate supply of serotonin. It is an over the counter supplement that has a low but therapeutic level of lithium. It may be helpful with depression, stress, and anxiety. **(R 187)**

I have tried it and find it quite helpful for me in coping with stress more gracefully. A friend of mine tried it as well due to extreme stress and found it very helpful. She gave it to her mother who was extremely agitated and confused with dementia and within a few days, her mother became calmer and thought much more clearly. She stated "right now Lithium Orotate is making her happy, conversational and cooperative." Prior to that, she was agitated, combative and hostile.

Some research on lithium orotate suggests that it is one mineral that has shown great promise in the treatment of Alzheimer's disease. The mineral lithium orotate, is a nutrient with established benefits for the treatment of mental health disorders. **(R 188, 189)**

Other supplements that help with depression include St. John's Wort and Sam-e. There is some strong scientific evidence that it is effective for mild to moderate depression. **(R 190)**

However, St. John's Wort has side effects of blood thinning so consult with your physician always before taking anything new. Research has shown an association with increasing the blood thinning effects of some drugs.

With regards to depression and panic attacks, Psych-K, hypnosis and the use of essential oils can be helpful. According to David Pryce, he had suffered insomnia and panic attacks two years ago. Although he tried various methods to get help including seeing a doctor and getting therapies to resolve this crippling problem, he continued to have it. He began searching for alternative solutions and that journey led him to the world of essential oils. He discovered that by using a special blend of essential oils from Young Living Oils, he was able to navigate through his attacks much more gracefully and get the much-needed help and resolution that he desperately needed. Simultaneously, he was able to finally sleep well again. He started with just one essential oil (Lavender) but after a few months of using it, he began blending it with other essential oils. He puts it in a diffuser. He stated that diffusing them improves the air quality he breathes and enhances his environment. He further stated that "essential oils saved me. It heals me in a way I can't explain. It is a perfect way for me to relax and refresh my mind and emotions." He highly recommends Young Living Essential Oils. David was so happy and excited about all the benefits of the oil that he offered so generously to share some of what he has learned from using them. Below are some of the essential oils he has used from Young Living Oils and what benefits he experienced.

Essential oils used by David:
    Lavender- calming and relaxing
    Peppermint- cooling, focusing and stimulating
    Stress Away- peaceful and comforting
    Copaiba- relaxing, grounding and moisturizing
    Frankincense-spiritual and grounding
    Lemon- cleansing uplifting and brightening
    Thieves- cleanses and purify the surrounding

With regards to his own health regime, the following blend is what has worked well for him. (Each person may vary on what works best for them):

Blends
For Sleep
1. Lavender- 3 drops
2. Copaiba-2 drops
3. Stress Away-2 drops

Calm and Relax
1. Lavender- 2 drops
2. Frankincense- 2 drops
3. Stress Away- 3 drops

For Work and Concentration
1. Peppermint-3 drops
2. Lemon- 2 drops
3. Thieves- 2 drops

Immune System
1. Thieves- 3 drops
2. Frankincense- 3 drops
3. Lemon- 1 drop

David cautions that when one is using a diffuser with essential oil, it is important to not exceed 15- 30 minutes. Using it for a prolong period may result in headaches or other undesirable effects on the health.

Post-Traumatic Stress Disorder (PTSD) is an illness that afflicts so many people and animals all around the world and is not just reserved to those in the military but also to those who had severe physical, mental or emotional trauma from other sources. (Animals also suffer from PTSD.)

The glucose in fruits is needed by our bodies for energy and also helps us in coping with life's challenges. In his book, *Medical Medium*, Anthony William has written about the importance of fruits in helping us cope better with severe stress and creates a protective veil for traumatic events. He noted how people respond to severe trauma differently depending on whether one is consuming a healthy amount of fruits that give us the good glucose we need for our body and brain. Those who did not eat fruits, or had low glucose were more likely to develop PTSD. On the other hand, the individual getting enough healthy glucose was able to handle the same situation much better and did not perceive the situation as a threat that would haunt them for life. He does list the specific fruits to eat that would help in his book *Medical Medium*. **(R 191)**

Many health practitioners have written about the importance of super foods, especially those high in vitamin B-complex, for treating PTSD and other forms of high stress. One is Anthony William who has written about many supplements, including Hawaiian Spirulina, GABA (GAMMA-Aminobutyric acid), Ginkgo biloba, (Note: Ginkgo is a blood thinner, so caution should be used) and B-complex. I also find it helpful when I eat enough fruits and raw organic honey.

Other alternative methods that can be quite effective with depression and PTSD include **Rapid Eye Technology/ Tapping**, **EDMR** (eye movement desensitization and reprocessing), **Psych-K**, and **Hypnosis**. They are very powerful methods that can give freedom from emotional issues that are sometimes based in issues that are extremely complex and intertwined with our subconscious mind. This can control our behaviors and how we react to things for decades until they are addressed properly. I have experienced some forms of tapping, Psych-k and Hypnosis and have found it extremely helpful for releasing trapped and repressed emotions. They are powerful tools for healing emotional wounds, traumas and issues. After I was healed by these various methods, I studied them as well and found that they were indeed powerful tools for helping us to integrate and deal with deep seated emotional issues. **(R 192, 193, 194, 195)**

Many of us have experienced great pain or injury at an early age. Unless completely cleared and healed early on, the emotional trauma and pain from such occurrences can linger within us and become a part of our subconscious. When this happens, it often affects our behaviors, how we perceive the world and how we relate to one another.

It can be hard to see all the layers of pain and suffering we have endured throughout the years. And it can be even more difficult to break free from the bondage of our subconscious reactions to situations unless we address and heal the issues within our subconscious mind. In my experience I have found that the best tool for breaking free from the clutches of our subconscious is **hypnosis.** When done well, it can help us to see more clearly those situations that may have contributed to our negative subconscious programming. It can also help us to replace bad programming with more positive suggestions thus resetting the subconscious and allowing us to be our higher, more Divine expression.

Sometimes our emotional and physical sufferings have origins in a previous life, in which case, hypnosis combined with **past life regression therapy** can be of great assistance in understanding the origin and cause of trauma. This conscious awareness can then open the way to deeper more complete healing. Past life regression with a qualified hypnotherapist can result in dramatic and transformational changes within us. I have done past life regression hypnosis on several occasions and the awareness of the various incarnations led to my greater understanding of the various aspects of my personality. That led me to a journey of self-healing and integration.

The Violet Tara and the Violet Consuming Flame or Ray

After reading Peter Mt. Shasta's book, *I AM the Violet Tara*, I began attending his meditation group to learn more about the Violet Tara and Meditation practice. I started to learn how to invoke the assistance of the **Violet Tara** and use the **Violet Flame or Ray** more and more in my life

to clear away physical and emotional pain and suffering. I once had a terrible headache in the middle of the night but immediately invoked the assistance of the Violet Tara to clear my headache with the violet flame. I quickly felt better and fell asleep. At other times, I suddenly felt sad for no reason that I was aware of. (In retrospect, I now realize that various reasons can contribute to how I would feel – such as, planetary energetic shifts, psychic attacks, or negative entity attachments). I didn't like how I felt, so

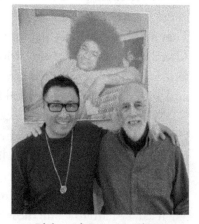

*Blake with Peter Mt. Shasta
beneath a picture of Sai Baba*

I invoked the assistance of the Violet Tara to assist me with clearing the negative energy in my emotions. I often ended up making a decree for the Violet Tara to clear the toxic energy within me. Within a short period, I would feel a complete shift in how I would feel and the positive feeling would stay with me the rest of the day. I now use the Violet Flame, Ray and Energy during U.U.M.M. when working on planetary clearing of negative energies.

Excellent Methods to Promote Emotional and Mental Harmony

Meditation, Tai Chi, Yoga and Qi Gong are techniques that work on our body, mind and spirit. They work in a holistic way to bring integration and balance within us. They also utilize various breathing techniques to improve the Qi, prana or energy flow throughout the body for wellness. I have also experienced great benefits and relaxation from Yin Yoga and Iyengar Yoga and highly recommend them with a qualified Yoga instructor.

Shen drops herbal tonic elixirs are a great support which you can order from www.dragonherbs.com. Shen drops are effective because it supports the Shen energy within us. It is one of the three treasures or energies within us that supports our Divine self and elevates our mood, feelings and psychological well-being.

One revolutionary method of helping with depression is receiving a **Neuro Light healing** session. It is a light therapy co- developed by Guy Harriman, an inventor. It is a systematic use of various patterns of flickering light and the usage of the healing frequencies of various types of music for to create brain fitness and wellness. I have tried it and found it extremely helpful for shifting negative and emotional thought patterns within a short period of time.

During a dark moment in my life I was gifted a complementary session by Marian Brandenburg, a body healer, an intuitive massage therapist, Chi Nei Tsang Practitioner, and Ajna and Neuro Light Practitioner. After the session, I felt extremely upbeat, energetic and blissful. I have recommended the treatment to others who have had similar benefits. It can also help with anxiety, mental focus, memory and other cognitive issues, as well as helping clients to recover from the effects of a stroke. It is awesome for what I call a brain tune up.

Exercise (cardio), Forest Therapy (based on Shinrin Yoku), Biofeedback and dancing can do wonders with depression and stress. You can learn more about how I overcame it from my first book, Dare to Imagine. Finally, have a physician, pharmacist or other qualified healthcare practitioner review all the supplements, herbs and medications you are taking and see if any of them is predisposing you to depression.

The Gifts and Challenges of Being an Empath

Empaths are people with highly attuned and sensitive feeling bodies. For them it is another ball game when it comes to dealing with emotional pain. Unless they have and apply spiritual tools to assist them, they deal with their own inner turmoil plus absorb the inner turmoil of others. A true empath (we are talking about someone who is empathic, not just empathetic) can literally feel what others are feeling.

Most people are empathetic to one degree or another, but a rare few are so sensitive to others' pain and emotions that it can even become debilitating, especially if they do not understand and do not know how to deal with those feelings. **(R 196)**

If untrained in how to keep their energetic fields (especially the feeling body) clear and strong, empaths can become overwhelmed by the energies of others sometimes finding them unbearable. They can also feel so alone because most people find them odd or weird because they do not realize the gift of being empathically connected to the world.

Empaths can learn how to ground themselves to Mother Earth and learn how to protect all the energies they feel from being absorbed into their energetic space. They can learn how to create a shield of white light or bubble around themselves to separate their energetic space from those of others. They can ground by visualizing themselves actually connecting energetically to Mother Earth. They can imagine themselves energetically anchoring to Mother Earth. With regards to creating an energetic field, the empath can visualize a white light surrounding them. They can even make a decree like, "I AM the presence of Jesus surrounding me with God's highest vibrational light of love, protection, purity and perfection."

Wearing a grounding stone can be can helpful as well like tourmaline, obsidian shungite, moldavite, etc.

Here is a quick exercise cheat sheet:

> *Visualize sending an energy column from your body down to Mother Earth then anchor it there.*
> *Visualize your being surrounded by a bubble or shield of white Light; you can even visualize creating three layers*

of white light like I do for protecting me from outside sources of toxic energy.

You can make a decree to activate your I AM Presence to protect you. You can say something like "I AM the Presence of Saint Germain surrounding me with the violet consuming flame that burns away any negative energy that is not for my higher good." When you say, say it with conviction and emotions. Visualize it to manifest that energy channel through you and around you.

Wearing a grounding stone when in public may be quite helpful.

Clearing Emotional Pain with Violet Flame

Dr. Mikaelah Cordeo, Ph.D. reports that in her private spiritual consultation practice, the most common problem her clients exhibit is unconsciously taking on other people's negative emotional energy and often not even being aware that it is a huge source of their problems. She suggests that it can be easily resolved with the following exercise.

"Imagine a small campfire in front of you (but, sometimes you need a bonfire). Ask the Angels to use the Violet Flame in this campfire and know that it will transmute all the negative energies you will release.

"Ask the angels to assist you to release all emotional energy that is not yours. See it moving out of your body from head to toe into the Violet transmuting flame. When all is cleared out, imagine a beautiful golden sun over the top of your head and allow it to descend into your heart. Allow the Golden Sun to gently fill the spaces you have just emptied with Golden Light from head to toe. Then continue to fill the space around you (the layers of your auric field) with more Golden Light. This can be repeated every day if needed.

"After clearing yourself (or another, your home, your land, or even the whole planet), it is helpful to remember this important physical law. **"Nature abhors a vacuum."**

175

*Something will come to fill it up if you don't choose it yourself.
So, call the Angels to refill the space with a positive light. It
can be Golden Sunlight, the Light of Unconditional Love,
Healing Light, the colors of a rainbow – reflecting many
Divine qualities, White Light of the Christ, the Gold Light
of the Buddha, and so forth.*

*"When working to heal the planetary emotional and
mental bodies of a particular issue, also call for your highest
intention for a healthy alternative to what has been cleared. For
example, calling for clearing of issues of abuse, you might ask that
interactions between adults and children be based on Divine
right action, unconditional love and holding an Immaculate
Concept of what is for the highest good for all concerned to
replace former accumulations of error, abuse, distortion,
selfishness or cruelty." (More exercises for spiritual clearing and
transformation and further information on the Angels, the Rays
and the Violet Flame is in Mikaelah's book,* **Live in Love**
– A Life Handbook for the New Golden Age.) **(R 197)**

According to Italia Oliver, RSSP (Reiki, Shamanism, Shekinah
Light, Pranic Therapy) Master Level Practitioner and M.Sc.in Education
has worked in the field for almost twenty years as a teacher, instructional
coach/specialist, and facilitator, the following are grounding stones for
Empaths: black tourmaline, lepidolite, black obsidian, malachite, hematite,
and amethyst. **(R 198)**

Once the Empath is grounded and has learned how to create an
energetic shield or bubble, it behooves them in learning Tai Chi and Yoga
to help them feel more grounded. Meditation will help too with calming
the mind and emotions. Trying some of the former mentioned supplements
will also help a lot.

Other things that lead to our sadness, anxiety and discontentment
include our attachment to material things or people. Once we learn to
release our attachment to things and people, we will begin to feel a great
surge of freedom.

According to Marian Brandenburg, one of the biggest issues that lead
many to addictions of various types including addictions in shopping,

social media, dysfunctional relationships, etc. is our lack of self-love. I concur with Marian and feel that when we love ourselves and become one with God's Love, we can end all our sufferings and addictions. Loving your inner child is an important part of emotional growth and maturity.

When we learn to release our expectations of people and learn to love and give freely without anything in return, it empowers us and elevates our consciousness and reveals more of our Divine nature.

The sooner we realize that everything is so impermanent and so unreal, the sooner we can begin our search for that which is eternal and Divine within us. Once we discover that and our true nature and live in love and compassion, our lives become much more meaningful.

Many of us are so anxious and apprehensive about what tomorrow brings while others are pre-occupied with their past which may be full of sadness and regrets. Both ways of living, keep us away from our true nature and full potential and keep us trapped in the world of duality, illusion and ego. There is no tomorrow and yesterday. It is only this moment's awareness that is real. Our moment with our here and now is the only reality that truly matters. Yes, we can plan for the future and reflect on the past but learn to live in the present with great mindfulness and you will be set free from the illusion of the future and past.

What helps when an individual is so pre-occupied with his or her worries of the past or future is instead to focus on what you are doing at this moment; to become present in the now (*The Power of Now* by Eckhart Tolle). Focusing on your breath for several minutes will begin to severe the ties to your worries. Focusing on your spouse, boyfriend, girlfriend, work completely, etc. will also bring you to living at the here and now. Being Here and Now is so healing, important and powerful. **(R 199)**

Take time every day to be mindful and live here and now. Meditation can help you experience the here and now awareness as can the conscious choice to be in peace and to be aware of your breath.

The Zen of Living can also help one sever ties to all past and possible future emotional turmoil. When we become one with what we are doing be it dancing, singing, writing, walking, meditating, or swimming, our body, mind and our soul become one. This creates harmony and freedom from the limitation of time and illusion and allows us to be in the here and now.

"Sing from the depths of your heart.
Let your heart melt in prayer.
Leave aside all shyness and
Open your heart to God."

~

Amma

CHAPTER 7

PRAYER, INVOCATIONS
AND DECREES

Prayer, Invocations and Decrees

Prayers are a Universal form of communication with the Divine that can be utilized successfully in our daily practice regardless of religion, dogma and beliefs. It is our intention of Love being transmitted through the cosmic web of God's Consciousness or Energy to our point of focus. It transcends the limitations of the time and space continuum. The power of prayer can be extremely uplifting and transformative especially when it is done in a group or said in a decree from a pure and loving heart.

Some people make a distinction between prayer, invocation and decrees and call them the **Three Powerful Tools.** Prayers, invocations and decrees are all powerful in their own way, but all accomplish different things or things differently. All in one way or another are using the power of our voices to call forth assistance from God. This is true whether you are speaking the prayers, invocations or decrees silently or out loud, although the power of the spoken voice can aid deeply especially when giving decrees.

In general, the use of **prayer** is most common for people. Defined as a petition, request or communion with God it is often the initial step in "ask and you shall receive". For example, "I pray (request) that my friend's journey is peaceful and free of challenges", or "I pray for peace on Earth." Even songs can be a form of prayer, such as "Let there be peace on Earth and let it begin with me." The power of prayer has been demonstrated by both small and large groups the world over. Yet some also feel they are much less productive than invocations or decrees.

Invocations on the other hand are calling God or a deity into some type of spiritual or religious ceremony. For instance, "I call upon the Mother, Father and Holy Spirit, to join us this day and assist us in being in peace at all times." Or, "I call upon Goddess Kwan Yin to assist me in my compassion for others." They are a call for assistance from a specific higher power. Another example, "Archangel Michael and Saint Germain, I call upon you and your Legions of Light to remove all discordant energy from my home and return it - cause, core, effect, record and memory - to the Light for transformation."

Spiritual Decrees are energetically official orders that have the power of law. They are used to partner with God/Creator to bring something of the Light that is not currently in place on Earth into form here for the blessings of all affected. Decrees follow specific formulas to obtain their full power of manifestation: **(R 200)**

Spoken intention + focus + visualization + emotional energy or breath energy = Decreed Manifestation

I have done the exact formula above for years receiving great benefits for myself, family and the world at large. Part of the process is also tuning into my heart or I AM Presence as well to allow the Cosmic Energy to flow and manifest my decrees.

To me, I still consider the Three Powerful Tools as forms or expressions of communication with the Divine. Although each of the three tools are different, I feel that they are all still part of the Divine communication continuum and that they are just different ways of activating God's Love and support in our lives and those around us. Hence, I often use the word prayer quite loosely to mean one of the Three Powerful Tools.

Prayer to me is also a Divine tool that brings us closer to our Divine Self and God. I see the powerful tools as stepping stones towards God's Consciousness. We use one method or another depending on our level of spiritual maturity. The prayer or request is the most basic level of prayer. Invocations are an immediate form of prayer where we call upon God and or the Ascended Masters intervention. Decrees are the Master's choice of activation of God or an Ascended Master's Love, Energy and Healing through us in the absence of our ego. These are what I use to manifest healing and miracles.

When we decree it is helpful to be one with our I AM Presence focusing on the attainment of a high level of maturity and spirituality. I use all the three methods of Divine Communication throughout the day but when something is very important and urgent, I assert my Divine Nature by making a decree of merging myself with God's Consciousness or Presence or that of a particular Ascended Master like Saint Germain, Kwan Yin, Jesus, etc. and allow their greatness, love and healing to flow through me to my point of focus to manifest my intentions.

Many studies have been done that prove that prayer really works and that positive changes can happen because of it. The movie, *Inori: Conversation with Something Great,* talks a lot about the various scientific studies of prayer. I highly recommend this movie to any spiritual or religious group. It is in Japanese and has English subtitle but the special American guests are well worth watching including Dr. Deepak Chopra, Bruce Lipton, Lynne McTaggart, etc. The film was directed and produced by my friend, an award-winning Japanese movie director, Tetsu Shiratori.

Prayer is a common tool used in most if not all religions. It is a tool that we use to connect to God and with each other. As I have said, prayer to me is our way with connecting with each other and God through the Divine Cosmic web of God's Love, Energy and Consciousness.

Yet it can also be inept when done without heart or clear intention. I have seen many people praying but only doing it with lip service. Many of these people pray from an intellectual level with no emotional connection whatsoever. It is known that our feelings combined with intentions make them much more powerful and likely to manifest. So, while there is nothing wrong with praying without feeling, I truly believe we can turbo charge and amplify the power and effect of prayer if we just add a few additional steps.

Pray from the Heart

The Bible reports Jesus stating, "for when two or more have gathered together in my name, I am there in their midst". (Matthew 18:20) **(R 201)** Truly these are Divine teachings. However, if people are apathetic when saying a prayer, the effect may be weak. If people are day dreaming and disconnected rather than being present, the prayer becomes increasingly ineffective. Having said that, a small but focused group of a few or more people following some of the tools I will share can be so powerful.

Tools to amp up your prayers

- ♥ There is power in numbers but quality is more important than quantity of participants.
- ♥ Visualize the outcome of your prayers. When you perceive, you can achieve.
- ♥ Be in touch with your heart as you pray. Pray out of love and compassion.
- ♥ Learn how to activate God's Divine Presence in your heart.

You can do this by focusing in your heart or the center of your being. Imagine tuning into the Divine Spark of Light within you. This source of the Light is the Source of all consciousness-Divine Consciousness, God or Source. Focus your attention to this Light and begin to activate God's Divine Presence by making a decree like, I am the presence of God bringing forth Divine Light and Love to heal this person.

Whenever you use God's secret name, I AM, both the Mother and the Father are here with you. We then become the instrument that allows God to work through us to perform amazing miracles. What you are tapping into is the I Am Presence, God Presence, within yourself. When it is done out of love and compassion, the most extraordinary things can happen. Peter Mt. Shasta, spiritual master and iconic spiritual figure, has written extensively about how he activates this Divine Presence in his epic book, ***Adventures of a Western Mystic.*** **(R 202)** I highly recommend it!

- ♥ Pray from your heart and not from your ego. Erase any doubt in your mind about the outcome. God will bring about the necessary changes; so be the instrument and allow God to do what is required for the object of your prayer in accordance to Divine Will and Divine Right Action.

♥ Meditate - the more you do it, the more effective your prayer becomes.

I have had many miraculous things happen over and over again through the above methods, many of which I have written about in my books, **Dare to Imagine: 18 Principles for Peace, Happiness** and **True Success** and **Beyond Imagination: A Path to God and the Divine Realm**. Additional factors that can further assist the positive effects of prayer include your own spiritual evolution and maturity.

I have used spiritual props to further amp the intensity and power of my prayers.

Once I provided healing to an individual in India. She was a victim of black magic and had an energetic blockage created in her head for about a year. She was being psychically attacked by many negative entities. The individual sought help from a Catholic Priest, doctors (including a neurologist and psychiatrist), a reiki healer, and an oracle. She even went to get help from sadhus and other holy men in India but was unable to get any help that would free her from her suffering.

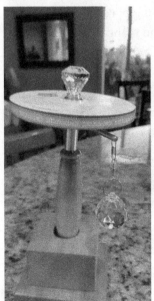

I tried my best to refer her to different experts because I felt this was not my area of expertise but despite her trying the above experts, she was still very distraught and in great turmoil. I felt great compassion towards her and finally decided to step in and help her out.

In this circumstance I decided to do an invocation to call God and the Ascended Masters to come and assist this woman who was tormented by black magic. I later made a decree like "I am the presence of Archangel Michael clearing away all blockages in Miss Jones' head and removing all negative energies and entities attached to this woman." I would

Tibet Tech Prayer Wheel

also say, "I am the Presence of the Violet Consuming flame burning away all blockages to Miss Jones' head and in, around and through her body." I also invoked and decreed the assistance of the Hindu Goddess Durga to clear the entities. She is known as the goddess of war. She has been associated with combating evils and demonic forces.

In addition to prayer, the tools I used included the most powerful prayer wheel in the world, the **Tibet Tech Hand-Held Prayer Wheel.** This prayer wheel contains 84,348,750,000 mantras. His Holiness Jigdal Dagchen Sakya, a High Lama who holds a position in rank third only to His Holiness the Dalai Lama, oversaw the design and construction of the prayer wheels, as well as the selection of the mantras used on each of the 8 DVDs. All the DVDs used in Tibet Tech prayer wheels are blessed and consecrated. H.H. Jigdal Dagchen Sakya has said, "As long as the Universe exists, the consecrated mantras will remain potent."

I also set up a group of healers that included my friend Matt Welke, a Reiki Master, to join me on this collaborative distant healing effort to further help my friend be cleared of the curse of black magic which created an energetic blockage in her head. The Reiki Master had asked some of his friends to help as well. Some of the healers also had Vogel crystal wands, while others used other energy healing methods. I also used my 13-sided Vogel Crystal wand to further amp up my healing prayers.

Using my prayers, visualizations, (decrees and mantras) in conjunction with other tools allowed us (the prayer team and God) to penetrate and break

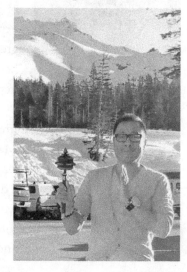

through the strong psychic and energetic blockage my friend had in her head.

Shortly after the prayer, the individual notified me that she felt a big shift and felt better. Her friend later told me she had not seen her so happy in a long time. With God, some tools, a support group, plus a compassionate heart, all things are possible. The last time I checked on my new friend, she is doing well and is living a relatively normal life.

I use the Tibet tech prayer wheel daily before my meditation and after it. I usually chant OM Mani Padme Hum and other mantras while spinning it. I have used it while blessing Mount Shasta as well as the waters that flow down from Mount Shasta at the Headwaters. I find it powerful to have and use.

I also use a traditional prayer wheel used by the Lamas like the one show here. They are about 18 inches long and contain scrolls of a mantra. Spinning the prayer wheels at home creates peaceful and harmonious energies at home.

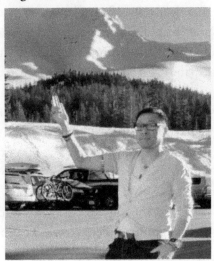

At other times I've used a Vogel crystal wand to amplify and project my prayer to a much higher level of intensity. Here I am shown using my 13-sided Vogel crystal wand to bless Mount Shasta.

The Vogel wand designed by Dr. Marcel Vogel is a powerful energy amplifier. He had helped many people heal with this wand. Many people have tried to copy his design, but an authentic wand sells

Blake shows Vogel Crystal he uses to bless Mount Shasta

for about over one thousand dollars and can go up to over ten thousand dollars depending on the size. I have also used this to clear stubborn energetic blockages.

My friend, a Master Healer and Shaman, uses it to clear entity attachments and practices weather shamanism. He was a part of my spiritual journey and awakening at Mount Shasta. Through his Vogel Crystal wand, decrees and energy, I experienced a higher level of consciousness and experienced a heighten sensory perception.

Additional Prayer Success Stories

Heal, **(R 203),** a 'must watch' documentary film directed by the talented **Kelly Gores.** During one scene in the film, a woman was battling with stage four cancer and her prognosis was poor. Despite doing yoga, juicing and eating well, she still had terminal cancer. One day she became very ill and had to go to the hospital. A friend arranged for a prayer group of 100 people from Facebook. All prayed for her and the next day, she woke up and experienced a miracle - her cancer was suddenly in remission and she has been well for the past two years.

Yes, yoga, eating and drinking well helped this woman but the power of prayer and love can often produce these amazing and incredible miracles that defy scientific explanation. Meditation enhances our ability to heal and create harmony for ourselves and with others. Let us explore further on how we can bring maximum harmony within ourselves and then begin expanding it to our planet, Mother Earth, and to the entire Universe.

An aunt of a colleague of mine had stage four liver cancer. She had a very spiritual Buddhist Monk pray for her on a regular basis. The last time I talked with the colleague of mine she stated, her aunt was suddenly in remission and the doctors could not understand why. My colleague, her aunt and family strongly believe it was the prayers as well as her own prayer and meditation practice that helped.

Once I was quite busy with work, family life, studying, and writing but had minimal sleep. I wasn't eating well, neglected to taking good care of myself and let my spiritual guard down. I began to suddenly feel sad, anxious and negative. I sensed a psychic attack was going on but was too busy to take time to slow down and spiritually protect myself. As I began meditating, I was somewhat distracted due to my fatigue but suddenly began seeing a negative entity in the inner realm. It was quite disturbing to say the least. However, my Divine Mother Amma, the Hugging Saint, suddenly appeared which she has never before. She was aware of the attack and suddenly gestured her arm and illuminated an extraordinary and radiant White Light that repelled the entity and shielded me. I was filled with awe, peace, bliss and gratitude. Unbeknownst to me my dear friend Lori, an Amma devotee, was secretly praying for me. She knew I was in trouble because of her clairvoyant abilities.

I later talked to her on the telephone and she told me that she was quite concerned about me and knew I was in trouble so she began to pray to Amma to help me. I was so flabbergasted that Lori was secretly praying for me during my attacks. Regardless how spiritual one is, if we let our guards down or live not in harmony and balance with God, we can subject ourselves to psychic attacks. Fortunately, such attacks are rare and if they do occur there are many methods we can employ to protect ourselves including praying to God, Archangel Michael, Jesus and Saints like Amma who have an extraordinary ability to help those who call upon them in prayer. Never doubt the power of prayer. Always pray with clear and good intentions and with a pure and compassionate heart. Visualize the prayer being activated and targeted to help manifest your caring intentions.

Learn to pray for yourself, your friends, family members, your community, your country and Mother Earth. Never underestimate the power of prayer! It has the power to change the world especially when we incorporate visualization, clear and good intentions and pray with a compassionate heart. What can turbo charge a prayer into manifestation by including the use of decrees which we will discuss later in this chapter. There are many ways to pray and all are valid. Below is a general prayer that I do in the morning before I meditate. It is my way of showing God my gratitude, love and respect. It is my way of asking for God's assistance and intervention into my life.

Morning Prayer

This is an excerpt of the daily morning prayers that I use:

Dear Heavenly Father, Divine Mother and friend,
To all great saints of all religions including......
Thank you for all your help with elevating the consciousness of the planet.
Thank you for helping more people to live an enlightened life.
Thank you for showing us how it is possible to live a perfect life and transcend death and the laws of karma.
Thank you for your help, support and guidance with my spirituality, meditation and writing.
Thank you, Heavenly Father for the gift of life.
Thank you for keeping my family and I safe.
Thank you for granting my family and I good health.
Thank you for using me as an instrument for serving your people.
May I be a beacon of Light for those who are lost.
May I be a bridge for people from all walks of life, uniting them in your perfect Love, Light and Energy.

May I be a vessel of love, compassion, kindness, patience, mercy, forgiveness, kindness, healing energy and Divine wisdom for all those who need guidance and healing.

Heavenly Father and Divine Mother, I pray that you join me in meditation where I abideth in you and you in me.

In the mighty name of Jesus, the Christ, Amen!

I pray daily for myself, family, friends and pets. I pray and meditate for all sentient beings, Mother Earth, and the Universe. It is important that we pray and decree daily and throughout the day as needed.

I pray (pray, invoke and make powerful decrees) daily and throughout the day when something comes up in my life, city, country or planet. I encourage everyone to pray and allow God's love to be shared and felt with every sentient being, and to do so daily

Thereafter, I expand that peace and bliss to my room and house. Eventually, I align my consciousness with the core of Mother Earth. I then repeat the process. I visualize my consciousness fill up the core of the planet. I then expand the energy from the core throughout Mother Earth and humanity. Next, I envision the entire planet and myself as one consciousness and make a decree of bliss and peace and allow that decree to expand to the Universe, then to God's Consciousness, then, I silently repeat Aum three times. I then hold my breath for a while, then I release it, I visualize the decree to expand from God's Consciousness to the Universe and back to humanity and myself. These are more advanced practices but are all part of U.U.M.M.

Combining Invocations and Decrees

After I meditate, I do what I call my **closing procedure**; during that time, I say another prayer of protection around myself before I go to work. It is important that we protect ourselves from absorbing other's negative energies or illnesses. It is also important we shield ourselves from what they call Energy Vampires. These are people who knowingly or unknowingly drain your energy. They leave you feeling drained while they feel radiant.

I sit in lotus position and visualize a light on my first chakra. I then gesture with my hands and create a circle from the base of my spine and surround myself with God's White Light.

As I am surrounding myself with this Light, I decree aloud, "I surround myself with God's highest vibrational White Light of Love, Protection, Purity and Perfection and repel all negative energies to be directed into the White Light to be transmuted into higher consciousness full of peace, love and harmony. I am protected by God's perfect Love, Light and Energy from all negative energies of body, mind and spirit including infectious illnesses, diseases, autoimmune problems, bacterial and viral infections and allergies.

I am fully protected by God's perfect Love, Light and Energy by his highest Archangels (Archangel Michael, Gabriel, Raphael and Uriel), my Ascended Masters, Angels of Mercy, Unnamed Angels and all my other Guardian Angels. As I finished saying that I will have completely formed a circle from my base to my crown chakra.

I then reach up and pull down an imaginary energetic cord to seal the protection. I then place my hands in prayer position in front of my heart and say, God is in my heart, mind and soul. I then inhale and illuminate my heart and I silently say, I am the presence of God filling me with Love, Compassion, Kindness, Patience, Gratitude, Mercy, Healing Energy and Divine Wisdom to guide those who need guidance and to heal those who need healing. As I exhale, I allow that Cosmic Energy to fill my entire being.

Once completed, I pick up my prayer wheel and chant Om Mani Padme Hum nine times; Loka Sumastah Sukhino Bhavantu nine times and end with Om Shanti, Shanti and Shantihi. Now, I am ready to begin my day full of Love, Compassion, Light and Healing energy.

Although prayer, invocations and decrees are very powerful, they become even more effective when we learn to meditate regularly. When we meditate regularly our consciousness, awareness, psychic abilities and healing abilities are raised to a higher vibration and we become more in harmony with the Universe and God's Consciousness. This is even more so if we visualize the outcome we desire before beginning our meditation and prayers/decrees.

Although we are Divine Beings who have chosen to experience human lives, we can begin having extraordinary experiences or what some call miracles when we begin to tap into our true and infinite nature through proper meditation. Let us begin our journey to discovering the great wonders within ourselves through combining breathing, mindfulness, visualization, affirmations, decrees as we explore meditation further and especially U.U.M.M. in the next few chapters.

189

*"While Meditating, we feel
a deep sense of intimacy with God -
a Love that is inexplicable."*

~

Paramahansa Yogananda

CHAPTER 8

MEDITATION

Deepak Chopra (author, public speaker, alternative medicine advocate, and a prominent figure in the New Age movement) stated that Meditation is the progressive silencing of the thought process until you get to the source of heart. And that is the first sutra actually in the yoga sutras of Patanjali. Meditation is a form of yoga, a mental form of yoga that allows you to get to the source of thought, the self of the individual which is also the self of the Universe because there is only creativity, infinite correlations, synchronicity and power. **(R 204)**

Peter Mt. Shasta stated that the word meditation means going to the middle, to the center of your being. This is a method that will by slowing the mind enable you to find that center that calm, still place, where you really experience the true nature of your being.

There are many health benefits that I have written about it in my two other books, ***Dare to Imagine: 18 Principles for Peace, Happiness and True Success*** and ***Beyond Imagination: A Path to God and the Divine Realm***. However, a few additional benefits of meditation that I will state here include helping with anxiety, stress, depression, high blood pressure, mental sharpness, memory, etc.

Many studies have been done about the medical, emotional, psychological benefits of meditation. In addition, many religions have some form of meditation in them including Catholicism, Buddhism,

Sikhism, Judaism, etc. Even some of the early Catholic Saints were quite adroit at meditation like Saint Teresa of Avila.

While meditation is a powerful tool to assist with the process of enlightenment, transformation and healing, the ultimate goal of meditation is for the individual to establish oneness with God and the Universe. It is also the ultimate foundational tool for bridging our consciousness with that of Mother/Father/God and Creation as a whole.

Most people are happy with using meditation as a tool to release stress and to gain a greater state of inner peace. While this is a great place to begin, meditation can do much more, even changing your perception and open your eyes to a whole new reality.

I have had many Divine experiences throughout the many years of meditation practice including being able to see some of my past lives, to seeing other faraway civilizations and ultimately to being one with the mind and Consciousness of God. It is through meditation that I connect with many of the Ascended Masters.

There are hundreds of meditation techniques out there and it is hard to know which to choose. Some of the more common ones include Zen Meditation, Vipassana Meditation and Transcendental Meditation. Others techniques that work on the Chakras and Kundalini include Kundalini Meditation, Kriya Yoga, and The IAM˙ - Integrated Amrita Meditation.

My Favorite Meditations

Vipassana Meditation was the type Buddha used to reach enlightenment and which Peter Mt. Shasta practices on a regular basis.

Kriya Yoga was brought to the world by the avatar, Babaji. Yogananda brought it to the west as a powerful tool to reach God in the most intimate way.

The IAM Meditation® - Integrated Amrita Meditation Technique is the technique which Amma has taught her swamis and she offers training to anyone at a nominal fee through her many great instructors. It is a powerful way to reconnect with your real center and thereby experience Divine Joy and peace in all aspects of our lives. Born out of Amma's deep resolve for our spiritual enhancement, this technique when practiced with dedication is designed to bring integration into our lives – an integration of body, mind, intellect and heart. Those who are interested in her method may visit her website at **(R 205)**

I like Vipassana Meditation because it is a pure form of meditation originally taught by Buddha and the type he did when he reached enlightenment. Even at its basic level it can be quite profound, therapeutic and healing. It purifies your mind for infinite possibilities.

The basics of Vipassana Meditation include: 1 - Either close your eyes fully or about ¾ closed. 2 - Whether the eyes are open or closed, the emphasis is on the breath. 3 - Though clouds of thoughts will invariably arise, the practitioner will identify them only as a thought and then return his or her awareness back to the breath. Sounds may be heard or perceptions felt, again, it is labeled as a thought and the awareness if brought back to the breath. The practitioner learns to still the mind and begins to perceive the various subtle sensations throughout the body, as well as become more aware of the rise and fall of the natural breath, noting its sound, quality and depth.

This practice leads to insight, awareness and detachment from the senses, thoughts and emotions. Ultimately it can lead one into enlightenment as it did for the Buddha. There are 10-day courses where an individual can learn much more about this beautiful and powerful meditation practice.

This is an excellent and powerful meditation practice that I recommend to everybody to begin with. More information on this approach is available at https://www.dhamma.org. **(R206)**

Peter Mt. Shasta has an excellent video on how to get started with this meditation method. You can view it on YouTube at **(R 207)**.

I like **Kriya Yoga** because it is a sacred method of meditation aimed specially to help the practitioner to achieve communion with God. Those interested in this method can get more information at **(R208)** or see **(R209)** for another group that teaches Kriya Yoga.

I like the **IAM® - Integrated Amrita Meditation** Technique taught by Amma because it is a kundalini type of meditation that raises your consciousness beyond the limitations of the confines of the body and helps the practitioner attain great peace and while integrating our body, mind, and spirit and heart. Like Kriya Yoga and other types of Kundalini Yoga, it focuses on breath work and the movement of energy around the spinal channels. It combines yoga, pranayama and meditation.

In my opinion, no one technique is better than another. They all serve their purpose and it depends on each individual as to where they are in their consciousness and life journey. One system may be good at one point in life and another may be more appropriate at a later point.

I have been meditating for quite some time as part of my relentless pursuit of the spiritual truth of better understanding God and the Cosmos. I have been striving to perfect my ability of connecting to the Universe for many years and have prayed over and over again for help in accomplishing these goals. After many years of search, meditation and prayers, the Universe blessed me with knowledge of a new system I call U.U.M.M. (Universal United Meditation Method). I do this daily in the morning and do either that or Vipassana Meditation in the evening. It has enriched my life in a very deep and profound way.

(Universal United Meditation Method) U.U.M.M. is a type of Chakra meditation method but different than anything out there. The purpose of it is for unity with God, the Cosmos, Mother Earth and all of humanity and creation. I unveiled that technique in my second book, **Beyond Imagination**. The more I do this technique, the more I am connected to that Cosmic and Divine reality. Each year my consciousness and meditation mastery evolve further as my practice deepens.

Beware of Naysayers

Beware of people who say that meditation or yoga are evil or from the devil. Those people usually have no clear idea what meditation and yoga is all about and how empowering it can be. Others do not want people to learn it because of their own ego or need to control others to stay in their group or church. Those people will keep you in your spiritual slumber or coma. Though the path of God realization may differ from one path to another, all paths that lead to the truth, our true nature and God require some form of meditation to attain that.

Meditation is the cosmic key to unlock our chakra gateway allowing us to have the cosmic union with God or the Supreme Consciousness. This union allows us to have harmony of the body, mind and spirit cosmically.

True Yogis have that cosmic connection with God; people like Yogananda, Sri Yukteswar, Babaji and many others including our own beloved Peter Mt. Shasta, Apprentice to Saint Germain, author of many spiritual classics, spiritual master, American Mystic, and student of Lady Master Pearl. I consider him my spiritual father and great guru. He would always respond that the true guru is within.

All great spiritual masters, gurus, spiritual teachers, enlightened beings are meditators including Buddha, Jesus, Krishna, Yogananda, the Dalai Lama, Sathya Sai Baba, Amma, Deepak Chopra, Oprah, Dr. Wayne Dyer, Teresa of Avila and many other great Catholic saints.'

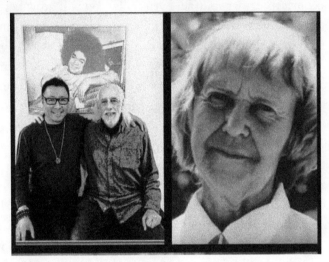

Blake with Peter Mt. Shasta   *Lady Master Pearl*
Sai Baba in photo behind

Discovering Divinity Within

Many people I have talked with have such a hard time stilling their mind and focusing within. They feel that their mind is like a monkey that cannot be tamed while others find it hard to visualize during meditation and end up giving up altogether. It is important to be compassionate towards yourself - doing your best at your meditation level.

Those of you who have such a hard time focusing, relaxing or visualizing might enjoy starting out with Dr. Wayne Dyer's **I AM Wishes Fulfilled Meditation** CD. James F. Twyman has put together enchanting music along with the sounds or tones that expresses the sacred and Divine sound of the name of God which is I AM that I AM. Listening to it can relax your mind and put you into a meditative state. You will be guided on how to create your own I AM mantra to manifest what you desire. This is the meditation method that Dr. Wayne Dyer and his family practiced. You can listen to it on YouTube at (**R 210**)

I used these tools when I first started to meditate and found them very helpful. The meditation is only 20 minutes. Using some type of guided meditation is a good way to begin building your practice, especially for those who have a hard time meditating. It is important to meditate daily until it becomes a regular routine. Eventually, you will grow beyond this to experience the Universe and God in a more divine and intimate way through more traditional meditation practices that focuses on your breath and kundalini energy instead of being guided through music or sound. The primary focus is being in stillness and quiet with your focus on the breath to allow the mind to quiet and your connection with your True Divine Self to be established.

Vipassana Meditation is the type of meditation that the Masters would like me to encourage most of you to study.

However, those of you who are ready for something new, different and quite powerful may find it very beneficial to *practice U.U.M.M. (Universal United Meditation Method).* After the Universe blessed me with the advanced system, I have worked towards breaking it down to a beginner's level as well as intermediate levels that are also quite powerful and transformative.

Through U.U.M.M., I have experience deep and Divine Cosmic bliss. It has opened the gateways to the Ascended Masters and God in the most intimate ways. I have come to discover the great guru within, the guru who is my all knowing I AM Presence.

It is through this meditation that I have come to experience what it feels like to be one with the Universe and one with God's Consciousness. By assisting me to continuously embody more of my mastery, it has allowed me to facilitate healing for my pets, family members, and me.

In addition, U.U.M.M. has contributed to the healing of our planet and beyond. It has helped me to manifest many great miracles in my life as well as in the lives of others that I meditate about. Regardless how much I write about it, it is more important that you experience it yourself.

It is my hope and wish that you experience the Universe, God and Divine Realms in your own special and intimate way after practicing U.U.M.M. for some duration.

In my previous book, ***Beyond Imagination***, I wrote about 27 principles for helping you reach God in the most intimate and sacred way. Practicing those principles and meditating with U.U.M.M. will lead you to your Divine journey within.

In Chapter 9 in this book, I expand these techniques even further allowing you to experience the Divine Realms with even greater benefits.

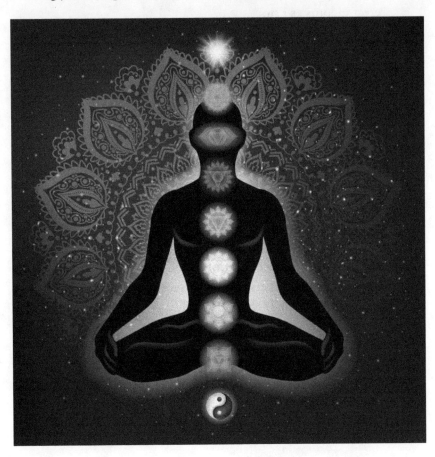

No Place Like OM*

There is a pandemic of red dust that fills the air and all around.

No one can seem to hide and run away from it.

Millions are stricken with panic, fear, and chaos as the dust abounds.

In the midst of all this, I focus only on my breath... breathing in ...breathing out slowly...OM, OM, OM... erect in lotus as I sit.

I begin to go within and travel through the sacred temples, portals and gateways that lead to the Divine Light, Love and Consciousness that dissolves and transcends all this dust, illusion and maya in this inner world of Divine Light and Sound.

I am no longer me, myself and my limitations but pure Light, Love, Supreme Consciousness
and its infinite possibilities.
It is truly a Divine Fit.

I am now a beacon of Divine Light that illuminates so brightly to help others also find their way back to OM where that Divine Light is always Lit.

Blake Sinclair

Poem inspired by Master Romio Shrestha, renowned modern master of Indo-Nepali-Tibetan Buddhist traditions of enlightenment art.

CHAPTER 9

U.U.M.M.— A METHOD TO CONNECT WITH GOD AND THE DIVINE REALMS

U.U.M.M. (Universal United Meditation Method)

This is a meditation practice that the Universe guided me in establishing with the blessings of the Masters. It is a system that utilizes affirmations, toning, mudras, visualizations, breathing in cosmic energy, and the energetic presence of the Masters at all the chakra centers. The pranic energy is guided to circulate around the body, going up and down the spinal channels and clearing blockages at each chakra and unleashing the cosmic energy in each gateway or temple. It is an energetic and kundalini meditation method.

The ultimate goal of this meditation practice is to attain God Consciousness and God Realization where the ego dissolves and gives way to the full expression of God's Love and Consciousness where the veil that separates God and I are gone. At the pinnacle of the meditation practice, the full expression of I AM that I AM is attained and realized. The meditation practice evolves as the practitioner's consciousness and mastery evolves. Before I get deep into the various levels of U.U.M.M., I like to share the other parts of the system that I feel are also important aspect of the meditation and devotional practice.

Below are steps I do prior the actual meditation part of U.U.M.M.:

1. I start by **drinking pure water** to clear my system. Sometimes I have it soaking in my Labradorite Elixir Dish prior to drinking it.
2. I light incense at my shrine and sage my meditation room to purify the area around the room of my sacred shrine.
3. I light a candle.
4. **Yogic Breathing Exercises** – I begin to still my mind and integrate my brain with alternating nasal breathing exercises. I alternate it with other Yogic Breathing Exercises.
5. **Chanting** - I usually chant a sacred mantra that was given to me by Amma. Those that do not have one can chant I am Holy, Pure and Perfect. I chant twice to the count of 108 mala beads to purify my mental, emotional and spiritual body.
6. I begin spinning my Tibetan Prayer Wheel and chant Om Mani Padme Hum for some duration.
7. **Prayer-** I pray for myself, family, canine babies, friends and our planet.
8. After ringing a pair of Nepalese Cymbals to clear the energetic field, I begin my U.U.M.M. practice. I sometimes use a singing bowl as well.

After I am done with the meditation practice, I begin spinning my Tibetan Prayer Wheel and chant the following mantras 9 times each:

1. Om Mani Padme Hum
2. Om Muni Muni Maha Muniye Soha
3. Om Ah Hum, Vajra Guru Padma Siddhi Hum.
4. Om Tare, Tuttare, Ture Soha* (*t pronounced d*)
5. Loka Samastha Sukhino Bhavanthu
6. I then say:
   May Peace Prevail within my inner Universe;
   May Peace Prevail in my household;
   May Peace Prevail in my city, state, country, planet, Universe, intergalactic Universe and beyond.
   Thereafter, say Om... Om... Om..
   Finally, say I AM PEACE that I AM.

7. I then chant Om Shanti, Shanti, Shantihi!

---

* Recommended by the Dalai Lama to chant for healing and protection from the virus.

There are many different forms of U.U.M.M., beginning with a beginner's level which I was guided to develop recently to various more intermediate steps that I will share here. The most advanced practice is reserved for private training since it is much more comprehensive and intensive but it is also very powerful, rewarding and transformative. I generally tell people to study some form of meditation for one year prior to studying U.U.M.M. The longer you have been meditating, the more effective and powerful your meditation becomes with U.U.M.M. Having said that, I have taught one individual the Temple of Divine Love method. This individual had little to no training in meditation previously. She had taken a one-day Vipassana Meditation intro course five years before but rarely practiced it.

I taught her the basic method and guided her a few times then made a recording of that meditation method. She listened to my voice guiding her through the meditation. Initially, she was only able to meditate 5-10 minutes using what she had learned in the past from different sources. However, after studying with me she was able to follow my method and meditate for 30 minutes within a short time. She excelled rapidly and made great progress. She began seeing lights (green, blue and white) while she meditated and began having greater focus and peace. After two months of practice of the Basic Level of U.U.M.M., she reached a state where she was detached from the confines of her body and was just consciousness in the state of meditation. Through this practice she feels more relaxed, happy and peaceful. Sometimes she cries during meditation because she feels overwhelmed by God's Love.

Beginner's Level Meditation Practice

Below is the **Beginner's Level Meditation Practice** which I have been asked to share with you to assist in creating peace within you in response to all the turmoil that so many of you are enduring.

Due to the complexity of my system, I will make an audio that can be downloaded or listened to on YouTube for the meditator to follow until he or she can do it without the guidance. An active participation with this system is important. I have written out the steps of the meditation practice so that you can read it and meditate or reflect on the message of each method. Try to visualize and incorporate what you learn from each method and that will make it easier for you to remember and integrate into your meditation practice.

Below is a very simple practice that anyone can do. I call it the A.O.L. (Activation of Light) meditation. It is best done outdoors during a sunny day and ideally done at the beach to incorporate the elements of Earth, Wind, Water and Fire. This is done to help the practitioner to imagine feeling and seeing the Light of God fill his or her entire being for cleansing and purification. It can be done for 5-15 minutes. It can be done indoors as well in a well-lit room or where there is a source of Light. The benefit of being outdoors is being able to feel the sun's rays and light as it radiates through your eyelids and skin to activate all of your cells. (Avoid doing it on hot days.)

Activation of Light Meditation

The following instructions will guide you on how to do this practice:

- Begin by assuming the sitting position of your liking. Make sure your back is straight and you are comfortable.
- Place your hands in a mudra position that is comfortable to you. (Ground yourself by imagining yourself connected with Mother Earth; imagine sending your energetic presence into the core of Mother Earth.)
- Start off with some deep cleansing breaths; as you breathe in, inhale all the positive energy from the Universe. As you exhale, let all negative thoughts, emotions or energy be released from your body.
- Begin your meditation by imagining the Light and Love of God flowing from the Universe down through your head and going to your heart or center of your being.

- Imagine the heart filling up with this Light and Love from God.
- Imagine it expanding and filling the rest of your being as it dissolves away any negative thoughts and emotions.
- Focus your thoughts on your breath and the Light that you are becoming until you are completely filled with God's Love and Light.
- Once your entire being is full of God's Love and Light, continue to be one with this Cosmic Light as you continue to slowly breathe in and out.
- Once you are done, slowly wiggle your toes and move your hands.
- Next, bring your hands in prayer position at the level of your heart and give thanks to God for bringing Love and Light into your being.

Once you have been practicing the above method or other forms of meditations for some time and gain more proficiency and comfort with meditation, you may consider venturing into the following methods the Masters have shared with me.

The above was just an entry level meditation practice but the next method is the beginner's level meditation practice which I have been asked to share with you to assist in creating peace within you due to all the turmoil that so many of you are enduring. Thereafter, I will share the other intermediate practices which have evolved since my last book to have more depth and impact on the practitioner.

Temple of Empowerment, Harmony and Energy

This practice is designed to help the practitioner attain peace within and to amplify feelings of wellness, joy and confidence in oneself and to share it with others. It supports one in stepping into the sovereignty of one's true and Divine Nature. It is also done to activate and support the energy of the Dantian. It takes about 15 to 20 minutes to do and can be quite calming. Breathing exercises before meditation is important but especially with this practice. I think it is very helpful to do the alternating nasal breathing for nine reps before starting this meditation to bring balance and integration to your brain. You can do it longer if you need it.

The following instructions will guide one on how to do this practice:

- Begin by assuming the sitting position of your liking. Make sure your back is straight and you are comfortable.
- Place your hands in a mudra position that is comfortable to you. (ground yourself by imagining yourself connected with Mother Earth; imagine sending your energetic presence into the core of Mother Earth).
- Slowly breathe in and out through your nose at a rate of five seconds in and ten seconds out. (As you breathe in, allow your abdomen to rise. As you exhale, allow it to go down.) If that pattern doesn't feel comfortable, you can change it to fit your respiratory needs. Once you find that comfortable rhythm, breathe in and out slowly for three to nine cycles of inhalation and exhalation
- Visualize the Light of God at a distance in front of you or above you whichever feels more comfortable to you.
- As you breathe in, imagine breathing in God's Love, Light and Source Energy flowing into the center of your solar plexus or third chakra (at the diaphragm, below the rib cage.
- As you exhale, silently say to yourself, Thank you for the gift of life; I process life well; each moment is an opportunity to learn, live confidently, give unconditionally, serve joyously and to live an empowered life full of love, compassion, mercy, forgiveness, and kindness to all that I meet.
- Visualize the Light of God at a distance in front or above you again.
- As you breathe in, imagine breathing in God's Love, Light and Source Energy flowing into the center of your third chakra.
- As you exhale, silently say to yourself, "Thank you for the gift of life; each moment, may I illuminate God's Love and Light to its full glory in all I do." Then imagine it illuminating from your chakra.
- As you breathe in, imagine breathing in God's Love, Light and Source Energy flowing into the center of your third chakra.
- As you exhale, silently say to yourself, "Thank you for the gift of life; may I be an ambassador of God's Love and Light leading others to find the Love and Light of God within themselves.
- Now take a moment to focus on your third chakra; imagine seeing and feeling the radiating Light and Love of God illuminating so brightly.

- Now direct that energy up the spiritual channels going through each chakra. As you go through each chakra, imagine seeing the colors of each chakra.
- Continue to direct the energy with your vision and breathe all the way up to the crown chakra which is at the top of your head, but do not stop there. Continue to go up into the Source of the White Light above you.
- As you descend back to your body through your crown chakra, visualize God's Love, Light and Energy flowing down through your crown chakra and continue down through the spiritual channels until it reaches the area behind your navel and below the rib cage.

(As you do this it should be done during the exhale and the energy being directed down the spiritual channel should go down the anterior part of the spinal cord).

- Once your energy and that of God's Love, Grace, Peace and Light arrives at the third chakra, visualize that energy illuminates and expands at that chakra.
- Thereafter, inhale and direct the energy back up towards the crown chakra and into the Source Light; going up the dorsal (back) part of the spinal cord and down the anterior part of it; repeat the cycle nine times or cycles.
- After you have completed the cycle nine times, focus on your third chakra and begin to slowly inhale and exhale. Next work on illuminating the Light and Love of God from the chakra and expand it to the Dantian (the area from your Solar Plexus going towards the navel, anteriorly) and the corresponding lumbar spine directly behind your navel. You may even allow it to warm up to activate that chakra and energy there. Slowly begin to increase the temperature and radiance of the Light within the chakra and Dantian area as you imagine your passion, joy, confidence, and love illuminating in service to others grows
- Slowly inhale and exhale and visualize yourself having peace and oneness with this Light and Energy. (Imagine that Light

illuminating so bright the love, passion, joy, confidence and positive energy to serve others).

- Next slowly inhale and exhale; as you do this silently say, "I am at peace with myself, my family, my friends and those who love me and those who do not."
- Slowly inhale and exhale again and say, "I have peace and oneness with Mother Earth, all of humanity and all creatures, great and small."
- Slowly inhale and exhale again and say, "I have peace and oneness with the Universe, all the planets, God, and my I AM Presence."
- Slowly inhale and exhale again and say, "thank you I am Divine Peace that I am. As you say it, visualize God's Love, Grace, Peace and Light illuminate and expand from your third chakra.
- Continue to slowly breathe in and out as you visualize the Peace and Light of God expanding to fill your entire being, your room, and your house.
- Once everything is filled with God's Love, Grace, Peace and Light begin to inhale for about 4 seconds then hold your breath for as long as you can in this peaceful state of being. Then slowly exhale and breathe again while enjoying this great peace, bliss and serenity. Finish by breathing in and out slowly and calmly. Continue this state as long as you need it.

The next method is more of an **intermediate step** for healing you, others and Mother Earth by opening and activating the gates of Divine Love.

Temple of Divine Love Meditation

The Temple of Divine Love is a type of heart chakra meditation; it is like the previous one I shared in my second book (Beyond Imagination) but this one is more advanced. This is one of four meditation methods I practice within U.U.M.M. This is what I consider the intermediate form in my meditation system; however, it is quite comprehensive and powerful just the same.

The intention of this meditation is to open the heart chakra, allow you to integrate the ego and allow you to be one with you I AM Presence. This meditation practice will heighten your ability to manifest and to help heal yourself, others and the planet.

The outcome of this practice is feelings of peace, serenity, love and compassion. The practitioner's vibrational energy will be shifted to a much higher frequency. Done regularly along with devotion, Seva or service and prayers, it will increase your ability to connect with the Ascended Masters and God. Miracles may begin to happen more regularly as well moments of synchronicities. The Divine Light within you will begin illuminating much brighter and those who are clairvoyant will see it and enlightened animals and creatures will be drawn to it.

Physiologically, your blood pressure will decrease as well as your heart rate. Your immune system will be strengthened; you may experience more energy and have a feeling of wellness as more endorphins are produced in your body.

The following instructions will guide one in how to do this practice:

- Begin by assuming the sitting position of your liking. Make sure your back is straight and you are comfortable.
- Place your hands in a mudra position that is comfortable to you. Ground yourself by imagining yourself connected with Mother Earth; imagine sending your energetic presence into the core of Mother Earth.
- Slowly breathe in and out through your nose at a rate of five seconds in and ten seconds out. (As you breathe in, allow your abdomen to rise. As you exhale, allow it to go down.) If that pattern doesn't feel comfortable, you can change it to fit your respiratory needs. Once you find that comfortable rhythm, breathe in and out slowly for three to six cycles of inhalation and exhale.
- Visualize the Light of God at a distance in front or above you.
- As you breathe in, imagine breathing in God's Love, Light and Source Energy into the center of your being.
- As you exhale, silently say to yourself, "Thank you for your Divine Love. May your Love fill the reservoir of my heart, mind and Soul. Imagine the Light of God filling your heart to become a Sun of God.

- Again, inhale the Love, Light and Energy of God to your heart or center of your being,
- As you exhale, say, "Thank you for your love. May your love bring love, compassion, kindness, forgiveness and mercy into all that I say and do."
- As you breathe in, imagine breathing in God's Love, Light and Energy into the center of your being.
- As you exhale, say, "thank you I am Divine Love that I AM". While you are saying that imagine God's Love filling your heart and slowly expanding and radiating from your heart like the Sun of God and then filling the rest of your body. As it radiates, it purifies every part of you.
- Breathe in God's Love, Grace and Complete Acceptance into the center of your being.
- As your exhale, allow that Divine Presence to fill and surround your entire being. Experience the peace that comes with knowing that you are loved just the way you are despite any wrongs you have done in the past or present. As you exhale, silently say to yourself, thank you for loving me and accepting me the way I am despite all my flaws, sins and imperfections. Thank you for seeing through the veil that obscures my soul and true self for within the depth of my soul, you see the true beauty that is holy, pure *and perfect*.

Forgiveness

- Inhale God's Love, Grace and Forgiveness into the center of your being.
- As you exhale, forgive yourself of all the actions you have done that may have caused you or others to go further away from God. You could say, "I forgive myself for all the things I have said and done to hurt others intentionally or unintentionally in this lifetime or previous lifetimes back to the beginning of time and any and all future lifetimes." You may even say silently, "I apologize for the wrongs I have done to others in this lifetime, previous lifetimes all the way to the beginning of time and any and all future lifetimes." Continue this for as long as you like to forgive

yourself and apologize in preparation for our holy communion. If you are having trouble forgiving yourself, you can practice what I call **Celestial Waterfall of Forgiveness.** Otherwise, you can proceed to the next step of the meditation.

• Inhale God's Love, Grace and Forgiveness to the center of your being.

• As you exhale, forgive all those who have done wrong to you. You may say in your mind, "I forgive all those who have done wrong to me in this or previous lifetimes and any and all future lifetimes." - or give specific names of individuals who have done wrong to you

Note: *If you have trouble with forgiving someone due to some traumatic experience and it affects your meditation change your inhalation and exhalation to a slower rate. and slowly exit out of meditation. Continue this until you are calm and relaxed before you end your session.* You may say, "*I forgive you for ...." then say, "I thank all" You may need to work with a counselor, Life Coach or Marriage Family Therapist on doing deeper healing before doing this part or you can skip the part about forgiving that particular person until you are ready.*

• Inhale and exhale while you visualize yourself forgiving all those who have done wrong in your life. You may say, "I forgive you for ...." then say, "I thank you for being a part of my life. Thank you for helping me to be who I am today. Thank you for helping me to see the things that are required for me to change in order to reach higher mastery. Also say, I love you and then visualize and send them a blessing of infinite love and blessings to them and their ancestors. Also, pray that they experience the Living Light of God. Or you can make a decree like "I am the Presence of God sending you and your ancestors infinite love and blessings and allow you to experience God's Love, Light and Consciousness.

• The next step opens you to receive **God's Love and Blessings** and is a continuation of the above steps.

• Inhale God's Love, Grace and Blessings into the center of your being.

- As you exhale, imagine God's blessings pouring forth from your heart and say, "thank you I am abundance that I am. I receive abundantly and give abundantly." Allow the abundant energy of God to fill your entire being. (If you are comfortable and ready, allow that energy to fill your room, house, neighborhood, planet, universe and into the Light of God's Consciousness).

Note: Advanced Step: *Those of you who are able and willing to expand that energy to Mother Earth and the Universe may do the following step:*

- Inhale God's Love, Grace and Blessings into the center of your being.
- As you exhale, imagine God's blessings pouring forth from your heart and say, thank you I am abundance that I am. I receive abundantly and give abundantly. Allow the abundant energy of God to fill your entire being.
- Next inhale and exhale. While you are exhaling allow your consciousness to go to the center of Mother Earth.
- Inhale God's Love, Grace and Blessings into the center of Mother Earth.
- As you exhale, imagine God's blessings pouring forth from the heart of Mother Earth and say, thank you I am abundance that I am. You can also add there is enough food, water, and shelter for everyone. Add whatever you like. If you want to go further, repeat the same steps and imagine the Earth as a Sun of God and repeat the previous steps to illuminate abundance from Earth throughout the Universe. You may want to also merge with the Source Light. If you do that, breathe in for a count of four breath when you are in the Source Light then hold the breath for 7 breaths then exhale with mouth open saying silently, I AM Abundance that I AM. Visualize the energy blessing the Universe and everything within it including you.

- *(I have also made decrees and enlisted the help of Ganesh, Lakshmi, Saint Germain and Kwan Yin to help manifest that abundant energy throughout my inner Universe and outer Universe. These are more difficult to do and private sessions may be needed to learn how to do this.)*

- Inhale God's Love, Grace and Blessings into the center of your being.
- As you exhale, imagine God's blessings pouring forth from your heart and say, "thank you I am bliss, peace, happiness and joy that I am." Allow that energy to fill your entire being. Then if you are comfortable and feel ready, allow that energy to fill your room, house, neighborhood, planet, universe and into the Light of God's Consciousness.

Note: Advanced Step: *After the above inhalation and exhalation, I make a silent decree of Hotei by saying I am the presence of Hotei manifesting bliss, peace, happiness and joy. While I am doing that, I raise my arms up and have my shoulders moderately externally rotated and holding the Gyan mudra above my head with hands on either side of the head. I make sure to put a smile on my face then go within and turn all my organs (heart, liver, spleen, kidney, colon, and lung) into happy Hoteis manifesting bliss, peace, happiness and joy. With my colon, I imagine millions of Hoteis all smiling and creating bliss, peace, happiness and joy. I expand that to my household, Mother Earth, Universe and into Supreme Consciousness.*

- Inhale God's Love, Grace and Blessings into the center of your being.
- As you exhale, imagine God's blessings pouring forth from your heart and say, "thank you I am Divine health and harmony that I am. I am one with God's perfect love and light."
- As you slowly breath in and out allow God's perfect Love and Light to fill your entire being starting with your body and working your way into your organs, tissues, cells, atoms and all the way to the electron, proton and neutron level. While you are breathing in and out, say, "I release all that is less than perfect back to the Universe formless and harmless. Visualize the toxic part of you

lift away from your body and going to the Universe and dissolved by the Violet Consuming Flame (or you can imagine it releasing down to Mother Earth and dissolved by the Violet Consuming Flame).

- Continue to slowly breathe in and out as you visualize the perfect Love of God filling your entire being including the spaces between the electrons, protons and neutrons. You can complete this segment by repeating, "thank you I am Divine health and harmony that I am" and imagine yourself as a perfect Light of God.

- The next steps facilitate the expanding your Consciousness and I AM Presence with that of the Universe and God.

- Direct your focus at three points - your I AM Presence anchored with you at the level of your chest or sternum (the heart chakra), the Sun of God above you and Mother Earth below you.

- Inhale the I AM Presence of all three to the center of your being or heart. As it meets at your heart, you may notice the Light in the center of your being is much brighter and more intense than earlier.

- As you exhale, allow that Divine Cosmic Light and Love of the I AM Presence to expand and fill your entire being.

- Next, as you inhale and exhale, allow that Light of Consciousness to expand beyond your physical body to fill the entire room, house, neighborhood, planet, space and ultimately to the Light, Mind and Consciousness of God.

As your Consciousness merges with the Source of God's Light, silently say AUM, AUM, AUM, and then surrender all thoughts, emotions, allowing yourself to experience deep cosmic peace and bliss while focusing on your third eye point. If you can hold your breath, hold it for as long as you can. If not, just breathe with slower respiration allowing your mind to empty more fully until you reach a state of blissful surrender with the Universe where you are one with the Universe. Stay with the stillness for as long as you can. Sometimes you may see colors but just remain calm and still. Do not analyze or react emotionally but just observe. Initially, you may see lights and colors. Eventually, you may begin to be visited by Angelic beings or Ascended Masters but continue to just focus on your breathing and remain an observer. Mystical experiences become more frequent experiences if you live in the fullness of love.

Note: *If you wish to meet with a particular angelic being or God, you must make your intentions known in prayer prior to meditation and do it on a regular basis. They will only come to you if you seek them and invite them.*

- When you are done, slowly become aware of the pressure on your legs and feet.
- Slowly move your feet and wiggle your toes, bringing your focus back into your body.
- When I am done, I proceed with my **closing procedure** as described in Chapter 7 on prayer.

This takes about 45-60 minutes to complete.

Those who have trouble with mental or emotional blockages interfering with forgiveness may integrate what I call the **Celestial Waterfall of forgiveness.** This is when you visualize the Love, Grace and Forgiveness of God flowing from his or her Consciousness down your crown chakra then down through your body to flush out and loosen up stubborn energetic barnacles or blockages. Visualize them slowly breaking down and being dissolved and flushed out of the root chakra and released down to Mother Earth; imagine purifying that energy with a lake of Violet Consuming Flames so that the energy is formless and harmless. I have also started to get more direct help from Kwan Yin. I visualize and pray that Kwan Yin pours healing energy from her sacred vase through me starting from my crown chakra, to my root chakra and down to Mother Earth. I usually do three rounds of healing cleansing energy with her. **The first** round I visualize Kwan Yin pouring a large body of healing water that flows through me to wash away all impurities of body, mind and spirit. **The second** round I see an energetic Light that pours forth from her vase to purge out all impurities. **The third** round I see a much denser and heavier energetic Light pouring forth from her sacred vase that slowly pushes out any remainder impurities in my body and auric field that were not cleared out previously.

You can do this a few cycles as needed to cleanse yourself. As you do this imagine those stubborn traits begin to dissolve, collapse, or fall off with the strong healing currents of the Celestial Waterfall, allow it to drain down to Mother Earth and dissolved by the Violet Consuming Flame.

Cosmic Kundalini

This is a system modified to allow you to experience cosmic oneness in a celestial way. It begins at the root chakra and connects you with Mother/Father/God, the Sun and Mother Earth in an intimate way. It is an intermediate level of meditation. Only do this if you are grounded, do not have any psychiatric disorders and have a good foundation with meditation (having practiced meditation for at least one to two years; preferably either Kundalini Yoga, Chakra Meditation or Kriya Yoga).

Grounding: Things you can do to get grounded include the following:
- Earthing
- Gardening
- Visualizing your being connected to Mother Earth
- Spend time with nature
- Walk in the park
- Walk on the beach especially without your shoes
- Practice Tai Chi
- Practice Yoga
- Go biking
- Dance
- Clean up the house
- Hold a grounding stone like tourmaline, hematite, shungite, moldavite, petrified wood, tiger's eye, black obsidian, etc.
- Practice the **5-4-3-2-1 Grounding** Technique. According to Dr. Sarah Allen, this is how you can do it: Open your eyes and look around you. Name out loud:
    1. Things you can see (you can look within the room and out of the window)
    2. Things you can feel (the silkiness of your skin, the texture of the material on your chair, what does your hair feel

like? What is in front of you that you can touch? A table, perhaps?)

3. Things you can hear (traffic noise or birds outside, when you are quiet and actually listening things in your room constantly make a noise but typically, we do not hear them).

4. Things you can smell (hopefully nothing awful!)

5. Thing you can taste (it might be a good idea to keep a piece of chocolate handy in case you are doing this grounding exercise! You can always leave your chair for this one and when you taste whatever it is that you have chosen, take a small bite and let it swill around your mouth for a couple of seconds, really savoring the flavor).

6. Take a deep breath to end.

Dr. Allen gives six other great grounding methods at her website that you can check out. **(R 211)**

Cosmic Kundalini Meditation

- Begin by assuming the sitting position of your liking. Make sure your back is straight and you are comfortable.

- Place your hands in a mudra position that is comfortable to you. Ground yourself by imagining yourself connected with Mother Earth; imagine sending your energetic presence into the core of Mother Earth. Slowly breathe in and out through your nose at a rate of five seconds in and ten seconds out. (As you breathe in, allow your abdomen to rise. As you exhale, allow it to go down.) If that pattern doesn't feel comfortable, you can change it to fit your respiratory needs. Once you find that comfortable rhythm, breathe in and out slowly for three to nine cycles (optimally nine) of inhalation and exhalation.

- Slowly breathe in and out through your nose at a rate of five seconds in and ten seconds out. (As you breathe in, allow your abdomen to rise. As you exhale, allow it to go down.) If that pattern doesn't feel comfortable, you can change it to fit your respiratory needs. Once you find that comfortable rhythm, breathe in and out slowly for three to nine cycles (optimally nine) of inhalation and exhalation.

- You will begin by surrounding yourself with three layers of white light to protect you as you begin to activate your kundalini energy. The following steps will guide you.

- Visualize the perfect Light of God at a distance in front of you or above you.

- Inhale God's highest vibrational white light of Love, Protection, Purity and Perfection or aka Cosmic Christ White Light into your root chakra.

- As you exhale, visualize God's perfect Light creating a powerful energetic bubble around your entire being. As you do say silently, "I surround myself with God's highest vibrational white light of Love, Protection, Purity and Perfection repelling away any negative energy directed towards me towards God's highest level of White Light and transmuted to a higher level of consciousness filled with love, peace and harmony." Imagine that light surrounding you in a protective shield that is 10 feet above, below, front, behind, right and left of you and all around you.

- Inhale God's highest vibrational White Light of Love, Protection, Purity and Perfection into your root chakra.

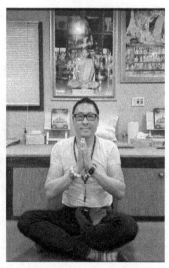

- As you exhale, visualize God's perfect Light surrounding you. As you do say silently, "I surround myself with God's highest vibrational white light of Love, Protection, Purity and Perfection protecting me against all negative energies of body, mind, emotion and spirit.

Blake sitting in prayer pose in front of picture of Master Lee.

- Inhale God's highest vibrational White Light of Love, Protection, Purity and Perfection into your root chakra.

As you exhale, visualize God's perfect Light surrounding you. As you do this silently say, "I surround myself with God's highest vibrational White Light of Love, Protection, Purity and Perfection. I am protected by God's highest Archangels (Archangel Michael, Rafael, Uriel and Gabriel), Angel of Mercy." Say your Ascended Master's name here (I usually say Saint Germain, the Violet Tara, Kwan Yin, Buddha, the Maha Chohan, Master Mun, Master Lee, Lord Shiva, Babaji, Sai Baba and Mother Mary) and say any other Angelic Beings you feel a connection with. (I usually say Angel of Faith, Unnamed Angels, and my personal guardian angel).

I realize that I have a comprehensive list but you do not need to make it that long. You can pick the one or two Ascended Masters or Cosmic Beings that you resonate with.

I have done two methods. The first is just with visualization. The second method is shown below. Those of you who are more physical or kinesthetic may like this next method. It is essentially the same as the above but with the movement of the arms encircling your energetic field and the method is described below:

- Visualize the perfect Light of God at a distance of 10 feet in front or above you.
- Inhale God's highest vibrational white light of Love, Protection, Purity and Perfection or aka Cosmic Christ White Light into your root chakra.
- As you exhale, silently say, I surround myself with God's highest white light of Love, Protection, Purity and Perfection. This Light repels away all negative energy directed towards God's highest vibrational White Light to be transmuted to a higher state of Consciousness full of love, peace and harmony. As you are saying

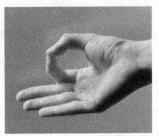

this slowly create a circle around you with your arms as you raise your arms up over your head. Continue to encircle yourself until the fingers are facing each other, palm is facing down, tips of fingers are touching and your hands are above your crown chakra. (If you were previously holding the Gyan Mudra or other mudra position you may continue to keep the thumb and index finger together to keep the circuit complete.) Thereafter, slowly bring your hands together in a prayer position and bring it downwards and stop at your heart chakra.

- Inhale God's highest vibrational white light of Love, Protection, Purity and Perfection aka Cosmic Christ White Light into your root chakra.

- As you exhale, silently say, I surround myself with God's highest white light of Love, Protection, Purity and Perfection. This Light protects me against all negative energy body, mind and spirit. As you are saying this slowly create a circle around you with your arms as you raise up your arms up over your head. Continue to encircle yourself until the fingers are facing each other, palm is facing down, tips of fingers are touching and your hands are above your crown chakra (If you were previously holding the Gyan Mudra, you may continue to keep the thumb and index finger together to keep the circuit complete Thereafter, slowly bring your hands together in a prayer position and bring it downwards and stop at your heart chakra.

- Inhale God's highest vibrational white light of Love, Protection, Purity and Perfection or aka Cosmic Christ White Light into your root chakra.

- As you exhale, silently say, "I surround myself with God's highest white light of Love, Protection, Purity and Perfection. This Light keeps me safe at all time. I am protected by God's highest Archangels, (Archangel Michael, Rafael, Uriel and Gabriel), Angel of Mercy," Say your Ascended Master's name here (I usually say Saint Germain, the Violet Tara, Kwan Yin, Buddha, the Maha Choha, Master Mun, Master Lee, Lord Shiva, Babaji, Sai Baba and Mother Mary) and say any other Angelic Beings you feel a connection with (I usually say Angel of Faith, Unnamed Angels, and my personal guardian angel).

- As you are saying this slowly create a circle around you as you raise your arms up over your head. Continue to encircle yourself until the fingers are facing each other, palm is facing down, tips of fingers are touching and your hands are above your crown chakra

- (If you were previously holding the Gyan Mudra, you may continue to keep the thumb and index finger together to keep the circuit complete). Thereafter, extend your hands up further and pull down an imaginary cord to seal in the energy. Slowly bring your hands together in a prayer position, bring it downwards and stop at your heart chakra and say God is in my heart, mind and soul as you slowly breathe in and out. I am the presence of God purifying my heart, mind, soul and spiritual body.
- Thereafter, slowly bring your arms down and place your hands on your lap in the mudra position of your liking.
- Next, focus your attention on your root chakra which is located in your tailbone or coccyx.
- Visualize the Light of God at a distance in front of you or above your crown chakra.
- As you breathe in, imagine breathing in God's Love, Light and Energy into your root chakra.
- As you exhale, silently say, "thank you I am safe and secure. I trust the process and have everything I need. I am always safe - body, mind and spirit."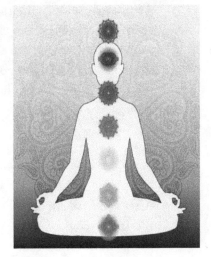
- Again, breathe in God's Love, Light and Energy into your root chakra.
- As you exhale, silently say, "Thank you, I am safe, grounded, focused and able to manifest my Dharma." Breathe in God's Love, Light and Energy into your root chakra.
- As you exhale, silently say, "Thank you, I am always safe to be one with my I AM Presence." As you inhale this time, inhale as you say Ah (while you are saying that visualize breathing into the root chakra the Ascended Master you want to connect with) and as you exhale say Aum…. As you say Aum, visualize the root chakra illuminating bright red. Do this 3 times.

- Focus your attention on your root chakra. Breathe in and out a few times to allow your consciousness to reside there.
- Next, begin to inhale, visualize and feel the energy rise up from the root chakra and going up the other six chakras until you reached the crown chakra.
- Imagine the energy rising dorsal to the spinal cord. (*General rule of thumb - energy goes up the back and down the front.*) As you go up each chakra, visualize the dominant color of each chakra being activated, 1st - Red, 2nd - Orange, 3rd - Yellow, 4th - Green, 5th - Light Blue, 6th - Indigo, 7th - Violet.

If you are able to inhale the spiritual energy to the crown chakra in one breath, that would be great (As you are going up the dorsal part of the spinal/spiritual channels,). If not, just breathe in a way that is comfortable to bring up the spiritual energy.

- As you exhale, imagine the energy coming back down from the crown chakra to the root chakra on the anterior (front) part of the spinal cord. Imagine the energy going down the anterior part of the spinal cord. As you go down through each chakra, visualize the dominant color of the chakra until you return to the root chakra.

You will repeat this cycle for a total of nine times but the last time you will raise the spiritual energy beyond your 7th chakra.

- After you have circulated the spiritual energy eight cycles around the spinal cord or what I call the spiritual highway, focus the energy back on the root chakra.
- During the ninth cycle, breathe in and out as you illuminate the root chakra. When you are ready, breathe in or inhale as you slowly raise the energy from your root chakra to your crown chakra. You can imagine a bright light spiraling up the central part of the spinal cord with a tail of rainbow colors being created by each chakra that it passes.

- If you are able, continue to bring up the kundalini energy up 10-15 feet above you to merge with your **Rainbow Body. If you do not see it, imagine this Rainbow Sphere of Light above you.** Once you reach it, allow all the kundalini energy and Consciousness to become one with your Rainbow Body.

If one breath is difficult, you can pause at the crown chakra to get another breath before going up to your Rainbow Body of Light

- Spend a few moments breathing in and out as your experience oneness with your Rainbow Body. When you are ready, look down at your physical body and now send a purple or violet light down into your body and enter through your crown chakra and continue straight down through the central channel of the spiritual highway or spinal cord. Continue down through the root chakra and extend all the way down to the heart of Mother Earth to anchor with her and ground yourself.
- Now focus on your Rainbow Body again and the Light in the center of it. Silently say, "I Am the presence of God guiding me to the Sun of God." Those of you who are more spiritually advanced and resonate to other Sun Beings may ask for guidance to go to another Sun of God for there are many and the sizes increases exponentially as we get further away from our solar system.
- Slowly breathe in and out as you journey towards the Sun of God
- Allow your Rainbow Body to ascend and drift towards the Sun of God.
- Enter the Sun of God and know that you are perfectly safe and secure in your Rainbow Body.
- Go to the center of the Sun and just focus on your breath; slowly breathing in and out.
- Silently say, "thank you for all your Love, Light and Energy you supply Mother Earth and all the planets. Thank you for your unconditional love and energy of creation" (and anything else you would like to say).
- Slowly breathe in and out and allow your consciousness to become one with the consciousness of the Sun of God. Next, imagine

connecting to all the Suns of God and the Central Sun or Source at the core of the Sun. Spend some time in peace, love and harmony there.

- When you are done with being one with the Sun/Suns/Source and experiencing that deep peace, allow yourself to return back to Mother Earth.
- Allow the energetic cord you created with Mother Earth to guide you back to your physical body.
- Descend slowly and peacefully back to Mother Earth and eventually back into your body.
- Enter your body at the crown chakra, and go straight down through the central spiritual highway all the way down through your root chakra to the center of Mother Earth where there is fullness of Light.
- Slowly breathe in and out and know that you are safe.

When you are ready, you can silently say, Thank you Mother Earth for all your unconditional love, kindness and compassion. Thank you for allowing us to live on your body. Please forgive us for not taking care of you and abusing you for so long. May I be a Light to bring about positive change to the Earth and her kingdoms in people's awareness of how to have Reverence for all of Life.

- Slowly breathe in and out and allow your consciousness to become one with the consciousness of Mother Earth. Enjoy that peace of oneness for as long as you choose.

Aside: While you still your mind in the Sun of God or Mother Earth, you may hear a response or see a vision during your meditation, when you are ready, as I have on many occasions. If you do not it is perfectly OK. It is more important that you give thanks to both of these Divine expressions of God.

- As you breathe in, silently say, "I Am the Presence of the Sun of God and God blessing Mother Earth with its Love, Light and Energy."

- As you exhale, slowly visualize illuminating the healing energy of the Sun of God and God throughout Mother Earth.
- When you are done, allow your awareness to return to your physical body and then to your heart chakra. Allow yourself to ascend back to your body on your in breath.
- Breathe in God's Love, Light and Presence into your heart. Allow it to fill the reservoir of your heart and illuminate His Love, Energy and Radiance.
- Direct your focus at three points - the Father/God/I AM Presence - within your heart, the Sun of God above you and Mother Earth below you.
- Inhale the I AM Presence of all three into the center of your being at your heart chakra.
- As you exhale, allow that Divine Cosmic Light of the I AM Presence to expand and fill your entire being.
- Again, as you inhale and exhale, allow that Light of Consciousness to expand beyond your physical body to fill the entire room, house, neighborhood, planet, space and ultimately to the Light, Mind and Consciousness of God.
- As your Consciousness merges with the Light of God, say AUM, AUM, AUM and then surrender all thoughts, emotions and experience to deep cosmic peace and bliss while focusing on your third eye point. If you are able to hold your breath, hold it for as long as you can. If not, just breathe with slower respiration allowing your mind to empty more fully until you reach a state of blissful surrender with the Universe where you are one with the Universe. Stay with the stillness for as long as you can or when you begin to have your mystical experiences.
- When you are done, slowly become aware of the pressure on your legs and feet.
- Slowly move your feet and wiggle your toes and return your awareness to your physical body.
- When I am done, I proceed with my **closing procedure** as described in Chapter 7 on prayer.

This process takes about 45 to 60 minutes to complete.

223

Advanced U.U.M.M. System

In my advanced system, God and the Ascended Masters are inhaled at each chakra and the emphasis is on activating the Light of God at each chakra. Affirmations are made at each chakra to reflect the various themes of each chakra. The whole process works on purification of the body, mind and spirit and allowing Divine Love to permeate every cell, tissue and organ. More time is spent on healing Mother Earth and others.

I actually go within each chakra via the Yantra (a sacred geometric form) of each chakra and connect with its affiliated planet and connect with Source at each chakra.

Due to the complexity of the advanced method, chakra awareness and activation in this system, I have decided to only teach my advanced system privately for those who are ready to learn. Through my method, much time is spent at each chakra. Let us take a few moments to get more familiar with these amazing energetic temples, gateways or vortexes. The first, second, third, fourth, fifth, sixth and seventh chakras all have names and properties. I call each a particular temple.

The seven chakras are the most basic ones. However, there are more above and below the root or first chakra. There are many that say there are about 12 chakras- 4 above the crown chakra and 1 below the root chakra. (Others see 5 new chakras integrating between the 7 traditional chakras.) When I meditate, I rarely stop at the crown chakra when doing my advanced method. At some point I become detached from my body and the chakras in my body become like planets or stars. I circulate my pranayama around it, go to the Rainbow Light and into the Cosmic Light or Source. Other times, I just go through a beam of Light that goes to the Source. The point I am trying to make is that there are other dimensions or cosmic chakras that we travel through as we go to higher consciousness. I am sure there are more than 12 chakras as our awareness and perception increases. One spiritual master who is known as a prophet once told me that our acupuncture points are like chakras. If that is the case, we may have up to 361 points or chakras within our bodies.

With regards to chakras, what exactly are they besides what I call sacred energetic temples?

Chakras are conical shaped energy vortexes. The first extends downward and seventh chakra upward. All the other chakras extend

224

horizontally both to the front and the back. According to energy healer and teacher Barbara Brennan, those pointing forward are Feeling centers and those pointing backward are Will centers. More details are available in her book, *Hands of Light* and her website online. **(R 212)** (or search for: chakra images Barbara Brennan.)

The first chakra is the root chakra or **Muladhara**; I call it the **Temple of the Safe Haven.** It is associated with the planet **Mars.** It is located at the coccyx (tailbone). It governs sexuality and our sense of security. It is commonly associated with the **color red** and is an earth element. It is associated with four lotus petals.

The second chakra or Svadhisthana. I call it the **Temple of Passion (intimacy, sexuality, relationships, emotional body and creativity)** in my system. It is associated with the planet **Mercury.** It is located about 3-4 inches below the navel and the level of the sacrum. It is associated with reproductive organs, kidneys, bladder and sex hormones. It governs creativity, sexuality and intimacy. It is commonly associated with the **color orange** and is a water element. It is associated with six lotus petals.

The third chakra what I call the **Temple of Empowerment, Harmony and Energy.** It is also known as the **Manipura** and is associated with the planet **Jupiter.** It is located at the solar plexus or diaphragm - below the rib cage. It is commonly associated with the **color yellow** and is a fire element. It is associated with ten lotus petals.

Although the **Dantian** is located in the same general area, it is not the same as the second or the third chakra. First, a chakra can't store energy but the Dantian can. Secondly, chakras are vortexes where energy flows in an out. The Dantian is located at the navel area. This includes the navel, below the navel and the solar plexus area. Scientific studies also confirmed now that the navel area is regarded as the "Second brain," our enteric nervous system which handles some 100 million neurons and influences our mood more so than our neo-cortex. The enteric nervous system functions like the brain: it sends and receives impulses, records experiences, and responds to emotions. It is associated with the metabolic, digestive systems and immune systems, and with self-esteem, growth, joy, leadership, and power. **(R 213)**

The fourth chakra is the **Temple of Divine Love** or what is called the **heart chakra** or **Anahata.** It is associated with the planet **Venus.** It is located on the center of the chest. It is associated with love, compassion, joy, happiness, and kindness. This is where we can perceive our I AM Presence. It is associated with either **green or pink color.** (Pink is seen at higher dimensional frequencies.) It is associated with the air element. It is associated with twelve lotus petals.

The fifth chakra is the **Temple of Communication** or what is known as **Vishudda** and is associated with the planet Saturn. However, in my practice, I focus on Mother Earth at this chakra. It is located in the neck, ear and throat. It is associated with our ability to communicate, express ourselves and speak our Truth. It is associated with the **color light to medium** blue and connected with the space or etheric element. It is associated with sixteen lotus petals.

The sixth chakra is the **Temple of Divine Realms** or what is known as **Ajna** and is associated with the Sun. It is located in the pineal gland and extends forward and backward at the level of the third eye or between the eyebrows. It deals with our psychic abilities, intuition and inner visualizations. It produces melatonin and some DMT (Dimethyltryptamine). Although it is produced there, researched have shown that they are also produced in the Neocortex and Hippocampus even after the pineal gland is removed. **(R 214)** It is associated with the **dark blue color.** (I usually see more of a purple color when I meditate.) It is associated with two lotus petals**.**

The seventh chakra is the **Temple of Cosmic Consciousness** or what is known as the **crown chakra or Sahasrara.** It is associated with the Moon. It is located above the ear on top of the head and helps us connect to our Source, Supreme Consciousness or God. It deals with thoughts, awareness, decision making, and belief systems. It has been associated with **the color violet**. It is associated with one thousand lotus petals.

During the advanced phase, each chakra will activate the Divine Presence of different properties as listed below:

1. **Temple of Safe Haven –** This deal with our sense of groundedness, safety and security. It also governs our sexuality as mentioned earlier.

2. **Temple of Passion** - This deal with our sexuality, creativity, sensuality, intimacy, desires, pleasures, emotions and our ability to relate with others.

3. **Temple of Empowerment, Harmony and Energy** - This is about moving forward as a being of Light and Love in service of others. Joy, confidence, positive thinking and achieving peace and harmony with self, others and the Universe are all a part of this chakra.

   This is also about the integration and balance of the confluence of energies and channeled in a way to serve our I AM Presence, others and for the benefit for humanity. This is where we activate the mesentery system to create energy for the body and to balance out the various organs' stored emotional energies. (The mesentery is a web *of tissues attached to the intestines which also support blood vessels, lymph and nerve connections to the intestine.*)

4. **Temple of Communication** - This is about expressiveness, non-judgement communication, compassion and acceptance. It is also about speaking one's Truth and ultimately to speak Divine Truth.

5. **Temple of the Divine Realm** - This is about vision, clairvoyance, discernment, knowing, knowledge; it's also about being aware of how Divinity is in all matters of the Universe; it's about the inter-connection and having reverence for all of Creation and all Matters of the Universe.

6. **Temple of Cosmic Consciousness** - It is about Divine Mind, Divine Consciousness, Sacred and Divine Communion, Immortality and full Activation of all chakras.

This system integrates various mudras, toning and sacred words to activate and open the crown chakra as well as all the other chakras. It takes about 1.5 to 2 hours to complete.

This advanced system when done correctly will leave you feeling in supreme bliss and will open the door to the Cosmic Realm that will bring God and the Ascended Masters to you in the most intimate way. It is done to bring harmony, wholeness and oneness with oneself, others, our planet, our Universe and God. The more people that practice this system, the greater the positive changes we can have on our planet.

This system is quite effective for manifestation once we have surrendered our ego and allow God's Love, Light and Energy to flow through us.

U.U.M.M. system utilizes breathing and visualization to move the pranic energy and kundalini energy around the spiritual channels.

> *Breathing is a very important part of all*
> *meditation practice, for deepening focus*
> *and moving the consciousness*
> *from the outer realm to the inner realm.*

Proper breathing will lead one to the Master and Guru within and to the ultimate Source of Consciousness, Love and Light.

Let us explore further in the next chapter how this powerful breath of life can sustain us, help us achieve greater spiritual mastery and even lead to our enlightenment and salvation.

** You may reach me for a private appointment or training at www. blakesinclair.org

just breathe

CHAPTER 10

BREATHING (AIR ELEMENT)

D ue to the breath being our direct linkup with our I AM Presence
or God Self, it is through the breath of God that our Universe
was created. It is said that with our breath, with its inhalation
and exhalation, we are expressing the sacred words of I AM - Hum Sah
(the name in Sanskrit).

Because of this, how we breathe can affect our well-being and
spirituality. Breathing with mindfulness can help direct the pranic energy
within us for great spiritual and Divine experiences. Learning various
breathing methods also enhances our health and mental, emotional and
physical well-being.

If we breathe with normal respirations (12- 20 breaths per minute for
an adult at rest), our brain and body work normally and we get enough
oxygen and exhale the resulting carbon dioxide. In contrast, breathing at a
rate of under 12 or over 25 breaths per minute while resting is considered
abnormal. If that happens, our brain and body may not function at the
optimal levels due to insufficient oxygen being assimilated into the body.
(R 215)

If abnormal breathing is occurring on a chronic level, the usage of
a pulse oximeter device to measure the blood gas saturation level (the
amount of oxygen in the blood) may be indicated. Anything less than 90%
of blood oxygen is abnormal. If the oxygenation continues to drop much

lower than 90% and stays there, emergency care may be needed. If the breathing rate is too high and the saturation rate is too low, an individual can suffer hypoxia or some level of brain damage.

Pursed Lip Breathing

In the situation where an individual is hyperventilating or short of breath, doing what is called **pursed lip breathing (PLB)** can significantly improve that situation. **(R 216)** Many people who suffer with some form of heart disease (Congestive Heart Failure, Cardiomyopathy, etc.) or pulmonary problems (COPD, asthma, etc.) will have shortness of breath with exertion. Depending on the degree of severity, mild to moderate exertion might cause shortness of breath. Sometimes the oxygen level drops significantly during activity even with the usage of oxygen from a line connected to an oxygen tank or concentrator.

By doing the pursed lip breathing technique, it will improve our oxygen level to healthier ranges. During pursed lip breathing, the individual slowly inhales through the nose and allows the stomach to rise. When it does that it means the lungs are filling up and displacing the diaphragm downwards and pushing the organs and stomach to give way for all the oxygen to come in the lung.

Next, the individual exhales slowly through pursed lips. This allows the stomach to slowly lower. When this happens, the diaphragm is pushed upwards as the lungs begin contracting to expel the carbon dioxide that may be trapped within the lungs. This method of breathing is not natural for us unless we are a baby or a singer. However, most of us will need to be aware and conscious of how to do it until it becomes natural to improve our ability to get more oxygen. Some individuals may need to lie down on his or her back and place one hand on the abdomen to help bring it down during exhalation until it becomes natural.

The above breathing technique will help increase a balance of blood gas saturation, lower blood pressure and pulse rate. It will help the individual to feel more relaxed and energetic. COPD Canada suggests that using PLB has positive effects in treating stress and anxiety-related disorders.

Yogic Breathing

Although PLB breathing can be quite therapeutic, yogic breathing can help us experience greater peace, harmony and bliss.

Yogic Breathing is called Pranayama. Prana means the energy and yama means to control or master. Essentially the Yogi is a master at moving and controlling the flow of pranic life energy throughout the body, mind and spirit to promote wellness, attainment and spiritual mastery. Yogic breathing techniques can be so powerful and beneficial to our mental, emotional, physical and spiritual well-being.

4-7-8 Breathing

One type of yogic breathing is called **4-7-8 breathing.** It is a yogic breathing technique that has many health benefits. This is a technique that is frequently taught by Dr. Andrew Weil, M.D. In this technique the individual is instructed to ensure that the tip of the tongue is in the back of the front two teeth and the soft tissue above it. The individual starts off by exhaling forcefully to the count of eight. Next, the individual inhales for a count of four seconds, holds the breath for 7 seconds and then exhales for eight seconds. *(his video link on this is at (241) in the reference section.)*

This is to be done for four cycles and may be increased over time with a maximum of eight cycles. It helps with anxiety and stress. According to Dr. Andrew Weil, it can also help an individual calm down, sleep, cope with cravings. After two to three months of regular practice, there are very significant changes that happen in physiology- it lowers heart rate, it lowers blood pressure, improves digestion.

It is a very powerful anti-anxiety technique; in fact, much more powerful than anti-anxiety drugs that are commonly prescribed. I like to use it as my pre-meditation warm up breathing exercise or when I want to relax.

Voo Breathing

Another great method to deal with stress and anxiety is Voo Breathing. It helps to tonify the vagus nerve to relax you. You activate it by breathing in deeply and then exhaling with the word Voo and let it vibrate all the way to your diaphragm and gut. I have found it very helpful during difficult moments in my life. It was developed by Dr. Peter Levine. **(R 217)**

When I exhale Voo, I let it resonate in my entire being all the way down to my gut. I do it a couple of times or more as needed then focus on the stillness and peace that comes from it.

Alternate Nostril Breathing

Another powerful yogic breathing method is the Nadi Shodhana or Alternate Nostril Breathing. When I studied yoga, this was an exercise we did regularly. **(R 218)**

This breathing technique helps the individual to bring more balance to the body, mind and spirit. It helps with stress and anxiety. It also balances out the two hemispheres of the brain and helps the individual think more clearly and focus better.

The technique is done by flexing the middle and index finger of the dominant hand. Slowly seal the right nostril with the thumb and begin to inhale through the left nostril. Once you reach the end of the inhalation, place ring finger over the left nostril as you exhale through the right nostril. Keep the left nostril closed as you inhale through your right nostril. As you reach the end of the inhalation, slowly seal the right nostril as you exhale through your left nostril. This is considered one set or cycle. You can do this up to nine cycles. I have used this as a pre-meditation breathing exercise as well.

Holding Your Breath during Meditation

During U.U.M.M., there are various points through the meditation where there is some degree of holding the breath. At the climax of the meditation, the breath is held as long as possible to experience that peace, calmness, and emptiness that comes from the cessation of the breath. (Refer to Chapter 9, pp. 260, 268, 281)

According to HAA International Retreat, Hatha Yoga Pradipika stated that when the breath is irregular, the mind is unsteady, but when the breath is still, so is the mind still and the Yogi obtains the power of stillness. Therefore, the breath should be restrained. **(R 219)**

They also quoted Yogananda's great Guru, Sri Yukteswar, as he also once wrote about holding the breath. What is interesting is that he maintains that holding the breath creates such a calm in the autonomic nervous system that the inner organs get a rest, which they otherwise never do, whether during sleep nor during the waking state!

Although it is therapeutic to hold your breath during part of your meditative practice, it is not indicated for someone who has high blood pressure, cardiac problems or pulmonary problems like COPD, Asthma, Pneumonia, Bronchitis, Emphysema, or other chronic respiratory imbalances. It is important not to hold the breath too long unless you have had special training on how to do it safely.

Wim Hof Method

Another breathing method that seems to be quite effective in creating great health benefits and is getting much attention is the **Wim Hof Method breathing techniques.** It is based on Tibetan Tummo meditation minus the religious component. Hof claims that his Tibetan-based breathing method can help with or help alleviate symptoms of Multiple Sclerosis, arthritis, diabetes, clinical depression, anxiety, PTSD, bipolar disorder, cancer, etc. **(R 220)**

There are many variations of the Wim Hof Method. The basic version consists of three phases as follows:

Controlled Hyperventilation

1. **Power Breathing -** The first phase involves 30 cycles of breathing. Each cycle goes as follows:

   The individual starts by doing deep breathing at a rapid and steady pace in and out through his or her nose or mouth. The individual inhales fully but does not exhale all the way out. (When the individual exhales, it is passively released) As the individual breathes in and out, he or she should see and feel the abdomen or belly rise during the inhalation and it should go down during the exhalation as the diaphragm comes back down. It is somewhat like hyperventilating. Some sensation reported by Wim Hoffers from doing this included light headedness and tingling feelings in the fingers. These are common responses and are normal.

2. **Exhalation and Breath Retention** - After completion of the 30 cycles of controlled hyper-ventilation, empty your lungs and hold the breath for as long as possible.
3. **Recovery** - When urges to breathe emerges, take a full deep breath in. Hold the breath for around 10 - 20 seconds and let it go. The body may experience a normal head-rush sensation.

These three phases may be repeated for three consecutive rounds.

What I was taught at the San Francisco Wim Hof workshop was to breathe in and out for 30 repetitions. The in-breath was deeper and the out- breath was a shorter passive breath. The rate of the breath was like a slower form of hyperventilation. After doing 30 reps of breathing, we were instructed to exhale as much as we could then hold the breath for as long as possible. Thereafter, we would inhale for 10 seconds then breathe and repeat the 30 reps of breathing for 2 more sets.

A friend of mine, who is a Wim Hof follower, stated that the technique improves his ability to stay warm in extremely cold conditions. He has also been able to stay in ice cool water for about 15 minutes using the technique, and has even been able to hold his breath for 3 minutes using this breathing method.

Wim stated he is able to hold his breath under ice water for 5 min to 7 minutes with his breathing technique. This is especially helpful with meditation practices. However, one should never attempt to learn only the basics and try to swim under ice water or hike in the icy cold with shorts. This can be very dangerous and lead to your premature demise. I would also strongly discourage anyone from doing ice baths especially the elderly, ill or weak unless you have been thoroughly trained and given permission by your physician and Wim Hof. Those who are truly interested with the Win Hof Method should learn it at one of his workshops.

I see four parts within this method:
1. The breathing technique
2. Breathing exercises and physical exercises in preparation for cold water exposure.
3. Cold water/ice water exposure (this can help with inflammation, circulation, immune system and improving your mood).

4. And the power of the mind through visualization and focus to affect the energy dynamics within the body.

This method is purported to help people to boost their immune system, improve mental health, relief stress, to have more energy, to have better sleep, to increase will power, to boost concentration, to deal with depression, to have fibromyalgia relief, and to help with burnout recovery.

Wim Hof stated that we can positively affect our immune system and endocrine system through his system of breathing.

I have found his method helpful for improving the oxygen levels in my body so I could negotiate the high altitudes at Colorado. While hiking up to Hanging Lake at an elevation of about 7,000 feet, I was getting light headed and dizzy but after I rested and did the Wim Hof Breathing method, I felt rejuvenated and able to breathe well again and completed my hike up to the lake and waterfall. In retrospect, if I had been practicing the Wim Hof method regularly and especially before the hike, I would have handled the altitude sickness much more gracefully.

I also found it helpful to keep me warm in the early morning or when I am in a cold airplane. I found it especially helpful with improving one's ability to hold one's breath during meditation. It is a breathing technique that I believe we all should learn.

After learning this method and understanding the health benefits of it, I take cold showers daily regardless of how warm or cold the weather is. The cold shower is extremely invigorating and gives me a great jump start of energy to get me going in the morning. It also helps with stress, depression and anxiety.

While I attended the Wim Hof workshop in San Francisco, I was fortunate to speak privately with Wim during a break. I asked him about the effectiveness of the technique with depression and he said that it was very helpful and was even able to help people who were suicidal.

I had just lost my mom one week before the workshop and actually attended her funeral the day before attending the workshop so I was quite down during the workshop. However, after taking the class, hearing Wim's inspiring talks and learning the method and the various exercises, I started to feel better. Since then I started to practice his method on a more regular basis and found that it helped me to negotiate the mourning process much more gracefully.

After studying this method formally and learning the science behind it, I have come to realize that this method is probably one of the most effective methods for physical, mental, and emotional wellness. It challenges our system especially the thermo-regulators which improves core circulation and temperature. This system helps to oxygenate our arteries and tissues. It also helps to activate the periaqueductal gray which Wim believes will help us to activate our natural or endogenous opiates/cannabinoids which leads to feelings of wellness or bliss.

Besides the breathing exercises, there are various exercises done to improve rib, spine and diaphragm flexibility. There are exercises done in a horse stance that incorporate some rotational and diagonal movements which helps the individual better prepare for the ice pool and helps the individual to return blood supply to the limbs and body after enduring the ice water.

What I learned from the Wim Hof Method workshop is that regular practice of this method has been known to result in the blood being more alkaline, which, among other things, helps to turn off the nociceptors from perceiving pain. When the blood is acidic, the nociceptors are activated to process a threat of pain and hence the individual is more likely to feel and experience pain.

The Wim Hof Method has been met with much medical and scientific scrutiny but has emerged as a genuine and effective tool for improving our immune system, activating our core thermo-regulators and controlling our autonomic nervous system (which up until recently, science has concluded that it is beyond the grasp of our control). I highly recommend studying this cutting-edge tool of wellness from Wim Hof to obtain greater health and wellness.

As you can see, there are many blessings from mastering one's breath including greater inner peace, harmony, health and spiritual connection and mastery. When we detox with supplements, we cleanse and purify our body systems. When we meditate, we purify our heart, mind and soul. When we do proper breathing technique especially the Wim Hof Method, we release the health obstacles that are preventing us from being "happy, strong and healthy." Those three words are Wim Hof's motto for his system.

Our in and out breath is the mantra or Divine signature expressing our I AM Presence and Divine Nature. Management of this breath can affect our health, wellness, harmony and spirituality in such profound ways. Understanding the various breathing methods and being able to do them can help us to cope more effectively with stress, pain, depression and anxiety. When used in conjunction with intention and visualization, it could affect autonomic nervous system, Qi and kundalini energies. Learning how to control our spiritual or pranic energies by way of our breath and visualization may lead to higher states of Consciousness especially in the U.U.M.M. system.

Learning to still the mind and just observing the Divine breath, leads us to connecting with our True and Divine nature.

*"If you do not fast from the world,
you will not find the kingdom."*

~

Yeshua

(from *Essential Gnostic Scriptures*)

CHAPTER 11

PURIFICATION THROUGH FASTING

Besides meditating and breathing techniques to cleanse and balance our mental and emotional bodies, it is also important that we incorporate some form of fasting to cleanse our system. It is an important part of purification, detoxification and wellness. There are a variety of ways to fast: just water; juice fasting; and Intermittent Fasting. Fasting allows our digestive system to take a break and to allow our body to flush out much more of any toxins, damaged proteins, parasites and bacteria within our bodies. It helps to create new stem cells for our immune system. Let us explore how we can do this more gracefully.

All of us living in an ego perpetuated reality are imbued with toxic thoughts, emotions and toxins within our bodies. They limit us from achieving a harmonious and radiant health. We must purify ourselves in order for the Divine and Magical Presence to do what it does best within us which is to heal and bring harmony to our body, mind and spirit. In addition to the methods in previous chapters, we can also support our I AM Presence and body temple by fasting and detoxification.

Methods of Fasting

I have used three methods of fasting - one with water, one with organic detoxifying fruits and the other with eating a sensible and healthy meal along with getting enough water. The last method is called intermittent fasting. Studies have shown that **water fasting** could have health benefits. It may lower the risk of some chronic diseases and may stimulate autophagy, a process that helps your body break down and recycle old parts of your cells. Most water fasts last between 24 to 72 hours. You should not follow a water fast for longer than three days without medical supervision. **(R 221)**

Here are a few reasons why people choose to do water fasting:
- Religious or spiritual
- To lose weight
- For "detoxing"
- For its health benefits
- Preparing for a medical procedure

I do water fasting regularly once a month to clear myself of toxins and cravings developed from eating unhealthy food. I usually drink water for a 24-hour period from morning to morning the next day on an empty stomach. I often add some Himalayan salt and Fulvic minerals to give me some electrolytes and all the minerals and trace minerals I need for the day. This makes it more tolerable, especially when I am having an active day. I sometimes do a 48-hour water fast if I feel my body needs more cleansing to optimize my health and wellness.

The next day after my fast, I eat something non-greasy and mild like oatmeal. Greasy food might be too harsh after fasting and cause some digestive issues. I will have a light lunch and then a regular plant-based dinner to end my day.

Juice Fasting

Juice fasting is also referred to as juice cleansing. Pure juice contains most of the vitamins, minerals, and phytonutrients in fruits and vegetables. People who juice say it gives their digestive systems a break while allowing them to better absorb a greater deal of nutrients. Others swear by juicing as a way to:

- Boost the immune system
- Remove toxins from the body
- Lose weight

I find juice fasting much easier to do. I would juice various fruits and vegetables that are good for detox and drink it a few times a day and drink water in between. I usually will juice with cucumber, celery, and apples. According Anthony William, this combination has the right balance of mineral salts, potassium, and sugar to stabilize your glucose levels as your body cleanses itself of toxins. (R 222)

According the Anthony William, your juice should consist of celery, cucumbers, and apples. I like to also throw in cilantro and grapefruit for its detox ability and taste. I sometimes add oranges, beets and ginger as well to give variety of benefits and flavor. There are many detoxifying recipes you can find online or in his books. I have been able to fast for several days with this method due to the micronutrients in the fruits.

There are different ways to detoxify our bodies. The ones recommended by Anthony William are taking specific fruits and vegetables for healing different issues of our bodies. I think this is the best approach! You can learn much more comprehensively how he teaches the reader on how to specifically heal specific diseases and illnesses. He teaches the reader how to detoxify the metals within our bodies. He has a 28-day detox program you can easily follow in his book, Medical Medium.

Intermittent Fasting

What I do on a regular basis which I find quite easy to do is **Intermittent Fasting.** It is quite a popular method used for improving health, depression, weight loss, burning fat and (R 223) some people have found it helpful with curtailing their diabetes.

16/8 Method

In one type of Intermittent Fasting, you eat healthy and sensible meals but stagger the times you eat so that you have a gap of 16 hours between your last meal and first meal. One example is eating only between 11 am-7 pm. Some people find it easier to get through the 16 hours of non-eating by drinking healthy teas or water with lemon. I have done this many times and find it very helpful. This is known as the **16/8 method.**

I have also done it with the addition of **R's KOSO** to help me navigate through it much more gracefully. Koso is a fermented Japanese drink that is fairly new in the United States but Koso has been used in Japan for a hundred years according to **Ryu Okada, the Founder and CEO of R's KOSO**, Inc. Koso is made with many fruits and vegetables. R's KOSO has all that plus more to give its customer the best in nutrients for supporting our health and wellness.

Ryu stated that "Koso is rich in prebiotics, probiotics and enzymes that help digestion and gut health. It has been traditionally used by those who didn't have access to nutrient-dense foods but nowadays it has become a popular choice among the young and health-conscious individuals." The product is advertised as 100% natural, non-GMO, gluten-free and dairy-free. There are other Kosos in Japan but R's KOSO uses only the finest ingredients and the factory making it has been doing it for 70 years compared to other companies who have been doing it for a shorter time. According to Ryu, some of its competitor have additives, refined sugar, no lactic acid bacteria, no Koji and have less healthy ingredients in their Koso. R's KOSO have no additive, uses only natural sugar, ferment with a special combination of sake yeast, lactic acid bacteria and Koji and have over 100 different fruits and vegetables including seaweed and mushroom.

I have found it helpful during my intermittent fasting as well as with my gut support. R's KOSO provides guidance on how to use their product during intermittent fasting. **(R 224)**

I also alternate it with the **Eat-Stop-Eat** method where I do not eat for 24 hours. Regardless of which type you choose, drinking plenty of healthy fluids is important. I have many friends who lost a significant amount of weight doing this method. Intermittent Fasting burns your fat to be used as energy. I find this method a gentle way to detox and cleanse the system.

Three Most Common Intermittent Protocols

- **The 16/8 method,** is also called the **Leangains protocol.** It involves skipping breakfast and restricting your daily eating period to eight (8) hours, such as 11-7pm, or 1-9pm.
- **The 5:2 diet:** With this method, you consume only 500–600 calories on two non-consecutive days of the week, but eat normally the other 5 days.

- **Eat-Stop-Eat:** This involves fasting for 24 hours, once or twice a week, for example by not eating from dinner one day until dinner the next day.

Besides fasting your physical body to purify it, I urge all of you to purify your mind further by fasting from TV, radio and social media as much as possible. It is not only healthy but helps you to achieve much more focus, clarity and detachment to the ego manufactured matrix we live in. Ultimately, it will set you free to truly experience the greatness within and have healthier relationships with your family, friends and God.

Healthy food, organic fruits and vegetables, purified water, vitamins, supplements, fasting and detoxing can do wonders for us in creating great harmony within our bodies if used correctly. But is that all there is with creating harmony in the body? What about the power of visualization? If we can perceive it, we can achieve it- health, harmony, peace and healing within and without. Continue on to the next chapter for a discussion on visualization and its many benefits.

Other methods that are helpful for cleansing or purification include a liver, colon and kidney cleanse. There are 3-day cleanses, 2-week body cleanses and 28-day cleanses. You can get them at Whole Foods or online. Before trying any, always consult with your physician.

"Imagination is more important than knowledge."

Albert Einstein

CHAPTER 12

THE POWER OF VISUALIZATION

I f we can perceive, we can achieve. This truth is a combination of the Law of Attraction and our living in a reflective, responding Universe. When we perceive or focus on something with feeling we achieve it whether it is conscious or unconscious. The use of visualization is to bring our focus into a place of conscious intention.

The power of visualization is tremendous and is limited only by our imagination. It is utilized in every field of endeavor, from business, to sports, to healing and relationships. Visualization is one of the most powerful ways for us to co-create with the Universe as when we do it clearly, we are literally creating our desired outcome on the etheric plane of reality and then calling it into our physical, tangible lives.

According to Darshan Baba; Yogi, Author, Spiritual Mentor, Subtle Energy Healer, and Teacher of Online Subtle Energy and Meditation Courses, "it has also been shown in studies monitoring the neurons, that the brain essentially does not know the difference between what is seen with the eyes or internally such as in visualization and imagination. In other words, the same neurons light up whether we see something with our eyes or in our mind.

"Imagining or visualizing the body, cells, molecules, and atoms as being filled with Light or transforming to Immortal Light is the same as actually seeing it happen. The more consistently one focuses the mind in such a way the greater the effects and integration in manifestation

* * * * * *

Before we went from a Divine Being of Light to our human embodiment, we had the power to materialize and manifest through our intention, imagination and visualization. This was due to the heightened state of consciousness, harmony and overall frequency, in short, our Oneness with Creation. Some enlightened beings were able to bring that ability into the physical or earthly plane while most of us lost it due to the density and discord that we had co-created on Earth.

When we transition from this earthly plane and into the higher planes of Light, our ability to create, manifest and materialize returns. However, if we practice integrating our heart with our Divine Self, using our intention and visualization, we can begin to redevelop these skills in our current reality.

I have always been a very visual person which has been both my strength and weakness, especially when I was growing up. Now that I am awakened, visualization is now a greater asset than ever before. I visualize to consciously create in all aspects of my life and doing so has assisted me with healing, manifestation and meditation. I have facilitated the healing of many people including myself with visualization.

On its own visualization is quite effective, but when it is coupled with meditation, prayer and a compassionate and loving heart, it becomes increasingly powerful. Sometimes when I am working on a client, I will visualize healing Light and energy flowing over the injured area. Clients who are very in tune with their body energy can usually feel the healing energy flowing through them that is being guided by my mind and vision.

Many other times, while doing U.UM.M. I would visualize the illness of friends, family members or even my pets being healed. Many if not most of them were healed without them even knowing that I had even worked on them. For example, my dog's liver became normal after months of healing visions were held for him in U.U.M.M. He never took any medication or did any medical treatments for his liver dysfunction. However, it is important to note that due to free will, we can visualize and pray for other beings, but it is their choice whether or not they accept the assistance consciously or subconsciously.

Throughout my life, I would occasionally see pain in my body as a vibratory frequency with peaks and valleys. Depending on the type of pain and location, I would see a different configuration of the pain frequency. What I have done to rectify the pain is visualizing a healing frequency that is opposite to the pain and then I visualize merging them together like pieces of a puzzle. When the pieces come together the opposing frequencies negate each other and the result is that the pain is dissipated significantly or is eliminated.

The power of visualization can also protect us in our daily life as well as in meditation. One way in which this is achieved is whenever we are going somewhere, be it for a walk, driving, sporting activity or another activity, see yourself returning home or arriving at your destination safely and looking happy and at peace. This enables the Universal energies to align with you to create this outcome.

I was once involved in a car accident with a big truck. A truck made an illegal U turn and turned sharp left right in front of me and hit my SUV. The impact was huge but, intuitively, I immediately sent a protective Light around my entire body including my spine and body at the moment of impact. After the accident, I got out of my car expecting to feel hurt but was surprised that I felt completely fine.

This has happened again with another car and I did the same thing and visualized myself becoming fully protected. When I got out of my car, I was again fine. In both cases, it was the other driver's fault for the accident.

During U.U.M.M., I visualize and direct the kundalini energy up and down my spine. My body usually warms up when I am raising the Kundalini energy up my spine with my yogic breathing and visualization. Visualization is very important with U.U.M.M. for activating the chakras, moving the kundalini energy and connecting my Soul Energy with the Cosmic Energy.

Visualization and Manifestation

In the documentary film, **Heal**, a doctor is paralyzed from a bike accident. Instead of having surgery to correct his spine, he prayed and visualized how to systematically heal his spine. After he worked hard at rebuilding his spine through his visualization or imagination, he started to have a miraculous recovery in his motor skills. Eventually he had a full recovery all because of the power of prayer, visualization, intention and faith.

Before learning how to visualize and meditate, I would worry a lot about getting enough work. As a result, I would have to hustle to keep busy if possible. Now that I meditate, pray and visualize filling myself with the abundance energy, I no longer worry about work. I now have a thriving private practice that is overflowing with work and clients. I do not seek work like I use to; instead, new clients are now trying to do business with me.

Another example is how I have visualized abundance to all the relatives who have stayed at my house and every one of them has found a job despite being unemployed when they first moved in with me. In fact, all of them are working at ideal jobs that they enjoy doing.

At one time a relative of mine was hospitalized due to blindness of one eye. After many batteries of test were done and he was seen by many different types of medical experts, it was determined that he had neuritis of the optic nerve. With the normal course of treatment with steroids, the eye was expected to take several months to get better.

This would have devastated my nephew since he was a college student and working at two jobs. He was restricted from driving and that was a big blow to his independence. I was saddened by his turmoil and decided to offer him several healing sessions. The energy healing tools that I used to help heal the eye and optic nerve included a Vogel crystal wand, Tibetan Smoky Quartz, a special heart shape healing rose quartz crystal and a yellow calcite crystal.

Utilizing these tools, I taught my nephew how to visualize healing light from the Universe into his eye. In addition, I taught him how to use different color lights to help to cool the inflamed optic nerve. I placed the rose quartz over his eyes while I made a decree for healing his eye, decreasing the inflammation and opening the eye to sensory perception. While I did the decree, I would visualize sending healing light to open his vision and decrease the inflammation. I visualize different colors depending what I am guided to do or what is going on. In this case, I visualized a cool light of blue because of the inflammatory nature of the eye problem.

Many people memorize decrees but I often do what comes naturally or what I am intuitively prompted to say. I often decree for Archangel Rafael's, Saint Germain's, Kwan Yin's or a Healing Angel's healing energy. An example of my decree for this scenario is "I am the Presence of Archangel Rafael bringing cool healing light to Paul's optic nerve and bring harmony, balance and love to it." I would then visualize blue light to cool the inflammation and maybe white light for integration and healing.

After our first session, he began seeing light. The second session he saw even more light through the defective eye. In subsequent days while doing U.U.M.M., I continued to visualize healing to his eye. After a week of U.U.M.M. healing and my relative practicing the techniques I showed him, his eye began to improve even more. By the second week, his defective eye had improved even more dramatically and was actually seeing with greater detail. He told his doctor that he was able to see 90% better. After a few more weeks, his sight came back completely. Due to the accelerated healing, my relative did not have to miss school and work. Now he is back to his normal life again and was quite appreciative of the healing sessions and training that were given to him.

In another situation, I had a client who had spinal stenosis around the cervical spine and as a result had numbness of the hands. I worked with her on visualizing the Universal White Light entering her head and then down her arm to her finger tips. After doing this, she was able to start perceiving sensation on her fingers for the first time in a long time.

When our visualizations are strong and focused, others can sometimes pick up on it. There were two instances where I was focusing on sending my consciousness to two different spiritual masters. Both reported seeing me in their presence even though I was thousands of miles away from one of them and at least 30 miles away from the other. In another situation an enlightened being in the UK was able to feel me tuning into him while I was offering healing energy and prayers to him.

I once damaged my car after backing into a metal pole. The rear bumper was smashed in and I immediately filed a claim to get it repaired through my car insurance. Thereafter, I brought my car to a body shop to get an estimate of the cost of the repair. It was appraised at over 1,000 dollars to replace the bumper since the damage was beyond repair according to the gentleman at the body shop. I was a bit saddened by this and just prayed that the bumper would somehow reverse its damage. I visualized and prayed repeatedly after leaving the body shop. The next time I checked the bumper, the entire damage was completely gone. The only thing that remained was a small scratch or two. The car looked good as new. I then called the insurance company and the body shop to cancel the claim. I told them what had happened and they were speechless and in disbelief. Our vision and imagination are so powerful that it can sometimes manifest a miracle especially when done with a prayer and or decree.

Janet Doerr, Intuitive Nutritionista, explained that she was able to grow her Achilles tendon and heal her left hip through visualization, meditation and intention in her early twenties. She went to her doctor due to pain on her Achilles tendon. The physician examined it carefully and noticed it was thin as a pencil and stated she would need to have surgery but that it would break later anyways. Janet decided to heal herself instead. During a six-week period, she meditated on healing her Achilles tendon.

She visualized a man, brick by brick, rebuilding her tendon. She had the intention of her tendon growing, meditated on it and visualized it healing. She did it for about 10 minutes four times a day. After 6 weeks, she went back to her doctor and he examined her thoroughly but was flabbergasted and dumbfounded that her injured Achilles tendon was now the same size as the uninjured one and had healed completely.

She once also had severe osteoarthritis on both hips, the left was worse than the right but the right had severe pain that was so bad that Janet decided to undergo a total hip replacement on the right to find relief. The surgery was successful and the hip healed and rehabilitated well. Eventually she needed to do her left hip but at this time she decided to heal it like she did before with her Achilles tendon. She meditated on it and visualized it getting repaired with new cartilage. After some duration of time, her hip began to heal. She now can do everything possible with her legs including jumping with no pain and no longer needs surgical intervention to correct her pain issues.

Visualization done alone is powerful but when done in meditation and in U.U.M.M., the results can many times be as astounding and miraculous. Visualization is extremely important in U.U.M.M. because it is the key component to bringing the positive changes on our planet towards creating greater peace and harmony. If enough people practice U.U.M.M. and visualize the positive effects of U.U.M.M., the sooner and more effective we will be in helping Mother Earth and humanity with its spiritual maturity and advancement.

When our intentions are clear and altruistic and we are motivated by pure love and compassion, our visualizations, prayers and decrees can many times lead to amazing and miraculous outcomes. Let us start making more miracles, creating more harmony within ourselves and our planet and break down the invisible wall that seems to divide us so that all of us can find our way back home to our true nature for ourselves and our collective consciousness.

*"Only in love
are unity and duality
not in conflict."*

~

Rabindranath Tagore

CHAPTER 13

BREAKING DOWN THE WALLS OF DUALITY

Due to our own choices over the ages we currently live in a world of duality. In this illusionary reality things are not always that clear cut. One very clear example of this is in our global health care systems. Many people who are into holistic healing do not believe in modern medicine. Modern medicine may feel that many holistic methods lack the scientific research that proves their effectiveness even though many of them have been used successfully for thousands of years. Yet when we look deeply into the great variety of healing modalities, we can find blessings and validity to most, if not all dependent upon the situations for which they are being utilized.

Currently, the mentality of duality exists with the following: modern medicine versus holistic healing; rich versus poor; religion versus mysticism; God versus technology and science; the haves versus the have nots; one race versus another. However, if we choose to look without judgement, blessings can be found within each situation. This in turn can bring us to a greater state of gratitude and unity between the various comparisons.

Modern medicine has helped so many millions of people live and thrive. Many of my clients would not be here if it were not for some of the medicines they have been taking. Medicine is not evil. It is the judicious use of medicine that makes a doctor great or not. It is the art of knowing how much or how little to give and knowing what works and what doesn't and when to stop and try something new. My doctor has helped me to navigate through various medical challenges throughout my lifetime. My mom lived a rather normal life since her seizures had been controlled by medication.

Modern medicine is outstanding for emergency care, surgery and to some degree, acute care. It has helped millions survive and live and will continue to do so. However, in situations where modern or western medicine is not available, holistic modalities can be of great benefit.

Although Holistic medicine may not have as extensive scientific research as modern medicine, it is something that has been around for thousands of years and has helped millions to experience radiant health. Holistic Medicine includes but is not limited to Traditional Chinese Medicine, Ayurvedic Medicine, Homeopathy, Herbology and Chiropractic Medicine. Alternative therapy approaches include but are not limited to Acupuncture, Hypnosis, Psych-K, Craniosacral therapy, and a variety of energy healing modalities such as Reiki, Johrei and Theta Healing.

The above are all viable and great methods for healing. Holistic medicine or therapies are great for chronic conditions and things that are affecting harmony of the body, mind and spirit. It is also good for clearing energetic blockages and helping us dissolve stress-based illnesses. Many times, it can produce miraculous improvement in one's condition. Modern medicine and Holistic Healing each have their strengths and limitations. When integrated together we can have the best of both worlds; Dr. Andrew Weil coined the term Integrative Medicine. In this focus, the best modality is chosen for any given situation, giving respect for each component and what it has to offer.

Rich versus Poor

Many people think and accuse all rich people as being evil and greedy. Although there might be some truth to that for many but it is not so for all. I know a wealthy psychic who has set up a rescue operation for those who do not have money and need urgent medical care. She has a program that flies needy people to their doctors for free.

There is good and bad in the rich and poor.
Judge not, so you will not be judged as well.

Before Siddhartha became the Buddha, he was a prince and gave up his wealth to pursue enlightenment. Today in India, there is a siddha who was very wealthy and owned many businesses before he chose the spiritual path. He was considered by some the Steve Job of India. Now he lives a more modest life.

I also have a wealthy friend who travels to the Philippines to bring food and supplies to the poor and needy in the rural areas. These are a few of the thousands, if not millions, who give their time and money to assist those who are in need of healing assistance.

Then there are many of these so-called spiritual masters who are more interested in making money from people, having them follow them blindly and lure them in with promises of power, magic, and clairvoyant ability. True spirituality has nothing to do with opening the third eye, power or levitation. Many people who are not spiritual but practice some form of the dark arts can do those things as well. Then there are those who are spiritually and financially wealthy like Amma (or at least her non-profit organization) who have built schools, hospitals and houses for the needy. She has donated a great deal of financial resources as well as man power resources to help end the suffering of people around the world. Her service is not publicized but yet millions of people around the world have been helped by her.

Yet, it is not poverty that creates enlightened beings either, although I have met many very spiritual people who have very little means and quite a few are even spiritual masters. I have met many spiritual teachers who are more interested in making money than truly teaching the path to liberation and enlightenment. I have also met a few who are truly dedicated to sharing the Universal Truth like Romarishi Siddha and his Divine wife, Tara Leela, who teach it either freely to all who seek the Universal Truth or at a nominal fee at the Universal Fellowship of Light. **(R 225)**

Religion versus Spirituality

Religion has helped millions around the world find peace and harmony. They have helped the poor and needy all around the world by their various outreach programs. Religion has produced some of the great saints of our times like Saint Francis of Assisi, Saint Theresa of Avila, floating Saint Joseph of Cupertino, the many Dalai Lamas, and many Yogis who have even attained the Rainbow Body. Often, those that have transcended the limitations of religion and discovered the great Truths have become Mystics like many great Catholic Saints, Buddhist Masters who are also known as Catholic Mystics and Buddhist Mystics who include Padmasambhava and Milarepa. There are Christian Mystics as well. Another name of all God-realized beings or Mystics is Yogis.

Although religion was divinely inspired, man's ego often inserts itself into the religion which usually ends up in war and conflicts and keeps people living in the matrix. However, if we can learn to discern through man's ego like many of the religious Mystics, we can see the true Divine teaching wherever we go and in whatever shape or form.

The Mystic path is the path to liberation, enlightenment and God-realization but some in this path have misled many into a path towards the shadow self or ego self. A true Mystic and spiritual master will guide the individual in finding the great guru within to set them free with the Truth. Spiritual teachers are many but masters are few. With regards to those who have achieved God-realization are even fewer and far between. Even after Yogananda met many saints and Yogis in his life, he stated that few are what he considers to have reached a state of God-realization. One of those saints that he met and considered a God-realized being had few to no followers.

If religion and mysticism learn to work together and co-exist, imagine what great things can happen to the world. Many people follow so called gurus who are highly charismatic and have some mystical power but they end up never truly learning the true path of freedom or God-realization.

God versus Technology

Nowadays, many who are high tech or scientifically oriented seem to think that God is obsolete and only a myth. Many do not realize the true magnitude of God's Consciousness and Love. God is beyond the time and space continuum. God is real and beyond imagination and many, as well as I myself, have experienced His Greatness in the depth of meditation in what they call Samadhi. All great saints and Yogis have experienced this great communion with God in the most intimate way where our ego and consciousness are dissolved into union with God's Consciousness where we become one with God.

At the same time, many scientists believe in the Spinoza's God and that God is nature and has an order and harmony throughout the Universe. Unfortunately, that is only one aspect of the nature of God. The other aspect includes his Consciousness expressed in a beautiful form of Love.

In the late 1980s, Einstein's daughter Lieserl donated 1,400 letters written by Einstein to the Hebrew University. Below is an excerpt from one of those letters.

"There is an extremely powerful force that, so far, science has not found a formal explanation to. It is a force that includes and governs all others, and is even behind any phenomenon operating in the universe and has not yet been identified by us. This universal force is LOVE."

When scientists looked for a unified theory of the universe, they forgot the most powerful unseen force. Love is Light that enlightens those who give and receive it. Love is gravity, because it makes some people feel attracted to others. Love is power, because it multiplies the best we have, and allows humanity not to be extinguished in their blind selfishness. Love unfolds and reveals. For love we live and die. Love is God and God is Love."

Perhaps in the future more scientists will begin to accept the fact that there is a conscious and Divine Order in the Universe which is also known as God or God Consciousness.

Many worship the God of technology and find everything they need on the internet from news, weather, knowledge, play, socialization and even sex. We have become a civilization that not only worships the God of technology but are also addicted to it. Many millions of people are glued to their cell phones, iPads, laptops and computer from morning to night. We may try to escape the pains of the matrix we live in by diving into a virtual world of social media for comfort but become further trapped into a virtual matrix of an even greater illusion. This virtual reality is tearing apart friends and families all around the world. It has contributed to the depression of many people.

This addiction leads to a great disharmony and has social and emotional consequences. It also has adverse health consequences due to prolonged exposure to the radiation that we are constantly bombarded with. There will be cervical and possible thoracic spinal strains due to poor positioning with how we use our phones for long periods or how we sit when using on computer devices. The blue light from our computers or cell phones can cause eye strain and may possibly lead to macular degeneration, a very serious eye condition that can lead to permanent vision loss.

Perhaps technology is truly a double-edged sword but it is actually leading us towards our ego and away from God and others. Getting glasses with blue light protection will protect us. We can also obtain Swanwick Sleep Fit over Blue Light Blocking Glasses that fit over our frames to protect us from damaging our eyes, bodies and sleep patterns.

The EMF emitted from our technology (cell phones, cell phone towers, computers, Wi-Fi, routers, smart meters, etc.) can cause health problems. According to Jeromy Johnson (safe technology advocate and civil engineer), EMF pollution can affect us in the following ways:

- Headaches
- Difficulty Sleeping
- Heart Arrhythmia/Palpitations
- Tinnitus (ringing in the ears)
- Fatigue
- Depression/Anxiety
- Difficulty Concentrating/Forgetfulness
- Infertility
- Skin Rashes (facial redness)
- Vertigo/Nausea
- Reduced Immune System Function
- Cardiac, Nervous and Endocrine System Dysregulation

Jeromy gives us 7 ways of reducing EMF pollution that is extremely comprehensive and informative. I highly recommend the reader to go to his website and follow his recommendations. He also has information on shields you can place over your lap or put on your phone to decrease EMF pollution. **(R 226)**

Here are some tips I have given many people to decrease EMF pollution:
- Turn off the Wi-Fi when it is not in use and when we go to bed.
- Keep all electronic and small phone devices far from us when we are sleeping.
- Try your best to keep your phone away from your head and use speaker phones as much as possible.
- Avoid placing the laptop over your lap unless you have a special shield over your legs.
- Avoid long exposure to the computer or cell phone.
- Use an ear piece that plugs in the cell phone versus a blue tooth ear piece.

Other things you can do to reduce the EMF exposure. **(R 227)**
- Placing a Himalayan salt lamp near you or your computer.
- Wear a Nuclear Receptor around your neck. (This pendant was developed and designed by Dr. Fred Bell (a Quantum Physicist, Innovator, a former Nasa Rocket Scientist, and is a direct descendant of Alexander Graham Bell). **(R 228)**
- Some crystal therapists wear a shungite pendant around their neck and or shungite beads around their wrist. Some place a shungite ball or pyramid next to their computer.
- Some place powerful crystals next to their computers like Aventurine, Fluorite, Unakite, Amazonite, Jasper, Black Tourmaline, etc.
- EMF Solution is a tool that creates a coherent field, neutralizing negative effects of EMFs and supports deep healing and body balance. **(R 229)**

Although there are many bad things about technology, social media and internet addictions, many spiritual people (Yogis, Mystics, spiritual teachers, gurus, etc.) use it as a platform to help educate, motivate and empower people to raise their consciousness and awareness. Technology is not necessarily bad; how we use it and how we protect ourselves makes a difference with whether we are headed towards our ego along with its accompanied symptoms or illness or towards our Creator accompanied by a life filled with harmony.

People are still very discriminating and judge based on ethnicity, race or culture. If only we all realize we are different colorful expressions of God Consciousness, we will begin to love and have more compassion with one another. What we do to any of God's children is what we do to God. If we act out of kindness to God's most meek, poor and lowly child, we act in kindness to God.

The "we versus them" mentality of duality is the way of the ego. That way is divisive and only leads to greater suffering in the world. The way of the Tao, the way of harmony and Divine Love will lead to unity, wholeness and will allow our planet to continue to shift towards a higher level of enlightenment and consciousness.

We must realize that we are all one Divine Family, one Divine Mind and One Divine Consciousness of God.

Let us realize that and begin to have more love, compassion, kindness to people from all walks of life and to embrace and have reverence for all of Life through essential harmlessness. In the depth of all our Souls are the perfect Light, Divine Love, and Energy of God's individualized I AM Presence. Let us help each other discover that greatness so we can finally come together as one harmonious family or God's Consciousness and may God's will be done on Earth as it is in Heaven.

*"In the beginning
was Consciousness,
And that Consciousness
expressed itself as I AM.
"All that is Love, Light, and Life,
Came forth from the I AM."*

~

Peter Mt. Shasta

CHAPTER 14

I AM

I AM THAT I AM are the most sacred words in the Universe. Understanding these words and living in full expression of their essence is crucial to our spiritual maturity, advancement and salvation.

The words I AM are a powerful expression of Divine consciousness filled with the highest vibrational Light and Divine Energy of love, light, compassion, and God Consciousness. It is the breath and consciousness of God that created the big bang which manifested all material reality. All matter in the universe, including us comes from that Source of Energy, Light and Love. In effect, we are all Divine Beings or children of God and are one Divine Family, Mind, Heart and Consciousness.

Another name for I AM THAT I AM is AUM, pronounced as OM, the primordial sound of the Universe. The sacred syllable has been associated with different states of consciousness like awareness, dream and sleep. The Hindus also associate it as the three expressions of the Divinity-the Creator, Preserver and the Destroyer or Brahma, Vishnu and Shiva, respectively.

I chant the powerful, sacred and Divine syllable during my U.U.M.M. practice to activate and open each of my chakras. I also chant sacred I AM decrees to activate the Divine Energy to flow through my heart chakra and throughout my being and beyond for purposes of healing and bringing love and harmony to myself, others and Mother Earth.

For instance, I would sometimes say, "I AM the Presence of Archangel Raphael filling my entire being with healing Love, Light and Energy, releasing all that is less than perfect of body, mind, spirit and emotion… releasing it into the Universe formless and harmless." Once I have allowed that pure and Divine energy to fill me completely, I allow it to expand from me and into my household; I then expand further to Mother Earth and beyond.

When we say, chant or decree with the words I AM or I AM THAT I AM, we are activating our I AM Presence, Divine Spark of Light, Atman, Divine Presence, Higher Self or God into our being. I do this on a daily basis to access my Divinity and to assert my Divine Nature. When we call on the I AM Presence through our decrees, we are taking the first steps toward Oneness with our Creator.

We are all unique Divine expressions of God's Consciousness. When we learn to still our mind, integrate our ego and open our hearts to become one with God's heart and consciousness, our I AM decrees become so powerful to create and manifest our loving intentions through our sacred decrees.

The Power of the Words "I AM"

The words that we say after I AM are extremely critical due to the power of the words themselves. When we start a sentence with I Am, we call on God to create what we say next. The commandment, 'Thou shalt not take the name of the Lord Thy God in Vain' takes on a new meaning with this understanding.

The words I AM are words of Creation. So, whatever we say after them we create whether that is our conscious awareness or not. When we say I AM love, joy and happiness that brings the Divine nature of God more fully into expression through us. When we say I am angry or depressed, we diminish that active presence of God within us and accentuate these energies in our inner and outer realities.

Many of us do not realize how important it is when we use the words I AM in our daily lives. Developing an awareness that everything you speak after the words I am (I AM) have a powerful effect on your life both short term and long. Examples:

- I am sick versus I feel wonderful
- I am stupid versus I am bright and creative
- I am alone versus I am befriended and loved by many
- I am poor versus I am prosperous … and so on

Explore more of this concept with the teaching in *Conscious Language* by Robert Tennyson Stevens **(R 230)**

Being mindful of how we use the words that follow I am will allow us to becoming more empowered and positive. Here are examples of ways to use it to become more empowered:

- I am happy.
- I am peaceful.
- I am full of gratitude.
- I am surrounded by opportunities for growth. (instead of I am stressed out.)
- I am given the opportunity to learn. (instead of I am treated so unkindly by life.)
- I am resourceful.

The words that we say after I AM should generally be positive or empowering. However, it doesn't mean that we repel all negative emotions or thoughts that come up. They come up for a reason. If we continue to use them over and over in our verbiage, they begin to activate that negative emotion or thought in becoming a reality which may begin to permeate or saturate your subconscious mind until you become a walking manifestation of that emotion or negative thought.

When you find yourself saying negative emotions or thoughts after I am like I am dumb, I am depressed, I am worthless, etc., it is important we examine where it came from and why you are having it. It is generally the Universe's invitation for you to heal or integrate. We must then take measures to resolve it or integrate it better. Sometimes a professional like a counselor, clinical hypnotherapist, life coach, spiritual master or teacher can help you navigate through the dark sea of pain and suffering that we have pushed away from our conscious awareness.

Once you have begun healing yourself and begin understanding how important what you say after the sacred words of **I am,** you may want to then start learning how to say it in a way to activate the Divine energy to flow through you to bring about great changes around yourself, others and ultimately to Mother Earth and our Universe through decrees.

The Words I AM and Decrees

I am usually very specific with my I AM decrees since I have been working with (and serving with) different Ascended Masters throughout my spiritual life. I often decree to activate the Divine Presence of Kwan Yin, Saint Germain, the Great Divine Director, Archangel Rafael or God to help me be an instrument of love and healing energy to help those in need.

Other times, I would decree I AM the presence of the Angel of Faith, Healing Angel, Archangel Michael, or other angelic beings to help me in a specific situation that may require support, healing and protection.

I find that the more specific my decrees are, the more effective it is. Choosing the Divine Beings with the specific attributes you need and then doing decrees with their name brings their being, nature and presence into activation and action.

Examples of decrees are as follows:
- I AM the presence of Kwan Yin surrounding Mr. Jim with healing Light and Energy of compassion and love to allow him to experience greater peace and calmness within.
- I AM the presence of the Angel of Healing guiding me on what to do to help heal this individual.
- I AM the Presence of God filling me with love, light, compassion, healing energy and Divine wisdom to be shared with all that I meet.
- I AM the presence of Mother Mary filling me with patience, mercy and understanding in dealing with this person's anger.

Over the years, I have used I AM decrees with great and often amazing and miraculous results. Sometimes the results are instantaneous while other times it takes some repetition to build momentum to produce an outcome.

For instance, once a family member asked me to offer assistance to a nursing student who was going to re-take his licensing exam. The individual had failed the exam previously and was quite discouraged about it and was ready to give up. I encouraged the young man to take the test again after doing some more review before the next exam. During the exam day, I did decrees for giving the young nursing student support guidance and wisdom with choosing the correct answers and helping the young man remain calm during the exam. I did it over a period of about 45 minutes.

Shortly after the decrees, I was informed that the young man had finished his exam in about 45 minutes and was the first to finish. Mind you the young man was the last to finish during his last test. Needless to say, the young man passed his exam with flying colors and is now a successful registered nurse.

Another interesting story is about a time I was once traveling abroad and encountered a dilemma at the airport. Apparently, one of my bags was too large to be allowed into the plane. It didn't seem that much bigger than what was allowed by the airport standard but the staff was not about to let me through and he was quite serious and adamant about it. The gentleman was not one who would bend the rule and did not appear to have any emotions or compassion whatsoever. The other airport employees tried to reason with him but he would not budge. I decided to make a decree to open the gentleman's heart and mind to be compassionate and kind to let me go through without any hassle. Shortly after, the man waved his hand at me to pass through.

My decrees have helped me with all aspects of life from dealing with personal, spiritual and business matters. Many times, it has even helped me to find a parking space in San Francisco and we all know how hard that can be. My friends and family are always surprised by the great space I would many times find that is close to where we are going. Unbeknownst to them, many times, I would make a silent decree to find a space in close proximity to allow me and my group to have more quality time together.

For instance, sometimes I would make a decree like "I AM the presence of the Divine Director manifesting a parking space near the restaurant we are going to; this will allow me, my family, and my other relatives to have more quality time together."

Often when I get lost, I make a decree for guidance on finding my way back to where I need to be. Once I was hiking at Mt. Tamalpais with my family and we got lost. There was no one in sight and our cell phones lost connections. I made a decree that we would get guidance on how to get back home then suddenly a man appeared from one of the side trails and he was able to guide us back to our trail. I made a decree like:

"I AM the Presence of God guiding me and my family to the path that will lead us back towards the entrance of the park."

Many people memorize many decrees but I do not. I say what pops into my mind or what I am guided to say. It is my opinion that more important than the words are the intentions, emotions and visualizations that go along with the decrees.

More Life Examples

On November 16th, 2018 I drove to Mount Shasta. Unfortunately, the air quality was very poor because of the fires that were burning in the Bay Area (Paradise) as well as in Malibu for the past week. The sky and air were filled with smoke. In fact, many people wore special masks to allow them to breathe without inhaling the toxins in the air. It was not a good time to go to Mount Shasta but I receive inner guidance from Saint Germain to visit Peter Mt. Shasta.

It was truly a dismal and hazy day to be traveling. As I got within 1 hour of Mount Shasta, I decided to make a decree to invoke God's assistance in clearing the air quality as I went to Mount Shasta so that I could have a mystical experience without suffering any respiratory issues. While driving, I decreed "I AM the Presence of God, the Elementals and Mother Nature clearing the air of toxic fumes to allow me and many others traveling to Mount Shasta and those living in Mount Shasta to enjoy this sacred day." "May the airs especially at Mount Shasta be clear to allow me to have mystical experience without being distracted by poor air quality."

After the decree, I was dazed for a second or two but when I began to focus again, I couldn't believe what I saw. The sky in front of me was completely blue with no hint of smoke whatsoever. I looked at the rearview mirror and could see that all the smoke was now behind me. The weather at Mount Shasta was perfect when I arrived and remained that way even after I left. I had a wonderful time with Peter Mt. Shasta and later had a mystical experience on the sacred mountain. The conditions could not be more perfect.

On December 11, 2018, my wife called me and was quite distraught. It was her birthday and she couldn't find her car keys and eyeglasses. I talked with her to calm her down and gave her some ideas where it might be. She was quite exasperated and overwhelmed that she could not make it to two of her afternoon appointments. I felt great compassion for her so after we hung up the phone, I made a decree that St. Anthony would guide her to the keys as well as the glasses. I later called her and she had found both the items and was able to enjoy her birthday. The decree I made was "I AM the presence of St. Anthony guiding Cassandra on where she placed her keys and glasses."

I read that the Super Blood Moon Total Eclipse would be in the sky on the night of January 20th, 2019. Unfortunately, it was raining hard that evening. A friend contacted me and asked whether I was enjoying the eclipse. I told her I couldn't see it due to adverse weather conditions. It was raining hard and the sky was covered with rain clouds. Although I couldn't see it, I could feel a great lunar energy. I later made a prayer and decree to halt the rain and clear the sky so that we in the bay area could enjoy such an auspicious and Divine evening.

I made a decree like "I AM the Presence of God, the Elementals and Mother Nature clearing the clouds and stopping the rain so that the people in the Bay Area and I could enjoy the beauty and splendor of this majestic lunar eclipse." I could not sleep because somehow, I knew I was going to see the eclipse. Suddenly, I was compelled to leave the house and look up. When I did, I was pleasantly surprised to see that the Universe and the Great Masters heard my prayer and decree and blessed us with a surprise; the rain had stopped and the sky was suddenly all clear. There she was my beautiful, sacred and Divine Moon going through an eclipse with my Sacred Sun. It was a beautiful evening indeed.

I have done healing for individuals and animals near and far with miraculous results with the decrees. I find that the decrees work best when I visualize the outcome intensely as if it happened already, connect that vision to my heart, allow God's or the Master's Consciousness and Energy to fill my heart with much love and compassion, surrender my ego and then allow God and the great masters do what needs to be done.

I find it least effective if it is done for some ostentatious purpose or for the purpose of my ego. Sometimes we may not get the desired outcome because the Masters may have other more Divine plans in mind since they see the bigger picture. Whether you get the desired outcome or not is not important but learn to trust in God and always give gratitude and realize that God and the Masters are guiding everything to happen for a higher purpose.

Early Teachings about the I AM Presence and Decrees can be found in the Green Books, and particularly the first two books, **Unveiled Mysteries** and **The Magic Presence,** by Godfré Ray King which detail the story of his meetings with Saint Germain on Mount Shasta in the 1930s and the many mystical and wondrous experiences he had with the Ascended Masters.**(R 231)**

Peter Mt. Shasta has written extensively about I AM decrees and how to do them in his book I AM Affirmations. Additional resources for learning of I AM decrees include this book, **I AM Discourses** and Vlogs and books by Patricia Cota-Robles at https://eraofpeace.org. **(R 232)**

Here is a powerful decree that my friend, Kathryn Shanti Ariel, shared with me. I found it energetically powerful and wanted to share it with you. It assists us as individuals to align with our highest outcome every day:

I AM my I AM Presence,
and I AM the Resurrection and the Life
of the Immaculate Concept of my Divine Mission
now made manifest and sustained by Divine Grace.

The important thing to remember when giving these decrees or affirmations is to set your ego aside and allow the Divine Presence of God to work through you to help serve others. The I AM decrees or activations can be so powerful and miraculous when we learn to embody our I AM

Presence and unify our energy with God, the Masters and entire Company of Heaven.

I AM and U.U.M.M.

I am decrees and AUM mantra or chanting is very important with U.U.M.M. During the final phases of U.U.M.M., I usually decree I AM THAT I AM and allow my consciousness to expand and finally to merge with the I AM Presence of Mother Earth, the Sun of God, and God or Source.

All living matter is imbued with the I AM Presence at the center of its being or core regardless if it is an animal, crystal, mineral, tree, ocean, water, insect, Mother Earth, Sun of God, etc.

Once we gain mastery of the decrees and have reached a higher consciousness and attainment, we can begin co-creating a new Heaven on Earth within our multibody systems (physical, mental, emotional bodies, and spiritual or subtle bodies), which in turn creates our outer reality. We can begin helping to heal ourselves, others, humanity, Mother Earth and beyond.

Although it is important to activate our I AM Presence by decrees, visualization, affirmations and prayer with healing and loving purposes, embodying our I AM Presence fully and ongoing is the most important part of our spiritual mastery. Our I AM Presence, Divine Presence and Spark of Light is anchored in the center of our being in what is referred to as the trinity or threefold flame within our heart. On the right is a blue flame of Father God's Divine Power. On the left is Mother God's Divine Love, and in the center, the essence of Christ Consciousness.

We can feel it tugging at our hearts when we still our mind clutter and distractions in life. It's that inner voice or prompting that guides us towards a higher level of consciousness and spirituality. However, our shadow self or illusory self, often mimics our I AM Presence. Our I AM Presence prompts us to act out of love, compassion, kindness and for the betterment of others and humanity. It is the part of us that is altruistic and makes us a humanitarian. Following its path will lead to freedom or liberation. It seeks unity, harmony and global oneness. The ego, on the other hand, tugs at our heart too but wants to take care of itself only. It wants attention, love, kindness for itself.

It is only interested in self-preservation and fulfilling its desires, wants and lust. It is the "me world" where the ego is the center of this Universe. Following its prompting will lead to divisiveness and chaos. Adherence to this path is poison and toxic to the soul and will cause the individual to become a prisoner of the karmic cycle. How does one tell the difference? It is through observation and through discernment. The more you meditate the clearer you will be able to observe yourself objectively.

Listening to our I AM Presence will guide us to enlightenment and self-realization. Listening to the other will leads us towards the path of the ego. One path will set us free while the other will make us a prisoner of our own ego and karma. Following the Divine promptings within is like growing a new muscle or habit. The more you make this choice the easier it becomes and the rewards are enormous and eternal once we master it.

I have always listened to my I AM Presence but more so after my awakening years ago. It has led me to meeting many spiritual teachers and gurus who have guided me further in my spiritual mastery. It has led me to doing the right thing for healing and helping myself and others.

I was once at a social function at a park and suddenly a man collapsed into a seizure. A few of us ran to his assistance. Before long, he stopped breathing and became unconscious and we could not palpate a pulse. No one knew CPR, so 911 was called and emergency assistance dispatched.

I didn't know what to do but my I AM Presence guided me to hold the man's hand and send healing Light to activate and bring him back to conscious awareness. After several minutes the paramedics came and took the man away on a stretcher. I offered the man's family member a ride to the hospital. As we followed the ambulance, we could see the man regaining his consciousness shortly after he was brought to the ambulance. I was in bliss and the family member was just overjoyed.

Years before that, I worked at a rehabilitation facility. As I walked by a resident, I saw that he was unconscious, not breathing and completely jaundiced. I tried to find a nurse for help but no one was available. I was guided by my I AM Presence to take him to his room immediately and put him in bed. No one was available to help me but I suddenly had superhuman strength to just pick the resident up and toss him on top of his hospital bed. The moment the resident's body touched the bed, he became conscious and was OK thereafter.

In both circumstances, I was guided to do what needed to be done. It was beyond my comprehension but I trusted and surrendered to the Divine prompting and in both cases, a life was saved.

It was my I AM Presence that led me to many great spiritual beings and masters including Peter Mt. Shasta. It is important to note that all good things in our lives are brought to us through our I AM Presence. In contrast, all pain and suffering are the results of ego-based choices.

Once I received a strong message from within to visit Master or Venerable Panyavro Vachira, a Thai Forest Tradition Monk at Master Lee's Temple in Concord. I was planning on visiting him but somehow some family events came up and I did not go thinking I could go later. Later I contacted Master Relica about my interest to visit Master or Venerable Vachira, Unfortunately, he had an emergency in the family and had to leave for Thailand. Now I realize the urgency to see him.

When we listen to our intuition, which is the prompting from our I AM Presence or Higher Self, as well as trusting and following the great masters, things will flow in accordance of our highest plan. Unfortunately, this time I learned my lesson how if I ignore my I AM Presence's promptings, I can miss out on important opportunities and lessons that await me.

The Yellow Emperor and the Dragon Pearl

On October 19, 2019, I gave a lecture about Mysticism at the 16th Annual Taoist Gathering at the Zhi Dao Guan, The Taoist Center. I wasn't sure what to expect prior to the lecture since I was presenting to many prestigious people of the highest caliber; many or all of them were experts in their field. I meditated in the morning prior to the event and many great Ascended Masters appeared to me; they were my core Ascended Master Team. They do not usually manifest in a group this large of about 6 Masters except on rare occasions. I will usually see one of two at a time. They surrounded me and offered their love and support. They told me that something good would come out of my lecture.

After I delivered my lecture, various people met with me afterwards. Amongst them was a famous and legendary musician who is a friend of

Peter Mt. Shasta. Another was a medical doctor who flew in from out of state to attend this event. He was so happy that I gave that lecture and stated that now he knows why he came. The next person was a Sufi Master and Acupuncturist. We spoke for a little while but he suddenly surprised me when he smiled at me and stated "I know who you are!" He then silently blurted out who I was and I was flabbergasted since few truly see who I really am. (Those few who know include three spiritual masters including healers and a Buddhist Master). After his comment, I quickly dismissed what he said by smiling, patting him on the shoulder and giving him a wink. I won't share what he said to maintain my humility. I thought meeting these men of greatness were what the Masters were referring to; however, little did I know that they had something even more profound and special for me that evening. Dr. Alex Feng had invited all the guest lecturers to attend a dinner reception in Hayward. I had mixed feelings about attending it since all the guest were esteemed guests who were either doctors, masters or grandmasters. I felt kind of out of place and was contemplating about not attending. However, I felt a strong pull from my I AM Presence urging me to go and so I followed its guidance and went to the restaurant.

As I entered the private banquet room with my wife, I saw the host of the event, Dr. Alex Feng sitting with his wife Dr. Charlene Ossler and their friends. There were a few seats available but somehow my I AM Presence guided me to sit at another table with a bunch of strangers. As I began sitting, I was greeted by Dr. Paul Wang, the Key Note Speaker at the Taoist conference, Doctor of Acupuncture and Chinese Medicine and Wu Shu Master, and was drawn to sit next to him.

On his left was Rebecca-Danbi Kim, a Feng Shui Practitioner and Face Reading Expert and on her left was Grandmaster Yuanming Zhang. On his left were Dr. Steve Jackowicz, Mac, Lac, PhD, his wife and Dr. Hirsh Diamant, BFA, MFA, PhD.

Grandmaster Zhang was dressed in a beautiful, royal and mystical yellow robe and sported a magnificent black mane. He had this mystical, regal, majestic aura around him. He spoke some English but I felt a strong nudge from my I AM Presence to talk to him. I took a chance to reach out to Dr. Wang and to see if it was possible for me to talk to this man of greatness.

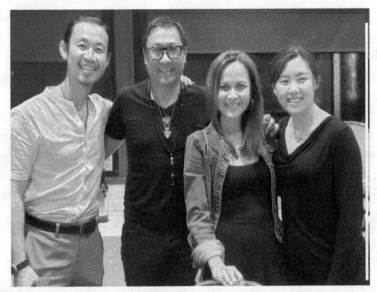

Dr. Paul Wang, Blake Sinclair, Cassandra and Rebecca-Danbi Kim

Fortunately, Dr. Wang happened to be the perfect person to translate our conversation. What followed was a mutually gratifying and amusing conversation due to Paul's superb Mandarin and English. We talked about different things including about some Chinese history, about the cave where the Yellow Emperor spent time cultivating himself, and about Sam Roi Yot, a mystical and spiritual mountain in Thailand. The great Master stated he would love to visit the sacred mountain of Thailand one day with me and welcomed me to visit the Yellow Emperor's cave as well.

Finally, we talked about the mystical and legendary Dragon Pearl. Its mystical origin has its roots with the Yellow Emperor of China. It was given to the Yellow Emperor through the blessings of the Heavens. Many of the artwork from China depict a dragon chasing after a fiery pearl with its claw. That Pearl is known as the Dragon Pearl. While Dragons represent the emperor, the Dragon Pearl is a mystical stone and is associated with many mystical powers.

The Dragon Pearl of the Yellow Emperor was passed down through the Yuan Ming Zhang's ancestors.

When the Grandmaster spoke, he sounded like an Emperor, an Enlightened Being and a man of true greatness. He also had an amazing sense of humor that I found so refreshing. After we conversed for a while,

277

it appeared a new and amazing friendship was born that evening. I knew nothing about Grandmaster Zhang until that evening. I found out that his lineage traces all the way back thousands of years to the renowned Zhang family in China and that he is the direct descendant of the Yellow Emperor.

It is said that The Yellow Emperor's reign in China began around 2697 B.C.E. when he united the tribes of the Yellow River plain under a single government. He was also a Taoist master and eventually retired from being a ruler to seek spiritual mastery and perfection which he obtained. It is also said that he attained Ascension and ascended to the heavens astride a dragon during daylight, for all his subjects to see. **(R 233)**

The Story of the Dragon Pearls

Master Zhang told the following story. *Right before the Yellow Emperor's ascension into the Heavens – as a transcendent immortal – a dragon appeared from the heavens and bestowed upon the Yellow Emperor (aka Huangdi) seven Dragon Pearls. These other-worldly jewels absorb energy from the sunlight during the daytime and cause the stones to glow like the moon during the night. They originate from beyond Earth and have the ability to help one's third eye as well as protect and enhance one's health. It also helps one's dreams and ambitions to come to fruition.*

The special energy of these Dragon Pearls was harnessed and utilized to help individuals become kings and emperors in the ancient past. However, these Dragon Pearls can only be used by employing a secret technique passed down to the Yellow Emperor's descendants.

The Dragon Pearls, secret methods, and mind cultivation techniques have all been passed down for numerous generations through the Zhang family. 2019 marks the 4,717th year since Huangdi ascended the throne and first passed down these gifts to his Yellow Emperor Hidden Transcendent lineage. Grand Master Yuanming Zhang is the descendant of Huangdi's grandson Zhang and is the 150th generation leader and lineage holder of the Yellow Emperor Hidden Transcendent lineage. Today Grandmaster Yuanming Zhang guards the stones and keeps them in safekeeping in several countries around the world, many of them being in the U.S.

Before his ascension, Huangdi bestowed the Dragon Pearls and secret techniques to one of his grandchildren. He also taught this grandchild, who received the name "Zhang", secret "wind fire" (Qigong) and "wind water" (Feng Shui) techniques." Today Grandmaster Yuanming Zhang teaches these subjects as Fire Dragon Qigong and Yellow Emperor Hidden Treasures.

I was flabbergasted when I found out about the Dragon Pearl, the Yellow Emperor and about Master Zhang; however, I felt like I was supposed to meet him and in fact, Grandmaster Zhang felt it was destiny that we met that night. I told Grandmaster Zhang I was very intrigued and fascinated with the Dragon Pearl. He asked if I would like to see it and I enthusiastically said, "Yes!"

He later invited me and my wife to visit him after dinner at his hotel in Jack London Square. So that night after dinner, my wife and I met up with him, Dr. Wang, Rebecca, his assistant and student, and Grandmaster Zhang at his hotel. The great Master spoke with us for a while in the lobby area next to a warm and beautiful fireplace. He taught my wife and myself some unique Qi Gong techniques, blessed us and told us to contact him regarding dreams we would have in 3 days. When he was done talking, he invited only me and my wife into his room while the other two remained in the lobby.

While in his room, he was preparing a ritual that would later change our lives forever. I was in suspense and had no clue what to expect but I began hearing a high-pitched Cosmic frequency in my right ear while he was getting ready to meet with us. I have heard this frequency on Mount Shasta when meeting with the Ascended Masters and most recently when I went to visit the Indian Saint Mother Meera in San Francisco.

Finally, when it was time to meet, the great Master guided me and my wife to stand towards the doorway. The lights were turned off while Grandmaster Zhang placed the mystical and legendary Dragon Pearls in our hands. It was quite an extraordinary and luminous stone. It glowed and radiated its energy in the dark and was extremely exquisite and mystical. I felt a strong connection to my heart from holding it. Meanwhile, my wife felt an electrical current from her head to her chest as she held it. Grandmaster drew together a pair of sacred Tibetan or Nepalese cymbals in the room early on and eventually around my wife and I to clear the room and our various body systems of negative energy and blockages.

I eventually had a vision of Gautama Buddha, Venerable Ajahn Lee as well as the Yellow Emperor in my meditative state as the great Master anointed me with some sacred and spiritual ointment on my third eye point and allowed me to smell it. Interestingly enough, Master Relica told me the night before that he (Ajahn Lee) had spoken to her and she wanted to give me something. A week later, she revealed to me that he wanted me to have a statue of him brought to me. These are her words – 'he told me to bring a small statue to you; it has been made at his temple recently. That temple will be released early next year. (Ajahn Lee attained liberation in 1961 but still keeps close communication with Master Relica).

Afterwards Grandmaster Zhang guided me to place the dorsal part of my hand on my wife's cheek while she placed her hand on mine. We began to download the Qi from our partner's face through the face, to the hand, up the arm during our in breath and we exhaled as we imagined the Qi flowing down the central channels. We did that 9 times then we kissed in a way to connect our Qi together through our tongue. What followed was an extraordinary mystical experience that would change how my wife and I would ever relate with each other again. As we hugged each other, I felt my wife's consciousness or soul merged into my body. We literally became one consciousness.

There was no me or her; it was just one soul. As we let go of each other, our consciousness returned to our respective bodies. We were instructed to continue to do our unique Qi Gong exercise daily and we have continued to do it religiously each day. The phenomenon where our souls merged together continued for three days. During that time one day while we were at church, my wife placed her hand on my shoulder, suddenly she felt her soul merge with mine.

Prior to that auspicious evening with the great Master, my wife and I had been having some marital conflicts and having issues about the Twin Flame phenomenon. I never shared that information with Grandmaster Zhang but somehow, he knew that we needed his help. He explained that what he did that evening and what adjustments he would do in the future based on our dreams would always keep the three of us connected beyond time and space. Grandmaster Zhang also stated that through tonight's process, we were blessed with longevity, joy and financial success. He also stated that my society status would be raised and my ability to help others would be greatly enhanced.

What he created for us that evening was the birth of our own Twin Flame. After that experience, Cassandra could literally feel what I felt although we were thousands of miles apart. The great Master had saved our marriage and gave us his blessings for *A New Beginning* and for that he has our eternal gratitude, love and respect.

This man of greatness had the aura of Jesus, an Ascended Master or a noble and enlightened Emperor. I have never met such a saintly, noble, Christ-like and royal man of utmost greatness before. He was full of love, compassion, understanding and mystical abilities. I was deeply touched by our friendship, his love and kindness.

After 3 days, I woke up from a dream seeing Grandmaster Zhang. I later meditated but began to feel the strong energetic presence of the mystical stone that Grandmaster once let me hold.

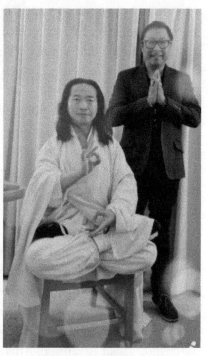

I was guided to place it in my third chakra and allowed it to circulate with my consciousness and kundalini energy around my chakras until I allowed it to exit through the crown chakras up past my Rainbow Body, into the Source Light and then into the void. I stayed in that void for some duration. Eventually, the explosion of Consciousness released it towards Mother Earth as my consciousness followed its journey as it landed in China where a royal and Enlightened figure picked it up.

Grandmaster Yuanming Zhang and Blake Sinclair on October 19, 2019

It was truly a beautiful adventure and I am thankful that my I AM Presence led me to this amazing and incredible journey.

In mid-July 2020, Master Mun (more formally known as Ajahn Mun Bhuridatta Thera) appeared to me. He discussed with me the importance of devotion and instructed me to spend more time studying Buddhist's teachings. After my Divine visit, I began to tune into my I AM Presence on what I should do next and was guided to read the Autobiography of Master Lee and another sacred Buddhist book. I began to take what Master Mun said seriously and dedicated myself to greater devotion and meditation. Little did I know that my obedience to Master Mun would further expand my consciousness, connect me more with the Masters and elevate my spirituality. A few weeks later, Master El Morya and Saint Germain appeared and asked me to visit Peter Mt. Shasta so I went ahead and made an appointment to see him on July 24, 2020. A few days prior to the appointment, Master Mun reappeared and told me to hold off on the trip for this week. Interestingly enough, my wife was not well at that time and was going to join me. I again complied with his instructions but deep within me my I AM Presence was prompting me to go and see Peter in the near future on August 1st. The next week, El Morya reappeared and asked me to now see Peter. Interestingly enough, my wife was well again at this time.

I texted Peter on July 30th and asked if I could come and visit him on August 1st. He stated that he was busy moving but that he make time for me.

On July 31st, I meditated. When my consciousness reached my heart chakra suddenly my Consciousness expanded beyond the confines of my body temple and beyond Earth into the Cosmic Universe where there was complete severance of my body, senses and worldly connections. I existed as pure consciousness and the Universe. I experienced a blissful state of pure consciousness known by many great masters as **"enlightenment."** It is beyond what I have ever imagined or read about. Many people believe it is about being awakened or spiritually knowledgeable but now I realize it means much more than that. I will discuss about it in more details in the chapter about Ascension. After I was done with my meditation, I went downstairs to the kitchen and saw two doves outside the window. They would often show up during my various spiritual advancements. I told my wife about my meditation experience and she was quite excited and responded that I was on the right path. I later went into my Zen Garden and was greeted by a beautiful and large Divine Monarch butterfly. It was flying around quite rapidly so I quickly grabbed my cell phone to capture this beautiful, mystical and Divine moment. I prayed that it would let me take its picture and after taking two shots, I got two beautiful pictures of it. I then looked up the meaning of the Monarch Butterfly and was quite flabbergasted by what I found and it means **"you are on the right path."** Bear in mind I have never seen any butterflies in my garden since moving to my house in 2001. This was a true message and blessing from the Universe.

The next day I was more than ready to visit with Peter and embark on my next spiritual adventure at Mount Shasta. Dr. Mikaelah Cordeo found out that I was going to meet Peter and wanted to join us as well so I invited her to join us. She drove down from Oregon to meet us.

We (Peter, my wife, Mikaelah and I) finally met and we had a wonderful time at Seven Sun Café. Our time together was quite spiritually uplifting for my heart, mind and soul. However, I soon found out why the Ascended Masters and my I AM Presence guided me to come today versus any other day. Peter told me that he had just finished moving out of his home and was planning to move out of Mount Shasta. This would be the last time I would be able to meet with him in this spiritual and mystical town until he would move back there. After we spent two delightful hours, we all went our separate ways.

Thereafter, my wife and I went to Mount Shasta and meditated at Bunny Flats. After blessing the mountain and the grounds around us with my chants, decrees, prayer wheel and Vogel crystal wand, we meditated next to a tree I was guided to sit next to. I did my U.U.M.M. Heart Chakra meditation. Within a short time, I was filled with God's Love and Light and began hearing that familiar high-pitched Cosmic frequency as the Ascended Masters appeared. Saint Germain and El Morya appeared first and then Sai Baba as well. Sai Baba began blessing me with his hands then the three began to hold their hands towards me transmitting Cosmic Energies to raise my consciousness and vibrational energies. That day was my first experience with El Morya at Mount Shasta and second time with Sai Baba. I have seen Saint Germain there multiple times. Needless to say, I was in supreme bliss and peace. While I was grounding and slowly readjusting my energies to come out of my altered state of consciousness, I saw a brilliant Violet Light while my eyes were closed. The first time I went to Mount Shasta I saw a beautiful violet ray emanating out of the center of the Sun. Twas beautiful indeed! After we were both done meditating, I saw a beautiful and Divine grasshopper sitting next to me. Grasshoppers represent good luck and are also an invitation to trust the inner voice/ I AM Presence. I have always trusted it and the grasshopper was a good reminder to always trust it for by doing so I would never be lost. Interestingly enough, after we were done meditating my wife asked if I felt the strong wind. She felt a lot of wind blowing by and was sitting directly behind me. I was filled with so much Light and entered into a different dimension that I had no awareness, perception or sensation of any wind. My wife is a new meditator and reports that she gets distracted sometimes but remarked how she was able to focus much better at Mount Shasta. Interestingly enough, I saw another orange colored butterfly flying around. I telepathically asked if I could take a picture of it. Within seconds it landed on the ground to allow me to take a close-up picture of it. My cell phone came as close as only a few inches away from it. The Divine Butterfly stayed on the ground until I left. It was truly another Divine moment and blessing. Trusting my I AM Presence and the Masters lead me to Peter and allowed me to have my mystical experiences at the mountain with the Masters and the Divine Butterfly. All the experiences lifted my spirituality and consciousness to a higher level.

After the mystical experiences, we left the mountain and went into town. We stopped by **Soul Connections**. As I was approaching the store, I was greeted by a beautiful picture of Gautama Buddha and Kwan Yin. They are both a part of my core Ascended Masters and this was a good sign seeing their pictures. I have been to the stores multiple times but have never seen their pictures out in front. As I entered the store, I don't know why but somehow, I was guided by my I AM Presence to bypass all the crystals and souvenirs I usually look at and went straight back to the shop extension on the right where there are singing bowls. Somehow, I was guided to a display case filled with Tibetan tools for spirituality. I was extremely drawn to the **Phurba** and had an instant connection with it. Dee, a clerk from the store, was helping me and thought I would be interested in their other Tibetan tools they had displayed in the front of the store window so she asked one of the managers or owners to assist me further. He showed a large and beautiful collection of Tibetan spiritual tools- cymbals, singing bowls, **Phurbas, Dorjes and Bells**. I felt a very strong pull from within and felt a strong connection with the Dorjes and Bells but most were in a set and were above my budget. I found one Dorje that I was drawn to but felt that without a bell I would not feel complete getting it. The gentleman helping me didn't feel that they had any separate bell but tried to find one anyways. Suddenly, he found a beautiful and exquisite bell that completely resonated with me and was priced fairly. The Universe blessed me with a complete set that was affordable. Little did I know that these powerful tools would soon change my spiritual practices. Incidentally, the **Phurba/ Kila** is a three-sided blade or knife which can be used for exorcism or to contain thoughtforms and negative energies. **The Dorje** represents the masculine energy and also represents the "method." It also symbolizes the thunder bolt and the diamond which is indestructible. It is said to be very powerful and clears negative energies. **The Bell** represents the feminine energy and "wisdom." Together they represent or symbolize enlightenment. I did not know that the first time I saw them.

After I purchased the Divine Gifts, I consecrated my Phurba and blessed it with the protective energies of Archangel Michael, Saint Germain, the Violet Flame, Buddha, Padmasambhava, Master Mun and Master Lee for my spiritual practices. Prior to meditating now, I draw up all the negative energies of my body, mind, emotions and body and bind them in an energetic ball which I place to my right in a small container of rice. I then make a decree to activate the Phurba and then pin down those negative energies. Thereafter, I meditate. I find it very helpful in keeping my mind clear. When negative things come up in the inner realms, I now can invoke an inner Phurba as well to pin down and remove all those energies to allow me to rise up in higher consciousness. By following my I AM Presence, I was guided to the tools to assist me in the integration of my previous Tibetan past life as well as increasing my spiritual practices.

Following the promptings from our I AM Presence will lead us towards the path that leads us following our destiny and callings in life and reveal great wisdom and insights.

All said, it is very important that we learn to tune in to our personal I AM Presence and better yet, to once again become One with our I AM Presence. What assists us in doing so is honing our relationship into a daily spiritual protocol of devotion, meditation and prayers. Living a life of love, compassion, kindness and service will make it easier for us to tune into our guru within, the Divine wisdom of our I AM Presence.

Once we discover it, find it and tune into this state of awareness, we will never be lost again because the Divine compass will always lead us to our Higher Self and God. And when that happens, we will realize the new responsibility we now have towards being a part of the Divine Team to help restore peace, unity and harmony on our planet.

Our Divine presence on earth is to be a beacon of God's Light, Love, Energy and Consciousness and lead as many people as possible on the path and journey to rediscovering their true nature and finding their way back home and back to God's Love, Light and Consciousness. This path will save our planet and lead to more of an enlightened civilization that lives in peace, harmony, and reverence for all life forms great and small. Being a Lightworker, Yogi, Mystic or God-realized being takes time, patience and hard work and may take many years to achieve. Hence, living a long life by taking great care of our body temples that allow us to be here will allow the individual to attain great spiritual mastery, cultivation, and healing abilities. This will enable us to make a bigger impact on humanity and Mother Earth.

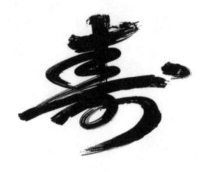

According to a Tibetan proverb,
The secret to living well and longer is:
Eat half,
walk double,
laugh triple and
love without measure.

CHAPTER 15

LONGEVITY

Longevity is a subject that has been around for many years, prompted by a desire within everyone to live as long as they can. The intention of this chapter is for us to explore the idea of longevity in more detail and shed some light from perspectives from various scientists, healers, a Stem Cell expert, spiritual teachers, Yogis, medical intuitives, a nutritionist, and a well-known Traditional Chinese Medicine Practitioner. We will explore some of the secrets from those who have achieved longevity and while also reviewing some of the contributing factors for the longevity of life of the Japanese people. In addition, I will share my ideas of how to optimize your wellness, which in turn will facilitate your longevity.

Some may wish to live long and healthy lives for vain reasons while others, like you reading this book, may want it for altruistic, Divine and spiritual reasons. Regardless of the driving force behind their interest, people from all walks of life have sought to unravel the mysteries of longevity including our scientists, doctors, shamans and health educators. Most of us have heard of the great tales of the searches for "the fountain of youth" and other legends that provide great longevity.

While no such external place has actually been found, there are certain races that seem to be quite successful in attaining longer lives, such as the Japanese people. Then there are those Siddhas and Taoist Masters who have mastered it to a level that is way out off the charts. Master Li from

China lived to be 256 years of age. Tapaswiji Maharaj from India lived to be 185 years of age. Although these two have died many years ago, there is a Siddha that is still alive and healthy today in India and is 130 years of age. My dear friends Romarishi and Tara Leela actually met this great Siddha a couple of times and know him personally. **(R 234)**

When I write about longevity, I am mainly referring to the physical body since the mental, emotional and spiritual bodies are eternal. However, in my opinion, addressing all our bodies as a whole and along with our elements is very important in supporting the success of our reason for incarnating upon Earth. If we reunite with our Divine Presence in unity, it would be able to optimize its ability to heal and repair our Earth body temple itself.

Longevity is not just about eating, drinking, and exercising well. It is also about achieving the harmony of our physical, mental, emotional and spiritual bodies. We must live in a way that enables our Divine Presence within us to be able to do its job efficiently. We can do this by way of ensuring that the elements (earth, water, air and fire) that Earth is comprised of are supporting our various bodies. Although it may seem that all this is so mechanical at face value, I will present elements in a way that is spiritual.

Until we return to unity with our I AM or Divine Presence, our body temple has a certain average life span depending on where we live and how we live our life. We can optimize our ability to live a long and fulfilling life by ensuring that the elements that support our various bodies are things that are pure, natural, organic and diverse in their impact on our physical, mental, emotional and spiritual bodies separately and as a whole.

In previous chapters we have discussed how environmental toxins that may be present in our foods, water, air and other elements can cause problems to our health. They create challenges for our Presence to fully embody and express our True Divine Nature as intended. The more we eat, drink and energetically take in that which is in harmony within our bodies, Mother Earth, Nature and God, the greater the well-being our bodies will experience. This in turn allows our Presence to embody more fully in, through and united with us upon Earth, allowing our lives to be longer and in greater joy and productivity.

We have also discussed how our ego perpetuated reality has created our individual and global suffering. We have co-created this reality and it has caused us to hasten our own mortality, aging and suffering. How we achieve longevity varies from who you talk to indicating there are various paths to this outcome. I will present information from different perspectives as well as my own to help you understand the complexities of this subject.

Scientific Theory

There is a scientific theory called Free Radical Theory of Aging (FRTA) that explains aging and was introduced in 1956 by Dr. Denham Harman at the U.C. Berkeley's Donner Laboratory. FRTA states that organisms age because its cells suffer free radical damages that accumulate over a lifetime and contribute ultimately to death of the physical body.

A Free Radical is an atom or a molecule that is missing an unpaired electron in its outer shell making it reactive and unstable. To regain stability, free radicals will steal electrons from its neighbor, initiating a series of chain reactions that repeatedly damage the delicate structure and function of living cells, allowing pathologies to initiate many chronic degenerative diseases, such as cancer, diabetes, cardiovascular diseases, dementia, Alzheimer's Parkinson's, etc. Free radicals come from within our bodies and from the outside environment.

The job of defending against free radicals belongs to "Antioxidants' a group of special compounds that are uniquely capable of quenching free radicals before they spread their destruction. Antioxidants literally sacrifice themselves by offering their own electrons and thereby become free radicals themselves. These newly created free radicals are relatively weak and do no further harm. There are hundreds of naturally occurring antioxidants - some are produced by our body and others come from our food or supplements.

Since we now know that it is the loss of electrons from atoms within cells that initiates the disharmony within our bodies, what can we do to replace it? There are two main ways of dealing with free radicals –

1. Antioxidants; and
2. Earthing.

Antioxidants

With regards to the strongest antioxidants, Andrei believes that the supplements **astaxanthin** and **glutathione** are two of the most powerful forms of antioxidants. Andrei stated that the glutathione level in Centenarians is much higher than in an ordinary person. His favorite one is Clinical Glutathione which he states can make it through to the gut unlike other brands which are affected by our stomach acids. With regards to astaxanthin, Andrei stated that it has a protective quality to the membrane of the mitochondria which may result in us getting more energy.

Astaxanthin

According to Dr. Axe, often dubbed the "king of carotenoids", research shows that **astaxanthin** is one of the most powerful antioxidants in nature. In fact, its ability to fight free radicals has been shown to be 6,000 times higher than vitamin C, 550 times higher than vitamin E and 40 times higher than beta-carotene. It is commonly found in Wild Salmon.

He and others also state that it provides the following benefits which improve Brain Health **(R 235)**

- Protects Your Heart
- Keeps Skin Glowing
- Eases Inflammation
- Enhances Your Workout
- Boots Male Fertility
- Supports Healthy Vision

Glutathione

Here is a summary about this important antioxidant: "What is Glutathione and Why Do You Need It?" **(R 236)**

- Glutathione is produced in the body and is a combination of three simple building blocks of protein or amino acids: cysteine, glycine, and glutamine.

- It is called "the master antioxidant" because it can regenerate itself in the liver (after each fill-up of free radicals) and go back to work.
- Research has shown that raised glutathione levels decrease muscle damage, reduce recovery time, increase strength and endurance, and shift metabolism from fat production to muscle development.
- Glutathione is critical in helping the immune system do its job of fighting infections, and preventing cancer and other diseases.
- Production of glutathione decreases as we age. Toxins also decrease healthy glutathione levels. The highest glutathione levels are in healthy young people, lower levels in healthy elderly, lower still in sick elderly, and the lowest of all in the hospitalized elderly.
- Certain foods help the liver produce more glutathione. These sulfur-rich foods such as garlic, onions, and cruciferous vegetables, premium, bioactive, whey products and colostrum.
- A number of supplements can help increase healthy glutathione levels including:
  o A good, organic, whole-food derived nutritional supplement
  o **N-acetyl-cysteine** (NAC). Time release NAC is the best option for keeping levels high throughout the day.
  o **Methylation nutrients**, including folate, vitamin B6, and vitamin B12
  o **Selenium**
  o The family of **antioxidants** which includes vitamins C and E (in the form of mixed tocopherols) work together to recycle glutathione.
  o **Milk thistle** (silymarin) helps increase glutathione levels and it is famed for its ability to cleanse, protect, and regenerate the liver.

C60

One antioxidant which has been gaining much attention is **C60.** According to some research with mice taking C60, the researchers noted the rats lived up to 95% longer. C60 is purported to have myriad other health benefits including decreasing inflammation and pain. It also has been linked with improving our immunity against viral and bacterial infections.

Although human studies may be lacking, there is a plethora of testimonials regarding its benefits. Further scientific studies on humans would validate its effectiveness on health, wellness and longevity.

In addition, Dr. Lester Packer and Carol Coleman state, there is a dynamic interplay among at least five major Network Antioxidants

- Vitamin C
- Vitamin E
- Glutathione
- Lipoic acid
- Co-enzyme Q10

So, when you are choosing to create greater health and longevity for yourself and family, it is critical to have antioxidants in your diet and do activities to assist your body in creating greater amounts itself. **(R 237)**

These five antioxidants have an amazing relationship with one another in recycling one another to be antioxidants again. According to 4longlife.com, these super antioxidants save each other and their recycling capabilities help maintain the critical and delicate oxidation-reduction balance of all our body's molecules.

With the exception of Coenzyme Q10, all of these super antioxidants can easily be obtained from foods. Eating foods that are high in antioxidants can be very helpful as well. Regarding antioxidants, the wild blueberry is touted as having the highest level of antioxidants. This berry is able to thrive in extreme conditions and therefore contains the nutrients for those who consume them to do the same. The Wild Alaskan Blueberry has five times the potency of a regular blueberry due to its ability to survive harsh weather patterns in Alaska. This is one of the major ingredients in Kyani's products and is on the *Medical Medium*'s 'eat daily' list.

According to *Active Beat*, there are 7 superfoods:

1. Dark green vegetables (lettuce, leeks, kale, broccoli, and collard greens)
2. Sweet potatoes
3. Red berries (like strawberries and raspberries)
4. Blueberries

5. Organic grapes
6. Walnuts
7. Pomegranates

The more we incorporate foods from these superfood groups, the more we support our well-being and longevity.

This is one viewpoint. Most nuts, berries, greens and many seeds are super foods, not to mention spirulina and chlorella. The best rule of thumb: eat the rainbow of colors every day.

Summing this up, when an atom loses its electrons, it begins a chain reaction that affects the cells and begins to perpetuate disharmony and leads to diseases. I believe that stress, physical, mental and emotional toxins, and environment exposures all accelerate that deterioration process.

How Do We Stop the Deterioration Process?

How can we stop this process? Although that may seem like a million-dollar question that no one can truly answer except an advanced Yogi, Taoist Master, a good functional medical doctor, a knowledgeable scientist and a good nutritionist. However, deep within our heart our individual I AM Presence/Godself knows the How. This knowledge is available to everyone through directly connecting to our Presence, asking for assistance and listening to, then following the guidance that we receive through our intuition and overall inner guidance.

It takes practice to get tuned in to our I AM Presence and listen to it. Many of us are bombarded with too many marketing stimuli to even be aware of our own thoughts, let alone that subtle and gentle prompting from within. Then there are those of us who are not spiritually evolved enough to do this yet as well as those whose time of awakening is only just arriving.

One thing I will again mention is that until we embody our mastery and become One with our I AM Presence again, longevity will not be about stopping the aging process but aging much more gracefully and then dying in Divine timing versus prematurely due to our ego perpetuated system that we have co-created.

However, in addition to antioxidants and overall nutrition there are many things we can do to optimize the harmony within and improve our odds.

Earthing

There is a simple way of getting more electrons directly from nature and getting grounded. According to *Barefoot Healing*, years of extensive research has shown that connecting to the Earth's natural energy, by walking barefoot on grass, sand, dirt or rock can diminish chronic pain, fatigue and other ailments that plague so many people today. This connection is referred to as Earthing or Grounding.

To put it briefly, when your bare feet or skin comes in contact with the earth, free electrons are taken up into the body. These electrons could be referred to as nature's biggest antioxidants and help neutralize the damage from excess free radicals that can lead to inflammation and disease in the body. The Earth is a conductor or free electrons and so are all living things on the planet, including us. The body is composed mostly of water and minerals which in combination are excellent conductors of electrons from the Earth providing there is direct skin contact or some other conductive channel for them to flow through.

Just by taking off your shoes and walking barefooted on sand, grass, dirt, or rock, can have healing effects on the body. It appears to be very effective with pain management and essential to our well-being. A thirty-minute walk in nature can do wonders for your body and facilitate in restoring greater harmony.

Herbs and Tonic Elixirs

Besides the above, herbal tonic elixirs can be a great support to creating great harmony within our bodies. According to Romarishi, herbal tonic elixirs can help us achieve radiant health and longevity. By taking various herbal tonic elixirs we can reap its health and spiritual benefits.

Romarishi Siddha (Ganga Nath) and his wife Tara are the co-authors of *Herbs for Spiritual Development*; an excellent book about tonic herbs and how it can help one achieve radiant health and longevity. **(R 238)**

According to Romarishi, the ancient sages were students of Nature and of the human body. They were scientists who conducted research on the body, mind and spirit in an attempt to maximize their functioning. After thousands of years of research, the sages of antiquity discovered that there were three basic energies in every human being. They called them Jing, Chi, and Shen. The three support the sages in their ability to reach a high spiritual attainment. The philosophy behind the usage of them has come to be known as The Three Treasure Philosophy. Romarishi refers to it as China's greatest gift to the world. According to him, there is a Chinese phrase that states that "The Three Treasures are the Entrance to the State of Conscious Immortality." The beautiful Chinese phrase is Jing Qi Shen Xuan Guan.

Jing is our essential or primordial energy;
Chi can be thought of as our everyday energy and
Shen is our spiritual energy.

When the three energies are flowing in harmony our mental, emotional, physical and spiritual wellbeing is attained.

Herbal tonic elixirs can be purchased at https://dragonherbs.com. You can call and talk to an Herbalist or Master Herbalist for free. I have taken the Ginseng Sublime, Supreme Shen Drops and The Eight Immortal drops. (Eight Immortals is a supertonic antiaging formulation of the highest order.) All of the herbs in this extraordinary tincture have antiaging, immune strengthening, spirit lifting, mind strengthening qualities and have found them very helpful in supporting my health (body, mind and spirit).

I also drink their Spring Dragon Tea. It is touted as the healthiest tea in the world. I drink this tea daily as part of my health routine and find it quite relaxing and refreshing. It contains Gynostemma or what is known in China as Magical Grass. In 1972, Japanese researchers discovered that many Chinese octogenarians drank this herb.

I also drink tonic herbs and find it very holistic and supportive to optimal health.

Besides the herbal tonic elixirs, Romarishi extols the benefits of **Reishi** and **Chaga**. This is what Romarishi wrote about them:

"When I was the apprentice of Master Taoist Herbalist Ron Teeguarden, I discovered the profound health promoting effects of two mushrooms in particular, Reishi and Chaga. I take Reishi and Chaga every day of my life. I consider these two mushrooms to be essential for my health. When

Tara and I went with Ron Teeguarden to the Shaolin Temple in China, he invited us to accompany him to a meeting with the head of herbal medicine. As we entered the Medical Clinic, we noticed an altar with a statue of Buddha. On the left of Buddha was a large Chaga mushroom and to Buddha's right was a large Reishi mushroom. This indicated how highly revered these two mushrooms are at the Shaolin Temple.

"I take both of them as part of my health regime. Reishi is a great herb and adaptogen and has anti-aging properties. Chaga is known to have anti-inflammatory properties and supports our immune system. Just in the last century the Chaga mushroom's antiviral, antimicrobial, anti-inflammatory, anti-cancer, cardio-protective, and antihyperglycemic properties have become more widely known."

I take Cordyceps which is also a great adaptogen. It has some anti-aging properties and also gives me more energy. A friend of mine, Joycelyne Lew, takes **Reishi** and **Cordyceps** religiously. She has taken it for years and looks many decades younger than her age. She is extremely active and doesn't seem to need much rest. She takes a special blend made by Gano.

Jay is a friend of mine who is a Molecular Scientist. She was ill for a long time and could not find any help from her physicians. She went to an Herbalist in Berkeley, California who gave her some Reishi from Galen's Way. After taking it for some time, she regained her health and now swears by it. According to Jay, the best Reishi can be purchased online at: https://www.galenswaystore.com/.

Another herb, **Haritaki**, is known as the King of Herbs in Ayurveda and Siddha Medicine. It detoxifies the digestive system, increases the glutathione levels in the body and increases energy. It also supports brain function and contributes to our longevity. It is also used as part of Chinese medicine. Romarishi, I and many other health conscientious people enjoy this as part of our health regime.

Strategies for Stress Management to Facilitate Longevity

Stress is probably the biggest threat to our longevity. Although much of what I have written about earlier will help deactivate the production of the stress cortisol, there are additional methods that we can employ as well that tone our vagus nerve to activate the parasympathetic nervous system to support health and turn off our body's production of the stress cortisol which if left on will shut down our immune system.

According to Dr. Deepak Chopra, we can stimulate the vagus nerve to promotes a relaxation response and can do so by putting cold water on the face, singing, chanting, doing mantras, yoga (especially Cat Cow, Downward Dog and the sun salutation); meditation, social interaction where there is a lot of exchange of love, compassion and empathy; breathing slowly and deeply; breathing in for a count of four, then pause one or two seconds, then breathing out for the count of six; laughter, probiotics, exercise, massage, fasting, lying on right side while deep breathing, acupuncture, acupressure, eating a high fiber diet, and taking a little dose of sunlight every day. **(R 239)**

The Japanese People on Longevity

Japanese people have been known to have good health and longevity. Some say it is because of their seafood rich diet full of health omega-3 fatty acids. Others point out the high consumption of seaweeds that help by supplying a good source of protein, iodine, and potassium. Some research seems to indicate that it helps to regulate estrogen and helps with PMS. Then there are those who say that all the *karaoke* that they do helps with cardiovascular health and dealing with stress.

According to Ryu Okada, Japan's people are known to have a long-life expectancy. One of the reasons is food. Fermented food and drink are a part of Japanese traditional food.

What researchers are finding is some people are living longer in certain countries like Okinawa, Japan. They have found that there are a lot more centenarians there. What the researchers determined was that there are a lot of common denominators:

- People who are able to walk live longer.
- Most of these people are still engaged in culture and society. They still have "meaningful work in life." They are contributing in their community.
- They live in an environment of a community where people care about them and they care about each other.

- The researchers mentioned how their plant-based diet contributed to longevity as well.

Experts on Alternative Methods to Improve Health and Wellness

I believe that mastery of the **Wim Hof breathing** can contribute significantly to our health, well-being and longevity because it strengthens our immune system, alkalizes our bodies and improves our thermoregulators for health. It also helps with stress management and pain. The cold shower or bath part of the Wim Hof method helps with inflammation, immune system, circulation and our mood as we discussed earlier but it also helps to activate the vagus nerve to bring more calmness to us. Many beauty experts advocate doing it for improving our skin and hair.

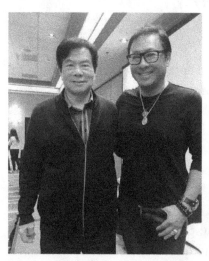

Mantak Chia with Blake Sinclair

Grandmaster Mantak Chia, a Taoist Master, talks about activating our **second brain – the mesentery.** The mesentery is a contiguous set of tissues that attaches the intestines to the posterior abdominal wall in humans and it is formed by the double fold of peritoneum. This aids in storing fat, allowing blood vessels, lymphatics and nerves to supply the intestines among other functions.

According to him, it controls all the digestion, absorption and elimination. By activating the second brain, we can increase our energy and overall wellness. In his video, he teaches exercises his viewers how to do this by instructing his viewer on a few simple exercises. I highly recommend studying his technique from the video or study directly with this great master and teacher. The one technique activates the cranial and sacral pumps to move the spinal and brain fluids as well as activating the Qi energy and flow. Grandmaster Mantak Chia believes that sickness occurs when those fluids do not flow.

In another technique, he teaches the viewers how to activate their energy centers such as the chakras and the Dantian which is in the abdominal area, to promote increased energy. **(R 240)**

I practiced some of the techniques I learned from the workshop Grandmaster Mantak Chia taught in the Bay Area for helping with digestive and stomach issues. I just massaged my abdominal area with some pressure in a circular fashion. It helped to release some of the trapped gases within me to provide instant relief. He believes that trapped gases in our organs lead to compromised health.

I also practiced his energy meditation technique and found it helpful for giving me more energy during the day.

Interview with Alexis

Alexis, her alias, is a parapsychologist and one of the top three Medical Intuitives to the stars according to *Billboard Magazine* a few years ago. She stated that there are many things we can do for longevity. She will elaborate more in her own book, but was willing to share with us a few important things that affect our longevity. These include stress, biochemistry (vitamin, mineral, amino acids (collagen and protein), and detoxification. However, like all health issues that arise, she would do a comprehensive session to assess the individual's issues to determine what the four feeders of the dysfunction are from the context of problems or reasons in the following areas:

- Physical (is there a bone spur, is there a hiatal hernia, etc.)
- Metabolic reasons (how your body metabolizes or utilizes vitamins, minerals and amino acids and etc.); It also includes looking at the metals in the body.
- Emotional
- Spiritual

She stated during our interview the following: "I am a big fan of basic biochemistry...especially in the alternative field there is a billion supplements out there. Everybody is overlooking just basic biochemistry. Because bodies just do not go wrong for no reason. In my work it's bringing the simplicity back to the body that has really supported me as a healer. Bodies go wrong for a few reasons:

- There's something in it that doesn't belong there and that needs to come out.
- Or there's something in there that you do not have enough of or you have too much of."

She further stated that "all diseases start at the gut." She sees a magnesium deficiency as a cause of colon issues for many of her clients. She also stressed the importance of liver health on how it affects our health.

Many clients, including medical doctors, see that Alexis offers a high level of success even those for whom traditional methods have not worked. Her treatment methods are quite comprehensive, holistic, individualized, eclectic and effective.

Dr. Alex Feng stated that there are four components with regard to health and longevity:

1. Elimination. Input includes environment, nutrition, personal relationships and spiritual connections. Elimination is physical, emotional and psychological.
2. Do you get enough sleep? Enough is defined as awakening and feeling refreshed. It may vary by person and across time. Accumulation of yin in sleep allows for healthy yang energy, for awake activity. According to Dr. Alex Feng, "sleep is the Ying that allows the Yang to be born; it is the nutritional component of life." When asked about how many hours of sleep is necessary, he replied, "it is not the hours but it's the quality; so I always ask my patients not how long they sleep, but do they wake up refreshed."
3. Are you having enough mental, physical movement in your body? With regards to mental movements, he believes that human beings need to be stimulated mentally. Studies have shown that when you play a musical instrument, learn a different language, do a crossword puzzle, or engage in things like mathematics and physics, your brain seems to be more functional, effective and more creative. You want to engage the mind as well as the body. Physical movement should not lead to exhaustion

4. Having a good attitude. Stay away from things that psychologically or emotionally injures you."

Dr. Feng believes that those four areas cover methods of self-care of longevity and give your body enough energy for life. He further stated that Chinese Medicine believes in upholding what we call Zheng Qi - upright energy, essential energy and constitutional energy.

Keeping these energies intact gives us access to Life Force. From that your body will take care of illness. The four components strengthen Zheng Qi (正氣).

He further said there are genetic issues involved as well and influences that affect our health and longevity with regards to illness and diseases but mentioned how modern science and traditional medicine are trying to address that. They are now doing in vitro DNA healing. They are doing some good research in this area. They can pull out cells, and they can play with cells in different ways and reinject it into the body. So, there are different ways you can look at genetic issues and try to resolve genetic problems. There is another whole new science that is involved in it, especially in Western medicine.

He mentioned that there are those in Chinese medicine who are doing research in China on meditation's effects on the Telomeres (which is your definition of your longevity). All this is at work!

According to **Lou Corona**, dubbed **the healthiest man in the world**, there are 4 principles that were shared to him during a near death experience that was quite Divine and Mystical. During his NDE, he was surrounded by White Light and a Divine or Ascended Being was at his presence and taught him 4 very important principles that saved his life and cleared all his health ailments. The principles are quite relevant to what we have discussed in this book thus far and will benefit all of humanity to help us attain a 'healthy and vibrant life."

1. Cellular Communication- He talked about the importance of clearing the emotional radar and dealing with past issues, and ultimately altering our way of thinking to become powerful individuals. He discusses the importance of listening to our body and possibly using muscle testing to tune into what we need.

2. Spiritual- "Maintain an attitude of gratitude. Stay present to the beauty and love of living."
3. Mental- "Recognize we are electrical, infinite beings with spirit. Every experience is a lesson and an opportunity for us to grow and learn."
4. Emotional- "Learn to love life, be joyful, radiant, accepting and non-judgmental of ourselves or others, and create peace and harmony everywhere. Embrace prayer, meditation, and communication."

I was extremely touched by his interview at puralive.com/healthiest-man-in-the -world-creates-puradyme/. I was touched by his spiritual journey, conviction and vision for the world which is to help humanity in shifting its current paradigm. I find Lou very spiritual, conscientious, loving and is quite sincere and passionate. I support his vision and have already placed orders for his Enzymes. They are essential to improve the digestive process. "Enzymes cause the body's biochemical spark responsible for life." He further stated that "when we eat 'live', enzyme-rich food and add enzymes back into our diets, we change our experience and begin a life addicted to living."

Darshan Baba on Longevity

Darshan Baba offers the following suggestions for increasing our longevity. Become Mindful of how you use your Energy.

We can notice that some habits, ways of thinking, speaking etc. use energy. While other actions and habits may take energy to perform, but actually generate or return to us more energy than what is spent in the action. The key is to first become AWARE, or mindful of our Energy and how we are using it.

Start eliminating unnecessary habits which are a drain of Energy. Slowly and systematically eliminate ways of being and habits which are simply wasting or draining our energy.

Overbalance your expenditure of Energy with actions, habits, and ways of Being that Increase your Energy and Frequency of Higher Realm Energy. Examples of these energy increasing actions include the practice of Tai Chi, breathing exercises like pranayama, visualizations, connecting with the energy of nature, etc.

Channel Super Intelligent Light into your Life through:

- Blessing the water of your bath or shower and charging with Super Intelligent Light and Energy Frequencies.
- Charging the water you drink with Super Intelligent Light and Energy. Also turning the water to an alchemical elixir for healing, longevity, and immortal nectar through mantra, intention, and/ or visualization.
- Before eating express great gratitude. Then charge the food just as you would your drinking water with Super Intelligent Light and Energy - calling mantras for immortal elixir, siddha medicine for immortal light body or visualizing the same. So, the food is also seen and transformed into "Kaya Kalpa" immortal light, yoga body, siddha medicine.
- Singing to call in the Living Force of Super Intelligent Light and Energy. This can be singing in your own language. Such as "Infinite Light, Infinite Light, Super Intelligent Infinite Light...", or mantras, especially mantras which call upon and invoke directly the forces of Divine Light.
- Connect to channel and allow the Super Intelligent Light Energy to flow throughout the body through visualization, conscious breathing exercises, and sitting or moving meditation.

Further information about utilizing Super Intelligent Light to Charge food and Water:

This calling Super Intelligent Divine Light is really just a matter of Intention. Darshan Baba uses some simple Mantras.

Siddha Rama Linga Vallalar's: "Arut Perum Jyoti, Arut Perum Jyoti, Thani Perum Karunai, Arut Perum Jyoti - Omniscient Super Intelligent Supreme Grace Light, Omniscient Super Intelligent Supreme Grace Light, Come Now Supreme Light of Compassion, Omniscient Super Intelligent Supreme Grace Light of Life".

Darshan also uses simple Light Mantras he has received directly from Spirit such as:

305

"Om Sarva Siddhar Jyoti Om - Shining Here Now Illumination of the Enlightened Intention of All Perfected Masters Combined."

One can visualize the water for bathing, drinking, and food we eat being filled with a Living Super Intelligent Light. This Divine Light is the Light of Life itself, Realization, Love, and Presence of the Perfected Masters.

We can chant these Mantras mentioned above, or say affirmations in our own language such as:

- I Call the Super Intelligent Divine Light of Love - All Life as One.
- I call the Infinite Light Here Now into this [Body, Water, Food, etc.]
- Shining Here Now! Illumination of the Enlightened Intention of All Perfected Masters Combined.
- With each and every breath the presence of Infinite Super Intelligent Light of Life and Love increases within each and every cell, molecule, and subatomic particle of this body.
- Expanding space filling with light, expanding space filling with light, expanding space filling with light.

Utilizing this power of intention and visioning within the mind, Darshan Baba charges food and water as Kaya Kalpa (a legendary immortal elixir or medicine of the ancient Siddha Masters). Simply intending and seeing it in the mind's inner vision to be happening, combined with the use of Light mantras as mentioned above.

Longevity and Sleep

Sleep is also very important for our bodies to recover and heal. It is during our sleep time that our bodies can most easily be in a state of receiving the energies that promote healing. In addition, the body can place more attention on healing itself since our other body systems are in a greater state of relaxation.

According to the Sleep Foundation, the average young adult (18-25) and adults (26-64) need 7-9 hours of sleep. Older adults (65+) may need

7-8 hours. Individual needs vary but lack of sleep will make it harder to achieve harmony of the body, mind and spirit.

According to Dr. Alex Feng, it is not the hours of sleep but the quality.

4-7-8 breathing

This method, pioneered by Harvard-trained Dr. Andrew Weil, is described as a 'natural tranquilizer for the nervous system' helping to quickly reduce tension and allowing the body to relax and to quickly reduce tension facilitating sleep more quickly. For no more than four total cycles, the count is as follows:

- Breathe in for 4 counts
- Hold breath for 7 counts
- Exhale for 8 counts

I recommend that you watch the video of Dr. Weil as he demonstrates the details of the breathing process. **(R 241)**

The hormone **melatonin** is also beneficial in aiding us in our sleep. Melatonin is made by the pineal gland (part of the endocrine system), and assists the body in knowing when to sleep and when to wake up. Some people's body's make less that than is required to support an optimal sleep cycle and therefore supplements can be helpful.

Andrei stated that Pharma GABA can be quite helpful for aiding people to relax allowing them to sleep better.

I have met many people who suffered from insomnia but have benefited from **Terrific ZZZ***. It does not contain melatonin or valerian. Rather it is made up of various essential oils and is quite effective. I and two of my family members have tried it with incredible results. I wake up feeling refreshed after taking it the night before. **CBD oil** can be quite effective with helping give support to those who have insomnia.

Benefits of Sun Gazing

Sun gazing in the morning on a regular basis can help us sleep better as well. What is sun gazing?

Sun gazing is described as gazing at the sun during the safe hours i.e. within first hour after sunrise or the last hour before sunset when the sun's rays are most gentle, UV is zero or very much less, therefore it doesn't damage the eyes. It is done barefoot thereby taking in the earth's energy as well. **(R 242)**

Why do it? Here is what they have to say about it:

- Stimulates the Pineal Gland as the sun's energy moves through the eyes and charges the hypothalamus tract, which is the pathway to the rear of the retina leading to the brain.
- Powers the brain and boosts production of serotonin and melatonin (the feel-good hormones).
- Relieves stress and tension.
- Activates the third eye and perceive higher dimensions.
- Increases energy levels.
- Increases the size of the pineal gland – Normally, as we age, the pineal gland shrinks. However, brain scans of Hira Ratan Manek (HRM), a long-term practitioner of sun gazing, showed that this 70- year-old man has a gland three times as big as a normal man.
- Reduces hunger pangs since body is nourished by the sun.
- Improves eyesight.
- Opens the energy channels or Nadis (Ida and Pingala) in your body.

It's important to note that the process of sun gazing is begun with 10-20 seconds per day, slowly building over time as your eyes and body become more acclimated to the process. For more information about technique I suggest you explore the above link.

Intermittent Fasting and Longevity

When we do intermittent fasting the body is raised into repair mode. As discussed in Chapter 11, there are several types of intermittent fasting. Dr. Michael Mosley, founder of the 5:2 Diet (a type of intermittent fasting), believes that intermittent fasting can extend our lives. He had reversed many of his illness through this method and his method has helped many people improve their health throughout the UK and elsewhere. His method is probably the most flexible intermittent fasting method because it allows you to eat normal five days a week but eat ¼ of your calorie for two days a week while doing intermittent fasting.

Other intermittent fasting methods are done daily and can be quite challenging for many. In one method, the individual fast for 16 hours and then eats sensibly during an eight-hour period. In another method which is harsher, the individual fast for 20 hours and eats for 4 hours. It is important to always consult with a physician to see if this method is good for you or not. **(R 243)**

So, we see that the methods for achieving longevity are many but are achievable with some hard work and dedication. I feel that the purpose of longevity should not be one of vanity, but rather that we choose to live longer to be able to be of service to God in helping others to live with greater peace, health and harmony. When we learn to serve others is when we finally learn to live. By helping others, we help ourselves.

Longevity Tips from a Master and Siddha

Below are other things we can do to attain longevity from two of the currently known longest living people in the world:

One of the longest living being in our planet lived to be 200 years of age, (although other sources say that he lived to 256 years of age) His name was Master Li Qing Yuen. He was teaching classes of longevity in his late years and outlived his 14 wives. When he was 130 years of age, he met a 500-year-old Taoist while traveling in the K'ung–T'ung Mountains. Li asked him the secret of longevity, and the Taoist taught him an exercise called Ba-Kua (eight trigrams) exercise, similar to Tai Chi Chuan.

According to Romarishi, Li Qing Yuen stated that his good health and longevity were the results of three things: being a vegetarian, maintaining inner peace, and drinking Goji Berry tea. According to Andrei, he also took Panax Ginseng.

Li's other secret to longevity can be summarized by his motto- "Keep a quiet heart, sit like a tortoise, walk sprightly like a pigeon and sleep like a dog" in order to insure a truly long and healthy life."

Li also attributed meditation to helping him achieve longevity, as he would also sit in meditation for a few hours at a time. **(R 244)**

Most recently, Romarishi and Tara, met with a well-known spiritual master, Maha Ananda Siddha. He is 130 years of age and was full of energy and vitality. His mind was in good shape despite not eating any food. It is said that he produces honey and milk from his pineal gland that sustains him.

This nectar is known as **Amrita** - the liquid of immortality. It is like nectar and it exudes from the Chandra center in the center of the head, deep behind the eyebrows. The juice is salty, similar to ghee, with the consistency of honey which drips down the back of the throat during certain advanced meditation practices.

> 'Who swallows this clear liquor dripping from the brain into the heart and obtained by means of meditation, becomes free from disease and tender in body like the stalk of a lotus, and will live a very long life.' ~ Hatha Yoga Pradipika. **(R 245)**

He may have practiced an ancient Indian art called Kaya Kalpa which has its origins about ten thousand years ago in India. This practice includes a special diet, breathing techniques, ritual herbal baths and being anointed with sacred oils.

Maha Ananda Siddha is also practitioner of Kriya Yoga meditation which was originally given to humanity by Avatar Babaji. Paramahansa Yogananda has his Kriya Yoga lineage traced back to this great saint. When Tara Leela, co-author *of Herbs for Spiritual Development*, asked this great saint what was his secret to longevity and his response was brahmacharya (or celibacy), also just an intense, persistent focus on God and elevated thoughts. **(R 246, 247)**

A Medical Perspective

According to Dr. Paul Hannah, MD., Psychiatrist, Intuitive Professional Speaker, author and Lac, the following are some important things for attaining longevity.

1. **Stress Management** – he feels that relaxation and getting rid of the stress is very important and that it is the number 1 cause of diseases. It causes so much inflammation and manifests itself in multiple metabolic diseases, chronic disease and cancer. So, number one is to manage your stress.

2. You must **have a purpose in life**. You must have a purpose that you really enjoy. It helps to know what your gift is.

3. **Make sure you function from a higher standard of Love and Truth**. Let your actions be based in love and service. Serve with compassion.

4. **Plant-based diet**- Many of the centenarians I know and have talked to, eat a very simple and healthy meal that includes whole grains and plant-based food.

5. **Being Active**- Take care of your temple. If you do not maintain your body, it goes through what we call atrophy and it deteriorates. It is important to be active. Being active keeps your hormonal system in sync. That's why you see some people in their 70's, 80's and 90's still running, going on marathons, having sex because they are still active and their hormones are active. A lot of people get old because their hormones are not functioning due to their lack of activity.

6. **We need minerals and enzymes**. We live in the United States and much of the soil has been demineralized. We are not getting enough mineral and enzymes. We need them to make sure you have the catalytic responses in our body. I do believe in supplementation but number one if you can get it from organic things, certified organic would be better. The reality with people living in this country compared to people in Costa Rica is that supplementation is very important. In Costa Rica, they do not need to supplement themselves because they have plenty of organic things growing all around and they can readily eat it.

Dr. William Sears, M.D. has written one of the best books I've ever read about health and wellness that is based on good science. He teaches us how to regain good health by activating what he calls our internal pharmacy to create a '**fountain of youth**' through activating the endothelium within the blood vessels. He does this by teaching us the essential skills and wisdom for wellness. He teaches us how to optimize our health through L.E.A.N. (Lifestyle changes, Exercise, Attitude and Nutrition).

His book is called *Prime-Time Health.* by William Sears, M.D. and Martha Sears, R.N. Little, Brown Spark Hatchett Book Group, 2010.

Qi and Longevity

One of the most important things in sustaining longevity is improving the amount of Qi we have and utilize. Certain exercises harness the Qi, while others exhaust it.

Yoga, Tai Chi and Qi Gong are the best exercises to help support a long vibrant life versus hard work outs, but other exercises that affect Qi may help as well.

Dr. Feng mentioned a doctor by the name of Lin Hsien from UC Irvine who has been doing research in trying to identify what Qi is and what it is not. Dr. Lin Hsien used three criteria to identify Qi: 1. Blood flow; 2. Warmth of the body; 3. Electrical output. He has a measurement to be able to do that.

He has discovered that when you do slow repetitive movements like Tai Chi, Yoga or nurturing movements then you have those three characteristics improve in your body; you get better blood flow, better warmth in your extremities and you have more electrical output from the body. When you do aggressive kinds of work like triathlons and running, you actually do not get the effects that slow nurturing movements could give you.

I clarified with Dr. Feng then that it doesn't necessarily mean we have to do specific Tai Chi movements but as long as we do the slow movement patterns. He responded that the key thing is slow and 'nurturing'. "There is a component of nurturing involved. It is a meditative concept. You say to yourself, 'I am with my Qi, I am getting better. I am doing all these exercises to improve myself.' It is part of that mental construct as well as self-healing.

"So, if we understand what constitutes Qi in the body and realize that slow, repetitive and nurturing movements affect it, then we can be creative with myriad exercises that can activate that Qi for health and wellness.

However, Tai Chi, Yoga and Qi Gong are systems that have all perfected the art of activating the Qi in the body and learning from a qualified instructor can ensure we are cultivating our Qi to its optimal level."

Cutting Edge techniques for Health and Longevity

Stem Cell Therapy

There are two other things that we can do to optimize our wellness. One is **Stem Cell Therapy.** I had the privilege to interview David Granovsky, a stem cell expert, advocate, advisor, blogger, and author. He has been in the field for about 12 years. According to him, it can help a host of diseases and health issues including sports injury, health and wellness, vascular issues autoimmune diseases, congestive heart failure, strokes, Parkinson's Disease, ALS, spinal cord injury, autoimmune diseases, inflammatory diseases, pain management, Alzheimer's Dementia, immune system, degenerative joints, liver damage, etc. **(R 248)**

He is aware of many seemingly miraculous cases where the impossible becomes possible. They include the following improvements with a patient's condition which include but are not limited to the following: a patient who had spinal cord injury and was wheelchair bound began to walk after a series of stem cell therapy; one 11 year of girl cut off the tip of her finger but was able to grow it back with stem cell therapy; client's with stage 4 Congestive Heart Failure improved two to three stages; damaged organs like the liver begin to regenerate. Japan is doing research on improving wet macular degeneration.

He stated that the limit to what stem cell can do is almost limitless but each person's response to it is unique. He stated that "you have the potential to heal every part of the body. He also stated that in one company he worked they use to say "you do not fix the disease. The disease is like a runaway train. First you slow down the train; then you stop the train; then you reverse the train. It's a process that requires patience.

"Some people do better than others. Although results vary, many people are being helped by it." He stated that most of the conditions like Parkinson's disease, ALS and Alzheimer's disease have shown positive response to stem cells but are the hardest to treat. "You need more treatment longer."

"It is my understanding that stem cells can help in two ways: it helps to decrease inflammation and it helps to regenerate new cells. Although much of the early research was done with bone marrow, embryonic and fetal cells back on the infancy of this new field and created much moral controversy, now however they have figured out how to get it from our own blood, umbilical cords, urine, iliac crest, adipose fat from our stomach and buttocks, nasal passages, and breast milk as well.

"Stem cell's ability to become an organ is quite remarkable. Stem cells from blood can become arteries or the heart while stems cells from our urine can even be used to make a tooth. Interestingly enough, in one research stems were sent to the heart but in 50% of the cases, the stem cell did not concentrate on regenerating or repairing the heart; instead, the stem cell went to repair the pancreas instead resulting in the individual's improvement of the individual's diabetes."

It seems as though it has a Consciousness and directs where the help is needed and tells the stem cell to become what it is via the messenger cell.

"Stem cells can be injected into the body via IV intravenous, intrathecal (within the spinal column), and intra-articular (within the joints). The response to the treatment can happen within one week or a month.

"Things that help create a positive environment for the stem cell to proliferate, multiply and activate include the usage of vitamins and minerals infusion and hyperbaric chamber. Stem cell and hyperbaric chamber (2 atmospheres of pressure) really love each other. They both assist each other. Also, each one separately is very good for Autism, Alzheimer's and what have you but when you put them together it is even better.

"Some of the issues with stem cell therapy might include dizziness, infection, low grade fever and pain. However, David points out that the pain is not long lasting. Pain is from injecting stem cells through the spinal column or joint. Overall, it seems like a viable option to improve one's health."

The Apo E Gene

The other cutting-edge method for health and wellness is with our **Apo E gene**. The Apo E gene was discovered in the early 1970s. Depending on which variation of Apo E gene one has, one may be more predispose to certain illnesses and diseases.

There are three Apo E gene variations, or genotypes, that occur naturally in Humans: Apo E 2m Apo E 3, and Apo E 4.

Since genes come in matching pairs-we each have two copies of every gene, one from each parent, there are six possible paired combinations: Apo 2/2, 2/3; Apo E- 3/3 and Apo E- 4/2, 4/3, 4/4.

For optimal health, you need to match your particular genotype with the most gene-supportive environment (GSE) you can create. You do that through what you eat, how you respond to stress which is largely determined by how you think. **(R 249)**

By eating the proper food and diet for your Apo E type, you may decrease your risk factor of contracting certain illnesses that include Alzheimer's disease and heart disease. A friend of mine has a family history of dementia and with her Apo E gene type, she was at high risk for heart disease and dementia. However, she proactively went to get help from an integrative medicine Nurse Practitioner and was advised to follow a nutritional protocol to decrease her risk factors. After years of being on that diet and taking certain supplements prescribed to her, her heart risk factors had improved significantly and she still lives alone, drives and able to carry an intelligent conversation for a good length of time and shows little to no signs of dementia as well.

On the other hand, the Apo E gene can impair good health if the body is given the wrong foods and other gene-unsupportive environmental (GUE) situations.

Below are conditions that Pamela McDonald, Integrative Medicine Nurse Practitioner that has found **exceptional** success with dietary change related to an Apo E genotype: **(R 250)**

- acne
- gout
- depression
- chronic pain
- high cholesterol
- hypertension
- multiple sclerosis
- anxiety
- fibromyalgia

- insomnia
- glucose intolerance
- arthritis
- diabetes
- alcoholism
- ADD and ADHD
- cardiovascular disease
- severe premenopausal symptoms
- chronic obesity
- insulin resistance
- menopausal symptoms

In the 1990's, Dr. Shealy first discovered 5 rings or energetic circuits in the body including the rings of: Fire, Earth, Crystal, Water and Air.

Each of the rings has been proven with biochemistry and clinical outcomes.

- **Fire** - may enhance DHEA, the most important hormone for health and wellness.
- **Earth** - may enhance Calcitonin, for stronger and healthy bones.
- **Crystal** - may reduce Free Radicals which cause premature aging.
- **Air** - may increase Neurotensin and Oxytocin, the Neuro-chemicals that give you the feeling of bliss and sense of well-being.
- **Water** - may normalize Aldosterone, which helps with fluid balance as well as with emotions.

The combination of the 5 rings has even greater benefits including helping to regrow Telomeres, the tail ends of the Human DNA for Health, Longevity, and many other benefits.

Shealy-Sorin Wellness demonstrated that using guided imagery and vis-ualization of these rings can enhance the effect of the rings and may even result in similar benefits to the ring application.

Dr. Shealy has 5 MP3 downloads that can help improve each element or ring of energetic circuits. **(R 251)**

My Perspective I AM Wellness Method

Now that you have heard about what some of the experts have to say about health or longevity, this is what I like to share with you to help simplify things and make it easier to understand, follow and achieve.

I believe that there are many great systems out there for health and wellness like the ones for Traditional Chinese Medicine, Ayurvedic Medicine and those systems of other sacred and ancient cultures. Most of these systems in general look at our wellness holistically. Each are different perspectives and frames of reference for restoring harmony to the individual but most take into consideration the body, mind, feelings and spirit, each having its strengths and limitations.

So, rather than focusing on those systems, I will now present my perspective in a way that ties in all I have written to this point, into a system that is easy to comprehend and follow.

As a precursor to this discussion, I will state that I feel it is important to get a complete annual medical to assess all our body systems. Ideally this will include a complete blood workup (including a heavy metal test) to assess if you have any pathology or deficiencies in the body especially with minerals. If an imbalance or other challenge is discovered, you can take this as an opportunity to learn as much as you can from your doctor(s), and from doing your own extensive research about all the possible ways to restore your body to health and harmony. After you have identified any issues and have researched wellness programs with your doctor or healthcare advisor, I feel you are then ready for optimizing your wellness.

It is equally helpful to see a Traditional Chinese Medicine practitioner or other Holistic practitioner to assess the Qi flow through the various organs or assess any blockages in the various chakras or deficiencies that affect their respective organs.

Earlier in the book I mention about the different bodies that we have - physical, emotional, mental and spiritual. They make up our **sacred multi-body temple** gifted to us from God. While our emotional, mental and spiritual body is eternal, our body temple withers with time. However, it will age more gracefully when we are happy, full of joy and have a passion for what we do. It also can grow old beautifully and gracefully if we give it the proper care, love, nutrients, food, minerals and hydration it requires.

Our various energetic bodies and our Earth body temple are affected by five elements in the Traditional Chinese Medicine system. They are earth, wood, metal, fire and water. However, in my system that I call **"I AM" Wellness Method**, we focus on four elements that we are comprised of - earth, air, fire, and water. It also includes the fifth element (metal element) but I discuss it in a different way than Chinese Medicine. I will explain it in way that may be different than other systems but it is what I was guided to share with you what works in conjunction with the U.U.M.M. system. Let us get more into depth what each system is:

Earth Element

The **earth element** includes all the food, vegetables, fruits, minerals, fibers, probiotics, vitamins and anything we can get from Mother Earth. It also includes Mother Earth, her beaches, mountains and nature as a whole. It also deals with being grounded (Earthing), in oneness, safety and being focused. **The proper amount of vitamins and minerals** in the **body is very important** in providing the essential environment to be conducive in allowing the Divine Presence to create optimal harmony within.

The Gut and the **digestive system** are part of the Earth Element and needs to be maintained with a proper ratio of probiotics to have a healthy flora. I consider this flora the **Garden of Eden** within our body. Due to the digestive system being the basis of the body's immune system, taking good care of it with proper probiotics, prebiotics and good amount of fiber will bless you with a good system, elevate how you feel on an ongoing basis and help give your body all the nutrients it needs from the food and fruits you eat. **Our Gut Health Is One of the Pillars of Health and Longevity.**

Part of that gut health involves activating the energy centers in our Dantian and promoting the flow of the organs blood and Qi via exercises, Energy Meditation, Qi Gong or Chi Nei Tsang. This is part of the Earth Element and also the Fire Element in my method.

In addition to pro and prebiotics, **Herbal Tonic Elixirs** are an important part of the nutrients from Mother Earth that support our body, mind and spirit.

Supporting the Earth Element can be done by eating organic fruits and vegetables and taking only those minerals, supplements and vitamins that are deficient in our bodies. Taking care of our gut and elimination systems are also very important. It is also important to spend time with nature and Mother Earth to balance our body, mind and spirit. Time spent in nature could be done in meditation but additional benefits are reaped by walking in nature, and Earthing on a daily basis. Meditation especially with U.U.M.M. can connect you to the earth element.

Water Element

The **water element** includes the water we drink, the water in fruits, the water in our bodies, including our blood, cerebrospinal fluids, urine, our circulatory system, lymphatic system and any other liquids in our body. It also includes any body of water on earth like ponds, lakes, creeks, rivers and oceans. It represents wisdom, cleansing, purity, transformation and the flow and integration with life. Water is also conscious and will react to our thoughts and emotions. It is important we choose positive, divine and noble thoughts to be in alignment with our Divine nature.

The **Spleen** and the **gallbladder** are part of the earth element as well. According to Ron Teeguarden, the spleen controls gastro-intestinal functions and generates qi, blood and bodily fluids. The Spleen is also responsible for the distribution of the chemical, fluid, and energetic constituents of food to all the appropriate parts of the body. (**R 252**)

Supporting the Water Element may be done by drinking only high-quality water that is filtered well enough to remove most or all toxins and contaminants. It is important to activate the water with fresh fruit juice, or minerals if the water is deficient of natural minerals due to processing in order to hydrate the body to allow health and wellness to be optimized. Since water is conscious, we can further activate the water we drink with our thoughts, energy and vision to empower it with our prayers, decrees or affirmations.

It is important to flow like water until you become one with the source of all life. Flexibility, adaptability, forgiveness, letting go, immortality, birth and rebirth and balance are important with this element. Issues with this element may lead to stress, fear, illness, weakness, low Qi and anxiety. Learning to surrender to your I AM Presence will bring greater integration, peace and harmony. (**R 253**)

<small>A New Beginning</small>

The kidney, bladder, reproductive organs and the lymphatic and circulatory system are part of the water element.

Qi Gong, U.U.M.M., Tai Chi, Yoga and Kriya Yoga supports this element. Chi Nei Tsang Massage and some of Grandmaster Mantak Chia's exercise are also very effective in moving the fluids and Qi through the various organs and spinal canal.

Fire Element

The **fire element** includes the kundalini energy, Qi, pranic energy, temperature of the body, the thermoregulators, and all electrical impulse in the body. It also includes the Source, Sun and anything that generates heat and warms the body. This element represents the passion and dynamic energy in life. At the core of all the energy is the Divine Spark of Light or I AM presence which is anchored to our heart. Our heart, in my opinion, is also the center of our **third brain**-the **Cosmic and Divine Brain** that animates our entire being.

Supporting the Fire element can be done by maintaining a healthy body temperature at a degree that is normal for you. Normal range is from 97 degrees F to 98.6 degrees F. Of course, there are variations. Higher ranges may be indicative of an infection while lower ranges may be indicative of an illness or hypothermia. **(R 254)**

The circulation of **kundalini** is important for wellness. Learning to activate and harness the Qi in the body through slow nurturing movements and the practicing of the Wim Hof Method supports this element. Practicing the Wim Hof method activates the thermo-regulators in our body and thus is associated with the fire element as well as the water element.

Living life passionately, having fun, playing and being creative also activate the fire element resulting in the promotion of health and wellness. Practicing the Wim Hof Method, including taking ice baths or cold showers, sun gazing, and meditating in the sun activates the fire elements or thermoregulators. Practicing Qi Gong, Tai Chi, or U.U.M.M. activates, supports and illuminates the fire element. Regular aerobic type of exercise can also be very supportive to brain and heart energy and health.

320

Herbal tonic elixirs like The Eight Immortals, Qi drops or Ginseng Supreme may be quite helpful for the supporting the Three Treasures of China (The Jing, Qi and Shen energy). Spices such as ginger, cinnamon, and various peppers can also assist in bringing the fire element into balance within our bodies.

The heart is a part of the Fire Element. Activating the **Divine Light anchored to it illuminates the Light and Energy of God's Love, Energy and Consciousness in its individualized form. The brain** is part of the Fire element due to millions of electrical activities of the neurons. The **pineal gland** is also part of the Fire Element and helps us see through our third eye, generate melatonin for sleep and in advanced Yogis or siddhas create spiritual nectar called Amrita to sustain life. Living out of Divine love, compassion, service, kindness, mercy, and forgiveness further supports this element by adding fuel to that Divine Light within that illuminates. Those that are clairvoyant as well as animals can see that light.

The **mesentery system and Dantian,** because of its ability to store energy, per Dr. Mantak Chia, is a part of this system. He calls it our second brain.

Although the **kidney** is part of the Water element, I include it in the fire element also because according to Ron Teeguarden, Master Herbalist, the kidneys are the great reservoir of energy for the entire body. **(R 255)**

Air or Wind Element

All aspects of Spirit are a part of the air element. The air or wind element includes the air we breathe and our breath. It includes our mouth, nose, lungs and respiratory system.

The Air element also represents the I AM Presence or the expression of one's truth or true nature. In the air element, the I AM Presence is expressed through basic breathing and vocalizations, especially when we utter words in alignment with love, compassion, kindness, mercy, forgiveness and open mindedness. When we sing Divine or positive songs, chant sacred mantras, pray out loud, do yogic breathing exercises and meditate, it further supports the expression of our I AM Presence.

When disharmony arises in the air element, respiratory illnesses like asthma, respiratory infections or other more serious illnesses may develop.

If we work towards resolving any grief issues, that would keep our lungs healthier and support our air element.

Supporting the Air Element can also be done by breathing in clean purified air, marine air or air in nature and then stilling the mind and being one with the breath to experience the oneness with our Divinity and true nature.

Purchasing a high-quality air purifier can improve your ability to breathe, sleep and meditate. It may also result in many other good health benefits.

I have a **Coway Airmega 400 Smart Air Purifier** that I find quite effective for clearing the air. It covers 1560 Square foot area and has a True HEPA filter that clears the air up to 99.97% of particles 0.3 microns in the air, including pollen, pollutants and other allergens. It also reduces more than 99% of volatile organic compounds and reduces fumes such as NH3 and CH3CHO. It also includes washable and permanent pre-filter to catch larger dust particles. **(R 256)**

I suggest adding an **air humidifier** in the home or room to give more moisture since I find that air can be a little dry when using my air purifier. A **vaporizer** during the winter is also very helpful according to Dr. William Sears. He recommends running a warm-mist vaporizer in our bedroom. It helps with adding humidity to our nose during dry winter months and it is also a healthy heat source. He wrote that "Steaming sterilizes the water." **(R256.5)**

There are also plants that can help purify the air and remove some of the toxins in the home. With regards to how to detoxify or purify the air of your home, Neha Kandwal, Environmentalist and Eco-blogger, has written that there are 12 plants that Nasa has recommended to help purify the air in our residence. They include:

1. **Areca Palm-** it helps to remove dangerous chemicals like formaldehyde, xylene and toluene. Best placement: Livingroom (**Note: nontoxic to dogs and cats** according to the American Society for the Prevention of Cruelty to Animals).
2. **Snake Plant-**removes benzene, formaldehyde, trichloroethylene, xylene and toluene. Best placement: The Bedroom (**Note: not pet friendly**).

3. **Money Plant**-removes benzene, formaldehyde, xylene and toluene. Best placement- any room (Note: **not pet friendly- keep away from children, cats and dogs** since it is toxic if ingested).

4. **Gerbera Daisy (Gerbera Jamesonii)** removes benzene and trichloroethylene- Best placement: The bedroom (Note: **safe with pets).**

5. **Chinese Evergreens**- removes benzene (found in varnishes, floor finishes and detergents), formaldehyde and other toxins. Best placement: The living room (**not pet friendly-toxic).**

6. **Spider Plant**-removes carbon monoxide and xylene. Best placement: the bedroom or the living room (**Note: pet friendly but if a cat consumes it, the cat may have digestive issues, diarrhea or vomiting).**

7. 7. **Aloe Vera**-removes formaldehyde and benzene. Best Placement: Any window sill or any well-lit corner (**Note: not pet friendly).**

8. **Broad Lady Palm**- can help reduce ammonia in many cleaning products. Best placement: The bathroom, the entrance or the Living Room (**Note: pet friendly).**

9. **Red-edge Dracaena or Dragon Tree**- helps to remove trichloroethylene and xylene. Best placement: a place where there are high ceilings. A well-lit corner of the living room or balcony (Note: **Not pet friendly).**

10. **Weeping Fig**-reduces formaldehyde, xylene and toluene. Best Placement: The balcony or a well-lit corner of the living room (Note: **not pet friendly;** can cause dermatitis).

11. **Chrysanthemum**-filters out a host of toxins including ammonia and benzene, which is often found in plastics, detergents and glue. Best Placement: Kitchen and Living room (**Note: not pet friendly;** toxic to pets).

12. **Rubber Plants (Ficus Robusta)**-their large leaves can absorb airborne chemicals and break them down. They also eliminate bacteria and mold spores in the air. Best placement: The living room or bedroom (**Note: not pet friendly). (R 256.5)**

For more info, you can check further at https://medium.com/@ iamgrenfield/12-nasa-recommended-airpurifying-plants-that-you-must-have-in-your-house-8797645054b9

It is important to breathe positive energy and exhale and release negative energies. Most importantly, we must get enough rest to nurture all the elements to be in good flow.

Qi Gong, Yoga, Tai Chi, walking, U.U.M.M., the Wim Hof Method and aerobic types of exercises are good for this element.

Metal Element

In Chinese medicine, the metal element is affiliated with the lung organ. Though is true I am discussing about it as not one of the original elements that we are comprised of but as a foreign byproduct of our ego perpetuated reality and not part of the original Divine plan we were created with. As we discussed earlier, there are good metals that we need for our bodies but there are also many toxic metals that we bring into our bodies through the food we eat, the water we drink and the air we breathe.

It is all around us and none of us can avoid it unless you live away from civilization like many Siddhas, spiritual masters and gurus. Once it is in our bodies, organs, tissues and brain, it generally stays and wreaks havoc especially when our immune system is shut down because of prolonged stress activated by the stress hormone cortisol in our body.

Viruses like the Epstein Barr Virus feed on it and their fecal waste and deceased bodies cause inflammation and pain in the body as we have discussed earlier. With this element, the individual needs to be more **mindful of the metals all around them and take methods to minimize exposure and do regular detoxing to release it.**

A discussion with your physician and holistic health practitioner can help guide you on what to do once it is determined that you have a certain metal toxicity. Hence, **regular fasting and detoxification is necessary in this day and age to rid the body of many of the heavy metals that compromise our health and wellness.**

However, minerals are a type of metal that is needed for optimal body function. They include: calcium, chromium, copper, iron, magnesium, manganese, molybdenum, potassium, sodium, and zinc. They are all important in creating overall health and wellness. A deficiency in any can lead to illness or disharmony in the body. More information about each mineral can be found at this Harvard study. **(R 257)**

Wellness revolves around the interplay and balance of the five elements and ridding the body of as much toxic metals as possible that is affecting our health. Remember, some metals like mercury may require a very specific protocol to release it from our bodies safely, so do your research. In releasing metals, it is important to have both binders and chelators to help remove the metal from our body versus being deposited elsewhere in the body.

Rest and sleep are also very important in supporting us in recharging our mind, body and emotion. The health and wellness of the four elements plus how much metal is within us will affect how the spirit is manifested within us. Disharmony of the one or more of the elements plus a surplus of metals will make it more difficult for the Divine Presence to create optimal health and wellness and may lead to illness, diseases and premature mortality.

Although I identify the five different elements, the reality is they all overlap each other and are interconnected by the Light of life that is animated by the Divine Spark of Light within or the I AM Presence by way of the meridians and nadis - energetic highways. These life force energetic highways are distributed to the various organs from associated chakras, and give us the blessings of wellness and harmony when there is no congestion and obstruction of energies. Also, it is important that although I wrote about how the Divine Presence exists in the Heart Element and the air element, it exists also in the Earth and Water Element as well. In the Heart, the I AM Presence exist as a spark of light of the Individualized aspect of God's Consciousness that illuminates, radiates and communicates with us from the core of our being.

How to use the "I AM" Wellness Method

When having issues in life, think in terms of the five elements of how you can attain harmony in your body again by activating the Divine Presence in all the elements. For instance, consider if you had a cold. Think of how to get well. With the Earth Element, there are many very good vitamins and supplements you can take to get better. Part of the earth element is also taking care of the gut which is 80% of the immune system. Also, ask yourself if you are you grounded enough, if you are not then you should work on grounding yourself more.

With the Water Element, one can make sure one is drinking enough fluids along with minerals and trace minerals (earth element) to make sure you are not dehydrated. Also, ask yourself if you are you like the water in its flow, nature and adaptability. Are you easy going or headstrong? Learn to be like water and your body, mind and spirit will thank you for it. If you hurt someone, learn to forgive them. If you did something wrong, learn to forgive yourself. You can further activate the Water Element by praying over a cup of water (with healing herbs like echinacea) with healing energy from your hand; afterwards, drink this blessed water for healing. This is a great way to further bring in the water element for healing.

With the Fire Element, it helps to activate the thermoregulators by practicing the Wim Hof Method. It will also help strengthen the immune system. Learn to tune in to your I AM Presence (Fire Element) for guidance on what you should be doing to get well. It may many times prompt you to rest, since you might be too much on the go or it may tell you to see a doctor.

Also, are you being kind and loving to yourself and others? Take time to nurture yourself and have fun with yourself and others. Too much work, will bring on the Yang energy and will lead to stress and melt downs. Rest and sleep are very important in recharging our body, mind and emotions.

With the Air Element, are you saying words that disempower you and keep you sick? Instead of saying I am sick, say something like I need some rest so my body can recuperate and recharge; I am well; I am harmony and I create more harmony now by doing…., etc.

Say words that empower your healing or make a decree of healing like "I AM the Presence of Archangel Raphael filling me with healing Love, Light and Energy." Part of the Air Element is resting so your breath can attain that rhythmic flow again and nurture the body, mind and spirit. If you are not congested or coughing, practicing Yogic breathing exercises can help to decrease the negative stress you might have and help speed up the recovery time.

The "I AM" Wellness Method is not set in stone but serves as a preliminary guide to giving the body, mind and spirit a surge of healthy support to allow the Divine Presence to be activated and mobilized to do what it does best- create harmony, peace and wellness. It takes into consideration the balance of the 5 elements and the 3 Brains working together in a loving and nurturing way.

Most people who are striving to be healthy will be tapping into the elements superficially by eating well and exercising but will have little to no regard to Qi, the Three Treasures, the Divine Spark of Light and the spiritual energies. In order to truly be in complete harmony and wellness, it is of key importance that we embrace the importance of them as well.

Many of the exercises that people focus on nowadays focus on speed or weight lifting for aerobic workouts or strength training. That is not a bad thing in itself but if that is the only thing for health and wellness then the essential part of health is missing. Furthermore, I wrote earlier in the book about very athletic and so-called fit people who suddenly drop dead. I alluded to the excessive loss of minerals as one possible cause.

Fitness and longevity do not go hand in hand especially with those who are weekend warriors who do extreme sports. Those utilize too much yang energy can deplete the bodies of excessive minerals. Sports drinks are unable to give us the sufficient minerals we need. Exercises that are slow, rhythmic and nurturing support our Qi and I AM Presence.

With regards to the Air Element, the modern exercise regime activates rapid breathing. But slower yogic breathing is needed to support Qi development and the movement of energy around our body for wellness, but certain fast, rhythmic breathing can even activate the thermoregulators like it does with the Wim Hof Method and offer many health benefits.

Yogic and meditative breathing techniques activate our parasympathetic nervous system and vagus nerve which are essential for dealing with stress.

It is important that we understand that what we are aiming for when thinking of the five elements within the context of the "I AM" Wellness Method. We are aiming to utilize those methods to activate Qi, spiritual energies and the I AM Presence in each element. The more we understand that, the more we can use this model to support that Divine Presence to bring about great harmony, peace and wellness within as well as without.

The "I AM" Wellness Method is a system that directs the practitioner towards connecting with his or her Divinity in creating that harmony within or what I call Heaven within. Adherence to the system and ensuring we take care of the five elements will significantly contribute to the longevity of the individual and allow the individual to live a fulfilling and enlightened life full of joy, meaning and purpose. It important that the three brains (brain, heart or heart chakra and gut, the inner of Garden of Eden) within our system are working together in unity and harmony for the best outcome of our health and wellness.

Besides the five elements from the "I AM" Wellness Method, the U.U.M.M. is a key component of activating wellness and healing of the self and others.

U.U.M.M. meditation supports all five elements. It utilizes the breath work, visualization and mudras to activate the kundalini energies to move through spiritual highways and canals in our spine affecting the air, fire and water elements. Its connection with Source, Sun of God and Mother Earth activates the fire and Earth element. The successful completion of the meditation practice allows all the elements to be activated to create a heavenly and blissful realm within as well without to those around your energy field.

Through U.U.M.M., the various chakras are activated and opened to allow the Divine Presence to flow cosmic and pranic energies from the Universe to the associated organs to support health, wellness and harmony.

The chakra system is very important in wellness and harmony. They are the energy vortexes or what I call sacred and spiritual temples situated from our tailbone to the top of our head. There are 7 basic chakras but there are actually more than that; there are chakras at the base of the soles of the feet, palms of our hands and further above our head as we have discussed earlier. However, I find that by keeping the 7 chakras activated and open, great health benefits can be experienced. We have described each chakra's attribute in the chapter on meditation.

Each chakra has different energetic attributes. How we support our five elements can affect whether the energy going through the chakras are blocked, stagnant or free flowing. What we say, do, feel or think affects whether or not our chakras are active and able to support our various systems and organs. In other words, our mental and emotional body affects our chakras for better or worse. Saying, doing, feeling and acting in alignment with God's Love opens the chakra. Conversely, saying, doing, feeling and acting in alignment with your ego may adversely affect the chakras, leading to their being blocked. Besides meditation, energy healing can also open blocked chakras but awareness, insight and integration of the problem will raise your consciousness to higher heights and help you to attain greater mastery.

Maintaining a balance of the five elements, minimizing the amount of heavy metals in our bodies and keeping the chakras activated and open through U.U.M.M. will support the mental, emotional, physical and spiritual body.

When issues are more complex, I find it very enlightening and insightful studying or following the Traditional Chinese Medicine 5 Element Theory and understanding the relationships between their associated Five Organs. Through understanding it thoroughly one can start to unravel the complexities of our health and wellness. It is beyond the scope of the book to get into depth with that system but having a general understanding of the emotions that are stored in our organs it can be quite insightful.

Each one of our organs represents a different emotion in Chinese medicine as we mentioned earlier in the book. The liver may store anger; the spleen may store worry; kidney may store fear, the lung is associated with the metal element and according Ron Teeguarden, it is associated with the ability to let go of the old while learning the lessons contained within experiences while the heart represents the Shen, the guiding spirit. When the shen is "shaky" or "disturbed," any emotion can become dominant. Frequently, a person whose shen is disturbed will experience agitation, nervousness, heart palpitations, insomnia, dizziness and fainting spells, uncontrolled laughter and grief, hysteria, deep sadness, fright, and mumbling to oneself. **(R 258)**

Those who want more of an in-depth system to learn about the relationship between organs and the about the five elements in Chinese Medicine may want to learn more about Traditional Chinese Medicine. One good book I highly recommend is ***The Ancient Wisdom of the Chinese Tonic Herbs*** written by Ron Teeguarden, Master Herbalist. Or you may choose to study with healing and wellness experts like Grandmaster Mantak Chia or Dr. Alex Feng.

The TCM (Traditional Chinese Medicine) practitioner or acupuncturist can examine the flow of energy in your body to assess whether your yin or yang energy is weak. If your yin energy is weak, you may age faster and your body's ability to heal may be impaired. If your yang energy is weak, you may have low back pain, energy and libido. **(R 259)**

Besides all the wellness methods I shared with you, there are other important **Principles with the "I AM" Wellness Method** and they include:

1. **Protection** – In order to keep ourselves strong and healthy, it is important to recognize the various ways that negativity of the physical, emotional, mental and spiritual variety can seriously impact our body, mind and spirit. It is important to take measures to protect our physical bodies as well as our auras and energy fields in order to be able to be our optimal selves and fulfill our divine purpose. (*The next chapter goes into more detail on the tools and methods for protection.*)

2. **Visualization** of your body and organs being well - When we visualize, pray and make decrees for wellness, we activate the Divine Presence or I AM Presence within us to direct healing light and energy to that body part of organ that needs healing. This is done during part of U.U.M.M. but may be done outside of it as well. I visualize my organs being in state of bliss and happiness to support my organs' health.

3. It is important to realize that the **connections of the I AM Presence exist in all five elements** and that all living things in our body and organs are conscious. We can talk to it and enlist its support in recovery. I was once very sick with a bacterial infection. I could barely breathe, I prayed to the bacterial infection to leave me and thanked it for teaching me how I must have more balance in life and have more rest versus work. I also made a decree to raise the bacterial infection's consciousness to a higher realm to evolve and ascend it to transform into a higher consciousness and become an enlightened bug so to speak – a love bug. One that infects everyone and every planet with a highly contagious love infection. After I made the decree, I visualized the bug leaving me and evolving, Suddenly, I was able to breathe normally again and slept well the rest of the evening and recovered.

4. Many of our stem cells are located on the rim of our belly button. According to Marian Brandenburg, we can visualize activating those and bringing them where they can be used to heal. Earlier in the book, I wrote about the stem cells and how they seem to have a consciousness and have the ability to heal, reduce inflammation and regenerate. You can also make a decree to try and activate the stem cells from your body to heal yourself with it. You can visualize and even talk to it to create or manifest whatever your body needs.

5. **It is important to have a balance of work, play, leisure and rest** Too much work can cause us to have a meltdown or be overstressed; too much play may exhaust our financial resources for the rainy days; too much leisure may result in many important things in life not being taken care of. Lack of rest may result in a deficiency of yin energy and lead to poor health and wellness.

6. **Proper Body Mechanics** - how we sleep, sit, lie down, walk and move affect our energy flow, how well our body functions and how well we feel. If we are sleeping in an old bed that is sunken, it will affect our spine and internal organs. We may eventually be suffering from various problems including low back pain. If our shoes do not have the proper arch support, we can have knee and hip pain. If we sit on chairs that are too low, it strains our backs when we get up. If we spend many hours on the cell phone texting or browsing the internet or engaged in social media, we may develop neck pain or strain on the cervical spine which can lead to a kyphotic posture and may possibly lead to nerve compression and sensory disruptions. Proper body mechanic especially during meditation will allow the pranic energy to flow smoothly and allow us to experience greater peace and bliss.

7. **Creating Heaven on Earth and Beyond** - Attaining health and harmony of our body, mind and spirit is only the initial phase of our spiritual evolution and mastery. As we evolve further in our spirituality, we will realize that the beautiful Universe within exists without as well and replicates itself into the macro Universe and Universes. Mother Earth also has lungs, arteries, body as well as a soul and consciousness. She also has chakras around her sacred body situated all around our planet that have similar attributes to

the chakras within us. There is also a relationship between the Sun of God, Mother Earth, Moon of God, and the various planets and us. Practicing U.U.M.M. helps us to expand that healing energy to our household, community, city, Earth and beyond.

True spiritual mastery happens when we exist beyond being a passive participant to being an active God-Realized being who is co-creating his and her Universe within and without and manifesting peace, love and harmony. We can truly achieve heaven on earth within our inner Universe and radiate and expand that to those around us, our city, country, planet, and beyond.

8. **Cosmic Pebble of Change** - We must realize that Divine Consciousness exists in all matters great and small. Our bodies, planet and Universe is conscious and reactive to input. It responds to our thoughts, emotions and energy. If we release our collective emotions of fear, anger and negativity on our planet, it will react in a way to express that collective emotion in a myriad of ways from volcanic eruptions, floods, earthquakes, abnormal weather patterns and other calamities.

   a. If humanity continues to display its disrespect, harm and rape to Mother Earth, she may eventually react to reset the planet and start a new beginning. However, when enough of us care enough to gain our mastery in our ability to infuse Mother Earth and humanity with love, compassion, kindness, and healing energies, we can begin to create Heaven on Earth and manifest a New Beginning of Divine, Empowered and Enlightened Beings of Light, Love and God Consciousness. May we embrace our Divine Nature and realize how we are all part

9. **Wellness Optimizer** - We can create change by educating people of one Divine Body and Consciousness about nutrition, wellness and about their Divine Nature and how we are connected with one another and with Mother Earth and the Universe.

10. **Stress is a Part of Life to Empower us to Learn, Grow and Thrive** - However, too much bad stress over a prolonged period can shut off our immune system as we have discussed earlier. However, there are good stresses called eustress that are beneficial for us and if we learn from them, it helps us grow, adapt and evolve

mentally, physically and spiritually. Our brain, body, organs, and muscles need to be exercised and challenged regularly for health and wellness. Meditation, Yoga, Tai Chi, the Wim Hof Method and Qi Gong all provide various levels of challenge to our body, mind and spirit and helps us to keep evolving into greater health, wellness and spiritual mastery.

Harmony

When all is in harmony, health is attained and the gates of longevity is opened for all sentient beings and all of humanity giving birth to this new Heaven on Earth.

Balancing the five elements in my system and/or the five elements in the Traditional Chinese System, detoxing heavy metals and toxins, keeping the Qi flowing through all organs, keeping the chakras opened and sleeping enough should be enough to create greater harmony, peace and radiance within, with the ultimate goal of creating Heaven on Earth within us.

However, those of you who are still having issues – chaos or disharmony of body, mind and spirit – may need to consult with your Allopathic doctor (physician) or one of the following:

1. Naturopathic doctor (holistic healing methods)
2. Osteopathic doctor (holistic healing methods)
3. Traditional Chinese Medicine Doctor (holistic healing methods)
4. Ayurvedic Medicine Doctor (holistic healing methods)
5. Chiropractic Doctor (holistic healing methods)
6. Acupuncture Doctor (holistic healing methods)

Other specialists that you may want to consult with if you still do not have a good resolution of your problem or if your health issues become so complex include the following:

- A Functional Medicine Doctor or Practitioner
- A Medical Medium like Anthony William
- A Medical Intuitive like Alexis or Janet Doerr

Sometimes our health issues become so complex that we need a special and gifted Medical Medium or Medical Intuitive to help us to pinpoint precisely what is going on and helping us to set up a protocol of food, nutrients and supplements to help restore the harmony within.

Unless we are good at tuning in to our I AM Presence, finding a Medical Medium or Intuitive, or getting a remote scan, we can help ourselves by learning the tools and principles that will support us in the mastery of our stewardship of our sacred temple of God.

I want to share a few basic exercises that stand out to me as being what I call the Spiritual Workout program for those who are on the go and can't always make it to the gym, beach, park or nature. They are done to address the five elements to activate them and exercise them.

1. **U.U.M.M.** (The Third Chakra or Peace Meditation) - should take 30 minutes for basic level.

2. **Super Brain Yoga** (helps to activate the brain centers and helps the brain to integrate; it also gives your digestive system some work out as well). It can be done for few minutes.
   The simple 3 minute exercise can be found at: https://www.youtube.com/watch?v=KSwhpF9iJSs

3. **Wim Hof Method and Cold Shower** (the exercise itself can be done in a few minutes). Can help with activating the thermo-regulators, immune system and support the body dealing with stress and pain). Start with warm shower and towards the last minute or so, you can try turning down the temperature as tolerated until you can tolerate it. Slowly increase time as you as you are able at cooler temperature. Each day try to take cooler showers for longer duration until you can do it completely without heat. Only do this if you have taken the Wim Hof class or receive approval from you doctor to do it.

4. **Tai Chi Warm up exercise**- slowly rotate torso to the right and left and allow your arms to lightly sweep to the right and left as you do rotate. Sweeping in the direction of rotation. You can do this for a couple of minutes with a relaxed mind and say I AM that I AM, I AM Compassion that I AM, I AM Love that I AM, etc. This helps to activate the Qi in the body and give your digestive system a work out

5. **Weight Shifting on an Acupressure Mat/Earthing** to stimulate the acupressure points on the base of the feet to clear blockages of all the organs in the body. You can march in place while brushing your teeth and washing your face as well. It can be done for several minutes. However, doing it in nature and having your bare feet I contact with Mother Earth is the best to take advantage of the free electrons from Mother Earth via Earthing.

6. **Practice one of the yogic breathing methods** daily depending on what is going on with you. 1-5 minutes as needed. You can do it as long as you need it without affecting your clarity of thought or consciousness. I once met a man who did it for one hour a day.

7. **Practice Mantak Chia's Second Brain activation exercises** and what he calls energy meditation. An example can be found on YouTube: **(R 260)**

8. **Jumping on a Trampoline** can help in many ways, including helping the cells, heart, bone, core muscles, gut health, lymphatic drainage and immune system. But only do it if you have good balance and core muscles. Otherwise a light jumping jack program can be helpful.

9. **Jumping jacks and jumping rope** are excellent ways to get a good cardiac workout.

10. **A brisk walk** is a good way to exercise without taxing the joints.

11. **Yogic exercises or stretching** are important to keep us limber and flexible.

12. **Resistive training with weights or a theraband** is helpful in keeping our muscles strong and healthy. The latter is a safer way to strengthen and tone the muscles and can be easily stored in your case.

You can pick and choose which exercise or groups of exercise to give yourself an exercise from as little as 20 minutes to as much as one hour or more. Just pick the exercises you want to do at any given day. It is good to do some form of cardio exercise at least a few days a week and alternate other days with muscle strengthening exercises. Stretching, Yoga exercises, Qi Gong exercises and meditation are best done daily or at least 5- 6 times a week.

Exercise is the most important tool for wellness. It activates our cardiovascular, vascular, cellular, digestive, neurological and respiratory systems. Through exercising enough, we can actually turn on the endothelium (Dr Sears calls it the Fountain of Youth) to activate the release of nitric oxide or what is called the molecule of life. As we have discussed earlier, it will dilate, repair and decrease the stickiness in our arteries- all this leads to better heart, brain and vascular function. It also activates all 5 elements and helps us to minimize emotional, mental and physical and age-related issues. Exercise is the greatest tool for creating energy and repelling stress and depression. It also helps us with hypertension, pain, high cholesterol, diabetes, dementia and heart related issues. Talk with your physician, physical or occupational therapist, health or wellness coach of personal trainer on which exercises would be best for your needs and goals. Exercise is indeed an important part of longevity and a very integral part of the I AM Wellness Method.

Warning: If you suffer any low back pain, have spinal problem, have rotator cuff injuries or tears, have COPD, heart problems, equilibrium or vestibular disorders or other underlying medical issues, avoid any exercise unless you have a physician approval to participate with any physical exercise program. Depending on your unique needs, a physical therapist/ occupational therapist may be needed to help supervise the initial stages of the exercise program or modify it to ensure you are doing it correctly

I encourage all to make the time to do the following:

1. Yoga, U.U.U.M., Tai Chi or Qi Gong to balance the body, mind and spirit.
2. Sun Gazing.
3. Earthing in nature.
4. Swimming, dancing, and playing sports like Ping Pong.
5. Pray and have devotion.
6. Do something that gives you passion, joy and bliss
7. Watch a comedy.
8. Find ways to serve and help others, especially your family and friends.
9. Spend time doing some type of creative and slow movement exercise while saying kind and nurturing words to yourself.

When spiritual masters (Mystics and Yogis) talk about longevity, they are not so concerned with longevity than with fulfilling their dharma or life mission. They are only interested in living as long as they are needed on the planet. On the other hand, some Yogis have much to do in their lifetime in helping others so they are interested in longevity and engage in advanced spiritual practices that allow them to live beyond what is our current normal life span. Most spiritual masters are more interested in making sure they achieve high mastery that will lead them to ascension and transcend the laws of karma.

Some Taoist Masters are very much interested in the mastery of longevity as well as immortality. Historically, Taoist Masters have been able to achieve longevity through their spiritual practices and herbs and as you have read earlier can live even up to 256 or even to 500 years of age. However, Dr. Alex Feng, (also a Taoist Master and son of a well-known Taoist Master) warns us of the need to attain longevity. He sees that need or longing as a "desire". To me, desire can be an offspring of the ego if it is only for a selfish reason, however, if it comes from a pure intention and heart it reflects the longing of the soul for God.

When a Yogi, Arahant or Taoist Master has perfected complete harmony of body, mind and spirit and oneness with our Father or Mother who art in heaven as well as completed all their earthly duties, they can engage in spiritual practices to help them transcend death and karma in what we call Ascension. That is when they achieve what is called in Tibet the Rainbow Body (Small Rainbow Body, Medium Rainbow Body and Rainbow Body), Atomless body, or Light Body.

This is what was portrayed in *The Last Jedi* when Jedi Master Luke Skywalker, ascended at the completion of his mission in life.

He literally merged into his Light body and ascended into the next higher realm of reality and consciousness. He achieved a state of liberation and Ascension. Those who have attained this state of consciousness are able to move between realms of astral plane and the earthly plane like Saint Germain, Master Ajahn Lee, Sai Baba and many others who are known as the Ascended Masters.

The Nyingma Sect of Tibetan Buddhism has perfected this Rainbow Body phenomenon. Father Titov was even invited to observe a Buddhist spiritual master achieve Rainbow Body and wrote and talked about what he had witnessed. He saw rainbows and heard angelic voices during the Ascension. These Tibetan Masters practice a type of meditation called

Dzogchen Meditation. Their lineage includes Padmasambhava, the second Buddha, and many other great Yogis. After Padmasambhava ascended, he left physical carvings on the caves to give evidence of his ascension like many other saints. Many thousands of great Yogis practicing Tibetan Buddhism have attained Rainbow or Light body.

It is estimated that there are over 160,000 individuals from China and Tibet who have achieved some form of Rainbow Body already. Others have achieved what they call Vajra Body. In this phenomenon, the deceased body actually becomes younger over a 30-day period and also becomes hard like steel.

Many Buddhist Masters give evidence of their mastery and ability to achieve their Ascension, enter nirvana and transcend the laws of karma by leaving behind spiritual crystals or stone relics after they have been cremated. Relics are formed in the chakras of the Masters and are treated with great reverence by Buddhist Monks. Some Buddhist temples, Stupas and even Rinpoches have some type of sacred Buddhist Master's relics. These relics are not just the perfected remains of a spiritual master, they are something much more magnificent as I have had the beautiful opportunity to find out and experience.

Master Relica

I recently met a Buddhist Master who I will refer to as Master Relica, her alias. She is a Thai Forest Tradition Buddhist Master. She has a plethora of relics of various Buddhist Masters including relics from Buddha. She was given seven relics of Buddha by a Buddhist Master in Thailand who eventually attained liberation and ascension. She placed the relics in a special plastic container which was sealed.

Two years later, Master Relica attained great spiritual mastery. One day while she was meditating, she heard clicking sounds from the relic container and saw three orbs of Light entering it and began to notice that her relics had multiplied to 1,000 relics; It continues to multiply to this very day due to her mastery, merits and devotion to Buddhism. She has donated many of them to various temples and monks. Although she started with Buddha's relics, more and more relics of many other great Arahants began to manifest in her shrine. Sometimes they would manifest in a sealed container while other times they would manifest on an offering tray filled with flowers for Buddha.

The sizes range from a size that is smaller than a grain of rice to ones that are the size of a large walnut sparkling with crystals. What Master Relica notices is that sometime the relics that are given to people begin to disappear due to the recipient's life style. One individual lost all of her relics and later went to India and prayed that they would return and that she would change her lifestyle to be more spiritual and devoted to the practice of Buddhism. When she returned to the states, she was pleasantly surprised that they had returned.

Master Relica stated that in Thailand many of the Arahants were able to also manifest the relics but many have ascended already. I was given my first relic of Buddha in June 2018 by Master Relica. I prayed that I would be granted the opportunity to experience a physical manifestation of the relics multiplying as well.

After visiting Mount Shasta, Peter Mt. Shasta and a Tibetan Stupa there, I returned home and was flabbergasted to see that new relics had manifested in my sealed container on my shrine. I immediately notified Master Relica and she asked me to open the container and she verified that there were now 13 new relics that have manifested. What makes this even more interesting is that when I visited Master Relica's shrine a week before, she showed me the various relics she had at her shrine but I was drawn to the crystal ones from Buddha and the heart shaped ones from Pra-aa-non, the monk who was always with Lord Buddha. When I looked at my relics after they have multiplied, I was pleasantly surprised that the Universe blessed me with one heart shaped relic as well as some crystal relics from Buddha.

This supernatural event is extremely important because it helped me to validate my mystical and Divine experiences in physical form. It shows that these Ascended Beings exist, are conscious and are indeed somehow connected to these relics as well as the Cosmic Web that senses what is going on. These relics validate the ascension of the various Buddhist Masters.

Many great Masters throughout history have achieved some form of Ascension and they include but are not limited to Jesus, Kwan Yin, the Maha Chohan, Buddha, Yogananda, Sai Baba, Padmasambhava (the second Buddha), Saint Germain, etc. It is truly possible to achieve immortality in this lifetime. It only takes some hard work, effort, consistency and lots of love, compassion, service, helping those around us experience Divine Love and the preparation and integration of many previous lifetimes. Depending on the style the individual chooses to practice or learns for his or her Ascension or liberation, the outcome of the Ascension will vary. It is not important which style we choose but what is important is that we live a perfected, enlightened and fully self-realized life full of love and harmony of our body, mind and spirit. What is important is we reached a level of a Christ Conscious and God-Realized Being full of Light, Love, Compassion, Mercy, Forgiveness, Service and Harmony.

Mastery of meditation is very important with our liberation and is important in helping us navigate gracefully through the various phases and portals of Consciousness upon our physical death; successful navigation will lead to our ultimate freedom or liberation.

If we can navigate through all the chaos, toxins and illusions of our ego manufactured reality and have mastered the art of being one with our I AM Presence, we will be in an optimum level to transcend the laws of Karma and death. However, a life of Yogi is not only about self-empowerment and liberation but it is also about serving the greater good and helping others achieve the same. When we live for our own selfish wants and desires even though it may be for a noble and spiritual cause, we have not really lived if our lives are only dedicated to ourselves. Let us explore how we can further help ourselves and others achieve greater peace and harmony in the world. By helping ourselves and others, we are actually helping to unite our family and our collective consciousness to begin to dissolve the ego perpetuated reality and give birth to God's Love, Light and Consciousness to all of Humankind and all creatures great and small.

Before we go further with that, it is important that we are aware of some paranormal challenges that may be an obstacle to our health, harmony and spiritual evolution. I have written much about the Light in us and the Universe but there are also some dark energies and entities in our planet that are not interested in our ascension, well-being and mastery so it behooves us to be aware of it and learn how to deal with it. However, fear not for in the fullness of Light and Love, there is an absence of darkness. Learning the secrets of how to protect your spiritual fields and energies is all part of our journey towards greater mastery.

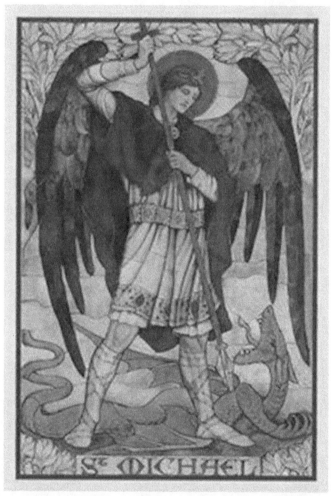

Archangel Michael Stained Glass Window Artist Unknown

CHAPTER 16

PROTECTION

The need for protection in our daily lives varies from dealing with other people's negative emotional energy and other negative influences through the media, technology, environmental pollution, physical traumas, accidents, disease, addictions, wars and natural disasters to physical and non-physical beings who seek to harm or control us.

We are constantly being bombarded by millions of toxic and negative news items, pictures, ads, commercials and energies from people. It doesn't take long before we start feeling fearful, angry, depressed and anxious. If we do not take measures to protect our auras or energy fields, we become a target of energy vampires or emotional atomic bombs that weaken our auras and can make us sick. It will compromise our abilities to help others as well ourselves.

Clearing yourself, your family and your home regularly with the Violet Flame is important. Clearing our personal life issues helps us stay in a positive frame of mind. Having a regular meditation or visualization practice, calling on the Angels for any needed assistance, setting our intentions to be safe and healthy, calling on the I AM Presence to hold a field of protection around you at all times and recognizing and avoiding negative people or situations whenever possible – all are valuable tools and can change a life of stress and fear to one of health, confidence and self-empowerment.

A number of people plug into others with an etheric cord to drain and take their energy. Most seem to do it unconsciously, but some do it on purpose. Empaths seem to be the most susceptible to this which can cause extreme exhaustion and can be a frequent problem, especially when around large groups of people, such as at parties, shopping or large events. Using Archangel Michael's sword to cut such cords and the Violet Flame to burn it back to its source is helpful in most cases. Spending a few minutes in gratitude can be a successful way to restore your energy after being drained.

People who overindulge in alcohol leave their fields open to attaching entities. This can also happen with the misuse of drugs. These can wreak havoc on their personal and work lives and make any addiction harder to stop.

Visiting hospitals, funeral homes, cemeteries and battlegrounds can allow those who have passed on and not made it to the other side to attach to us and cause a variety of troubles.

Many people very carelessly speak such negativity that it is actually a curse that harms people a great deal. Others intentionally seek to harm those around them. Lack of awareness of the reality of either cords, curses or negative entities, doesn't stop them from doing enormous damage.

People who practice black magic can summon elementals and demons to attack an individual or attach them with many entities. This can also occur with the misuse of drugs. The entities can silently break down and penetrate the auric field weakening the individual to become mentally, physically and emotionally ill or possibly even die.

Unfortunately, I have witnessed some very spiritual individuals being controlled by black magic. They were attached with entities and were totally oblivious of it. They were being secretly guided to live a life that keeps them trapped in maya, the matrix or an ego perpetuated reality. Some of these individuals have attained a very high level of spirituality but further growth has been halted by this process. Some are even used to promote teachings that are spiritually unhealthy. I have experience dealing with these matters, and hence I feel compelled to spend some time talking about this very important subject.

It is extremely important that we learn how to protect and shield ourselves. It is always a part of U.U.M.M. system to surround the practitioner with 3 layers of God's highest vibrational white light of love, protection, purity and perfection to keep the practitioner fully protected from the energetic and astral realms due to threats from negative entities and energies. Psychic interference from negative entities can occur. Learning how to deal with it with confidence and authority can be part of your soul's evolution. Included in this chapter are many tools and techniques to create a safe and sacred space and methods to work with angelic assistance to clear, transmute and protect you as you grow in the sovereignty of your Divine Nature. In extreme circumstances, you may need help from one with greater expertise.

For instance, if the individual has his or her auric field punctured by negative entities, the ability of the individual to protect him or herself can be compromised and limited due to the leak in energy or damaged chakra or aura.

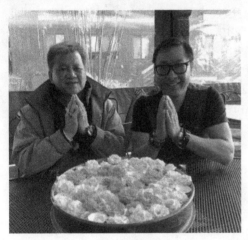

Felix Fojas with Blake Sinclair

Once the auric field is compromised and damage is done to various chakras, a specialized psychic healer will need to intervene and help repair the auric field and prevent further attacks.

Healers like **Felix Fojas** are the veteran spiritual warriors, Mystics, lecturers, teachers and healers that are able to effectively deal with such metaphysical matters and crisis. He is also famous exorcist from the Philippines (a Hollywood film has been made about his life and was recently released. It is called "Evil Takes Root".

He can remove any entities, including demons and neutralize its power. He then offers advanced spiritual rituals to prevent future attacks from a dark master. He is truly an authentic psychic healer who helps out of service to God and the **Ascended Council of Light** (formerly called the Great White Brotherhood).

Felix wrote a book about his extraordinary life called ***Supernatural and Beyond***. Few practice and understand the mystical arts like Felix. I am so blessed and fortunate the Universe has brought our paths together to help evolve me into a spiritual warrior as well, considering my own battles with entities and demons. Felix has been an important part of my awakening into my new role of a spiritual warrior.

Protection Tips from Felix Fojas and his wife Joanna Marie

- Fragrant plants or flowers are what should be placed around the house since the sweet scent is something that repels negative entities. Negative entities gravitate towards foul smells.
- Wearing special blessed amulets especially like those from the sacred Mount Banahaw in Philippines can be helpful and quite powerful. He once gave me an amulet he got from the mystical Mount Banahaw. It was made from an Amulet Master from that mystical mountain. Certain sacred mantras are said to activate it. It is carved from a mystical tree that protects the wearer from harm. Other amulets are also helpful like the St Benedict Medal and other esoteric pendants for protection.
- Listening to Gayatri Mantra by Sathya Sai Baba during your sleep can help protect you as you are resting. Chanting it three times will help as well.
- Books that can give you more instruction on how to protect yourself include the following: *Battling Dark Forces: A Guide to Psychic Self-Defense* and *The Eyes of Hierarchy* by Torkom Saraydarian; **(R 261)** and *The Supernatural and Beyond* by Felix Fojas. **(R 262)**
- If you have any objects that are infused with negative energies or entities, remove it from the house and bury it 2 feet deep. Soaking it in Holy Water can help (Alexis says that you can also put the objects in salt to neutralize it but best to get rid of the objects). Perhaps a combined approach might be even more effective.
- Prayers like the following can be very helpful: "*They Shall Not Pass!*" Decree by Elizabeth Claire Prophet of Summit Lighthouse. **(R 263)** Praying the Archangel Michael Prayer and Travelling Protection prayer "*Lord Michael before! Lord Michael behind! Lord Michael to the right! Lord Michael to the left! Lord Michael above! Lord Michael below! Lord Michael, Lord Michael, wherever I go! I*

Am His Love protecting here! Saying the *Lord's Prayer* is also very helpful.

- Calling upon Archangel Michael, Ascended Masters or other high vibrational beings like Sathya Sai Baba and Jesus can help.
- Asking Archangel Michael to Bind and Remove the entities is important. Otherwise they can slip away and potentially return or harm someone else. Ask that they be removed from the Earth and taken to their own right place for healing and transformation in the Highest Light of God.
- Always remember to refill yourself or the cleared space with new, sacred, healing light.
- Smudging a room with sage can help clear the negative energies. It should be done clockwise in a room 7x. As you enter the room call upon Archangel Michael to remove all that is not 100% Light.
- Tossing sea salt around the periphery of your house also helps to repel entities.
- Always cover your toilet after each usage; entities can travel through the sewage system and enter your house.
- During an active entity attack, affix pictures of protective spiritual symbols or esoteric symbols of protection on mirrors since that is also a portal of entry. Other places to post the picture is above the bedframe, in front of the bathroom door, master bedroom door and any other door with occupants.)
- When confronted with a demonic entity, a ghost buster, exorcist, or a specialized psychic healer who is well-versed in dealing with such matters may need to be consulted.
- Tawa, what Felix coined a Psychic photograph, may be used to verify the presence of an entity, element or demon. There are various forms of Tawa I have seen used, and they all seem to work. In **Beyond Imagination**, I wrote about the one that was used on me by an Albularyo, it was actually a Tawa made of alum. Others have used candle wax. Felix Fojas puts vapor rub on his client's third eye. He then utters a sacred, mystical mantra and places a bond paper over the third eye and gets an imprint. The picture can be quite startling and insightful but also may be quite disturbing.

It can reveal a picture of the entities or demons that are attacking an individual.

- Avoid purchasing antiques because it may be attached with negative entities. A Buddhist friend of mine once purchased a spiritual statue in India but after she got it, she became extremely negative and suicidal; she quickly gave it away and all negative thoughts went away. A client told me that her son did research on the occult and found that many times, those who practice the dark magic put a negative entity within a seemingly Holy statue in a popular spot.

- Unbeknownst to many worshippers, when they pray to the statue, they are actually praying to an entity within and giving more power to it. My client's son also found out that negative spells are often put in containers sold in antique stores. When a person purchases the item and opens it up, the negative energies and entities are unleashed. I have experienced this phenomenon from sacred pendants I have received. The entity was so powerful that it attacked my wife and wreaked havoc to my home until the pendants were removed from the house and depowered. My niece had purchased an antique piece but began having nightmares and began feeling very disturbed until her parents got rid of it. People like Felix Fojas are able to clear the entities from infused objects and neutralize it.

- If you suddenly fall in love with someone who is radically different than the type you normally like to date, try to think back if there was anything given to you prior to it. Love spells can be cast onto inanimate objects and renders the receiver in a complete spell of illusory love with the sender. It is important to properly get rid of all objects that were given to you. I also believe it is important to destroy or delete all pictures of the person who cast a spell on you. Just looking at the picture of the person may increase the likelihood of staying in the love spell.

- When going to historic places where there was lots of negative emotions, torture and deaths, always smudge yourself when you return home or where you are staying.

- Meditating with Mohan Ji's *Prayers for Protection*. The song *Siva Kavacham*, can also be uplifting and clear negative energies. You can find it on Spotify. **(R 264)**

Alexis – Views on Protection and Exorcism

Alexis, her alias, is a Medical Intuitive and also a modern Exorcist or what people call her - a Ghost Buster. She also makes a living clearing houses of dark entities or ghosts so that the owner can sell it. She uses a product called **Delete** to protect herself and recommends it to people who are constantly going places and meeting all sorts of people. It is an anointing oil that is designed to give us protection and a little breathing room from these malevolent forces, until whatever is going to happen, finally happens in this world. Delete is composed of nine essential oils in a base of high-grade almond oil. These work in a synergistic manner for this imbalanced state. It must be understood that the oils alone are not strong enough to do this work. It is the sealed frequencies that are prayers of protection in conjunction with the right oils in the right amounts that actually make this formula so powerful. **(R 265)**

Alexis also talked about taking Rosemary Salt baths to clear negative energy and entities.

According to originalbotanical.com, **spiritual baths** are exactly what they sound like: baths enhanced with spiritual power. They are a way to either infuse every inch of you with magic, or scrub away negative energy, illness, or bad luck. Cleansing baths are powerful tools for ridding you of unwelcome influences, while other baths can you attract love, money, success, or other blessings. **(R 266)**

She also talked about how we can avoid being attacked by negative entities by always allowing ourselves to be full of white light. Negative emotions like fear, shame, self-doubt, etc. draw the negative energies or entities to us. She stated that there is no darkness when there is light.

Note: *One of the ways to recognize the presence of negative entities is to notice that there is a significant increase in negative speech, emotions and behavior, chaos and/or extreme dirtiness.*

Protection Suggestions from Lori Guidinglight

My friend **Lori Guidinglight**, LCSW and Intuitive Healer, also has experience dealing with clearing houses of negative entities and gives the following tips in dealing with negative or dark entities:

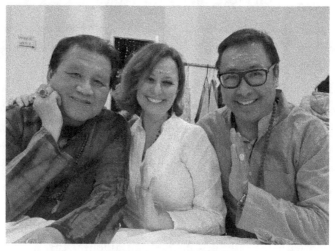

Felix, Lori and Blake

- Place fresh flowers throughout the house. They are sensitive to negative entities. The flowers wilting prematurely may be indicative of the presence of entities and further intervention will be needed. The flowers can help decrease the negative entity presence.
- Playing the YouTube video **Sri Lalita Sahasranama Stotram** can clear the negative energy in a room. I have done this in rooms with negative energies and entities and it shifted the energy significantly to more neutral energy.
- **Smudging** the affected **room with sage can help clear the energies but can be even more** effective when followed by smudging with sweet grass to add more positive and fragrant energy. Lori recommends also smudging the car, your body and pets when entities are suspected. See video on smudging at (**R 267**)
- Laughter helps shift the energy.
- Remove all things associated with negative energy or entities.
- Hug your loved ones and together pray for your **guides** and **protectors** to remove all that is not of the Light away then circle

both of you with extra love. She recommends **hugging** for 20- 30 seconds while bringing the two hearts in close proximity. She stated studies have shown that by doing that, the body creates **a** powerful hormone called **Oxytocin.** It acts as a neurotransmitter in the brain which helps you to create love bonds with the ones you love. It influences social interaction and sexual reproduction, playing a role in behaviors from maternal attachment to an infant, milk-release, empathy, generosity and orgasm. When people hug or kiss a loved one, oxytocin levels increase; hence, oxytocin is often called "the cuddle hormone" or "the love hormone." In fact, the hormone plays a huge role in all pair bonding. The hormone is greatly stimulated during sex, birth, and breastfeeding. Oxytocin is the hormone that underlies individual and social trust. It is also an antidote to depressive feelings.**(R 268)**

- Pray before each meal and pray or focus on blessing the food so that it can be energized and activated by positive thoughts and higher vibrational energies.
- Take an Epson salt bath. It contains magnesium to help to relax the physical body but it is also clearing the subtle body as well. A 1/4 cup - 1/2 cup of salt should be enough. She said it is best to soak in the bathtub for 12-20 minutes.

I recently met a very special woman, Michelle, her alias, who has a remarkable ability to communicate with angels but also sees dead people and lost souls. She gives the following tips on how to protect ourselves from negative entities:

1. Wearing amber, obsidian or tourmaline can be helpful.
2. Keep yourself clean - do not let other's baggage affect you; clear your vibes or vibrational fields (asks the angels to help **clear the energetic fields of negative emotions and thoughts**). Those negative thoughts or emotions create holes for entry for the entities.
3. Grow what is good within you. Do not focus on the bad. **Think about what is good and give it** power. She stated that we should allow compassion, love and kindness to grow within us.
4. Call for help from **Archangel Michael.**
5. Placing **selenite** under the bed or car seat can help clear the energies.

Star Santos speaks on Protection

I also was very fortunate to have a chance to meet and talk with **Star Santos** (Stargazer), a famous psychic, radio show host at ABS- CBN, as well as an exorcist and paranormal expert. She gave some important tips for protection against entity, hexes or demonic attacks:

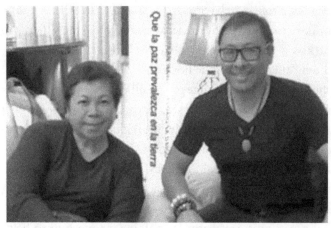

Star Santos with Blake Sinclair

- Call upon **Archangel Michael** for assistance.
- Wearing a **blessed St. Benedict's Cross, Medallion or Medal** can offer some protection. However, the cross should always be faced forward.
- The carefully arranged sequence of **specially picked protection stones** from Star Santos can be quite protective. Stones can be strung onto a bracelet and worn on the wrist. It is important that the beads or stone are touching the wrist to allow an energetic exchange to occur on the individual to cleanse the system and support the auric field for protection. It is important to wear the bracelet on as much as possible and it is **imperative to wear it on the right wrist.**
- It is important to **learn to shield yourself** if you do not have any protective bracelets or amulets. One technique is to visualize White Light to flow down the crown chakra, through your third eye, throat chakra, heart chakra and go through the root chakra down to Mother Earth to get grounded. Next, go back the spinal channels up to the crown chakra. Thereafter, imagine your body

covered with mirrors that repel and transmute negative energies but simultaneously absorb good and positive energy.

- Placement of **selenite, tourmaline and mica crystals in the four corners of the house** can give much protection with the occupants. Placing it around the bed can protect against attack during the sleep. Place rock salt in a bowl below where your head is, so it absorbs negative energies and bad dreams.
- It is important to surround yourself with white light before you sleep.
- It is very important that an individual avoids going to a funeral after an entity attack

Other Ideas from Lisa DeWitt

Another friend, **Lisa DeWitt**, offers a few important things to do as well:

1. Placement of a lime under your pillow for a few days can help. It absorbs negative energy and karma. Then take it out, cut it in half and throw it out. Be careful to wash the juice completely off of the knife and do not get it on yourself.
2. Vibhuti of Sathya Sai Baba (sacred ash miraculously created by Sai Baba) can be put on your third eye for protection and removing karma. Mikaelah Cordeo, Ph.D. relates that she once used it to close a portal to the lower realms, where entities continued to come in despite repeated attempts to close it. She stated, "I asked for Sai Baba's help and just rubbed the vibhutti on the wall where the portal was located. It closed instantly and did not re-open."
3. Tar Water can be used for removing negativity and is a spiritual cleanser. It can be purchased from eBay.

Protection Methods from Bella

Bella, CEO and Founder of Metaphysical Medium, Master Hypnotherapist, Life Coach, and Reiki Master, began her journey of being an exorcist unexpectedly, when a client of hers was possessed by an entity which began to latch onto her arm during a reiki session. (The entity appeared to be concentrated in the heart). She began to surrender and call out to the Universe for Divine assistance. Suddenly, Jesus appeared at the foot of the bed while

Mother Mary appeared behind her. Archangel Michael and Archangel Gabriel appeared as well as her deceased spiritually advanced grandmother.

Since this was Bella's first experience, she asked for guidance from all the Ascended Masters and her two favorite Archangels on what to do, **they instructed her to pray continuously.** She began saying the **Lord's Prayer** and the **Hail Mary** over and over again, and directed the energy towards her client. She began repelling the negative entity away from her arm and going down each chakra until she got to the heart. Suddenly, the Ascended Masters asked her to stop and she was directed to get some sacred tools; Bella was guided to get a cross, rosary, holy water, and other sacred and blessed objects from Rome to help her with her first exorcism. After getting the sacred tools, she began praying over the heart with hands on the chest, in a few seconds, the client's body literally shot off the bed in a state of levitation and a black entity exited the heart and was now in the room.

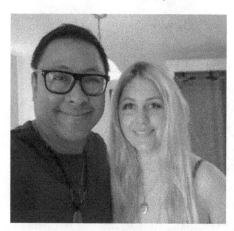

Blake Sinclair meeting with Bella

The Ascended Masters then gave Bella the exact words to say to banish the entity away from the house and planet. Bella literally could see the entity being repelled away from the house and out of atmosphere. Her client began crying profusely out of gratitude after the exorcism and no longer had any negative entity attachment.

Bella knows that if we surrender to the Masters and call upon them for help, they will help us and guide us on what to say and do. She said the most important thing is to **surrender and not be afraid since fear and limiting beliefs feed negative attachments of all kinds.** After many years of helping others, she offers the following suggestions for protection as well:

- **Make a proclamation or decree that your home is your sacred space** and that anyone who comes into the home has to abide by that or respect the sacred space. This is a spiritual concept that is commonly practiced in Hawaii. Bella stated that they do not use a lot of cleansing or saging because they do not feel they will be "attacked." They have a belief that they are Light and that if something is dark it cannot penetrate the Light.

This concept has a lot to do with intention: think about it, if you cleanse your house, do you want to spend your energy trying to "keep negative things out," or to "keep positive things in?" It's the intention that makes the difference. You can use the phrase "only that which matches my intention enters this space" for instance.

- From a psychological perspective, **consider how the unconscious mind works: it does not recognize negations or the word "not."** This means that if your intention is that you "do not want xyz," you are projecting into the universe that you actually "DO WANT xyz." Which is why people refer to the phrase "Energy flows where attention goes."

- "Keeping something out or away often requires low vibrations like hurt, anger, or fear. Another example is telling children not to touch a hot stove...9 times out of 10 they will reach for the stove after you told them not to because they are curious about it. What is it you wish to create for the space?

- "This is actually a very simple concept that many make much more complicated than it has to be. Every space is sacred, if that is what you choose to see, based on the Universal Law 'As above, so below. As within, so without'...because YOU are the creator of your reality."

- **Live in the Light 100%**, meaning avoid all sinful behaviors that do not feel as if they are totally in the Light, such as doing drugs, engaging in unhealthy or controversial sexual relationships with others, infidelity, hurting others, lying or being dishonest, or any other negative actions that could compromise your spirituality.

- **Solidify your aura and ground yourself.** Make sure your Aura is a clear blue line, 18 inches around your entire body, including below your feet and above your head. Grounding yourself pulls your soul entirely into your body leaving no room for entities. This connects it into the Root Chakra, as well as connects your Root Chakra to the stable Earth's energy (which comes from the Earth's core).

Note: there are a variety of grounding and protection techniques and with the new 5th Dimension energies transforming the Earth, even newer grounding techniques are emerging.

- **Surround your house or personal space (bed, office desk, chair, area of meditation, etc.) with sea salt.** You can put it across the barrier of the front door. The salt cannot be synthetic salt or Himalayan. Sea salt clears away all entities. You can also jump into the ocean and completely submerge your body in the naturally salty water to remove any negativity or entity attachments.

* * * * * *

According to my dear friend **Rob Thompson**, Host and Executive of Ghost Finders TV Series, Medium, Empath and Paranormal Investigator, one can help clear the house of negative energies and entities by doing the following:

1. Visualizing the removal of all entities and dark energies from the house.
2. Remove all objects from your house that were given to you which may have been cursed or activated via black magic to harm you. Toss it into the ocean. Throw it behind you over your shoulder without looking at it.
3. Smudge the house with white sage from top to bottom, room to room and including windows and door frames.

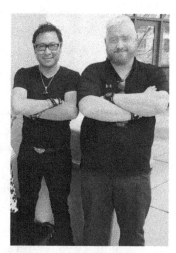

Blake with Rob Thompson

4. Put fresh cut white roses in every room.
5. Get a big bag of white salt and make a circle around your house with the salt. Make sure you so step one before closing the circle.

* * * * * *

We can also help protect ourselves by

- Meditating on a regular basis
- Serving others
- Praying and spending time in devotion
- Chanting sacred mantras
- Spending time with Nature
- Practicing random acts of kindness
- Singing spiritual or inspirational songs
- Hugging your loved ones for an extended time
- Volunteering
- Wearing high vibrational crystals
- Visualizing God's Love, Light and Energy filling you up
- Forgiving others releases us from dwelling in our lower mental and emotional body
- Listening to Christian, Buddhist or Hindu chants or prayers sung by beings of high virtue and spirituality
- Living in the fullness of God's Love
- Using of Metaform's 5-D Star Tetrahedron to help activate the heart chakra and help the user to reach higher dimensional reality. I have one that I hang down from the ceiling over my shrine and place of meditation. It is connected to a rotational device to further activate the cosmic energy and connection. It can be purchased at iconnect2all.com
- Placing or wearing an **I. Connect** in your room or wearing an **I. Connect pendant** to bring more balance in life. It is designed to provide a full range of integrative connections that enhance vitality, health and conscious awareness. Many people are connecting more to their "higher" self, experiencing joy, compassion, well-being, peacefulness, heightened meditations and physical improvements. **(R 269)**
- Placing a Sri Yantra symbol in your room can increase the spiritual energy and ambience of your room,
- Watching various aura cleansing videos can be very helpful. **(R 270)**
- Getting an Ajna Light and Neuro Light session can do wonders. Besides the above, I also wear a **golden obsidian bracelet** or various genuine **Thai amulets** of a famous Saint like **Khruba Siwichai** (he is well respected Thai Buddhist Master who is

believed to be a Bodhisatva with magical, miraculous power and has the ability to protect those who wear his pendant) which has been blessed by a Buddhist and Spiritual Master for protection. Many Thai people also wear high quality **Tektite** for abundance as well as for protection.

- A faithful adherence to your spiritual and devotional practices.

I also wear a sacred and powerful Timaru wood which is associated with the danda /staff of Shiva and is known to have protective powers banishing negative energies and entities. I got mine from Darshan Baba who blessed it before he gave it to me. He got this when he was in India from the forest of Haidakkhan and it was dipped in sacred waters like Kumbakonam Mahamaham Theertham which is said to contain the properties of all holy waters of India combined and blessed by Siddha Masters.

I many times wear crystal pendants and bangles blessed by Amma, the Hugging Saint, for protection. Things blessed by a Saint have high vibrational energy. A friend of mine who is a shaman, spiritual warrior and exorcist wears a Vogel Star of David pendant to protect him. It is made of amethyst. He gave me one during one of our mystical adventures at Mount Shasta. He purchased his pendant at Crystal Wings Bookstore in Mount Shasta. I usually wear mine during my pilgrimage to Mount Shasta.

Other forms of protection include **invoking or decreeing for Archangel Michael, Saint Germain and the Violet Tara's assistance in blazing the Violet Consuming Flame** to remove and clear the dark entity or energy.

Removing Entities with Archangel Michael and the Platinum Net

Dr. Mikaelah Cordeo, Ph.D., Mystic and Spiritual Teacher, shares this powerful method to remove negative entities or energies. "Call upon Archangel Michael (Say his name three times) and ask him to use a platinum net extending 300 feet below and 300 feet all around you (your house, work place or car) and then to pull up the net, **bind and remove** any negative beings and take away all the negative energy and entities away. Visualize the net being sealed and taken away by Archangel Michael and sent to their own right place for healing in the light for the highest good of all concerned.

Ask the Angels to refill the space with light filled with the optimal Divine qualities that will enhance the space and support the occupants, such as Divine love, Christ Light, health, strength, courage and abundance."

"Note: It is important that negative entities be bound immediately or they can slip away and come back to bother you or someone else. It is also a good idea to ask your Angels and I Am Presence to place you in a field of Cosmic White Light Protection before you start and set your intention that all that you do be for the Highest Good for all concerned and that you are free from any backlash or negative repercussions also unable to be traced."

* * * * *

Some have used **tourmaline and selenite** to clear the house or room of negative energies. I have both in my room including many other sacred stones and crystals. (You can get more info or resources from ***The Crystal Bible*** written by Judy Hall.)

Now that you have learned more than the basics of psychic self-defense, let us move forward and discuss about being a modern-day Yogi, being heroes of humanity and Mother Earth.

It is important to realize that what protections and cleansing we can do from a personal level, can also be done at a global level as well especially as we attain greater spiritual mastery as we begin to transform our lives into that of a modern-day Yogi.

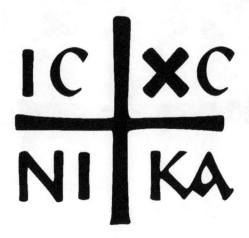

Christ Victory

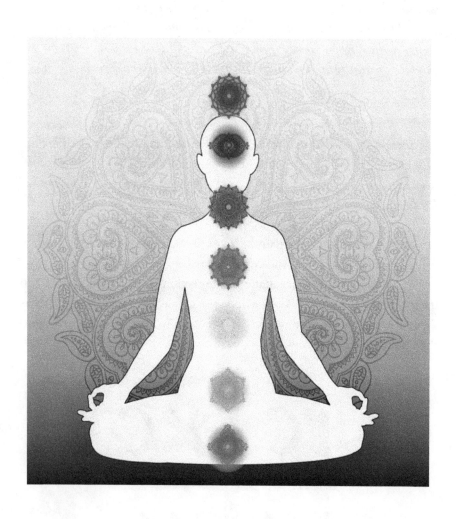

CHAPTER 17

THE MODERN-DAY YOGI

We have learned how to eat, drink, meditate and pray our way to being a modern-day Yogi. Hopefully what you have learned by now is that the path of a Yogi is ultimately about re-establishing that oneness with our Creator or Source, Mother Earth and Universe. Oneness is a critical part of our creating Heaven on Earth, as the journey is as within as it is without.

Many people have the impression that a Yogi is one who lives in a cave in the Himalayas or somewhere in India or Tibet and is an ascetic and meditates all day. Although this may still be true of many in these modern times, it is not true or required for all. Yogis come in all shapes, forms and practices and do not necessarily practice yogic asanas although they can be quite helpful with helping us perfect our meditation and spiritual practices.

Some Yogis or masters look nothing like what many of us imagine they should appear. While some may appear like Gandhi or Yogananda, they may also appear like an ordinary elderly woman like Master Lady Pearl or young and beautiful like Master Relica. Meanwhile, there are those who dress, look and act like an authentic Yogi and yet guide their devotees in a path that keeps them chained to the ego perpetuated reality or prison.

Some think that Yogis are people who eat healthy, are vegans, do meditation and do a lot of Yoga. Although that is true for many, it is not true for all Yogis. Some are vegans while others are a flexitarian. Many

Yogis do asanas but others do other forms of spiritual practices to heighten their connection with the Universe. Regardless, all Yogis meditate deeply as part of their spiritual practice. Doing so assists them in attaining the quiet within and state of no mind which in turn allows a deep connection with one's Presence/Divine Self and God to occur.

Yogis live a life in harmony with the body, mind and spirit and their way of life leads to God realization and oneness with God, Mother Earth, humanity and the Universe. However, nowadays many modern-day wannabe Yogis seem to be focused on flexibility, health, saying cool spiritual phrases and getting great abs or core muscles through exercise.

Yoga was designed to help the individual go within and eventually discover their Divinity or Creator. However, modern day yoga seems to be more into fitness, looking good and feeling good. More emphasis seems to be more on how to perfect the asanas, reap its health benefits, take awesome pics with complex yogic poses, becoming a yoga instructor or starting a yoga business or practice than actually training on how to go into the deeper stages of the yogic practice which focuses more on inner spiritual energy work, cultivation and communion with God. Although the above may be true for some, I have known others who practice Yoga regularly and are quite spiritual and enlightened. Ultimately, it is up to the individual to strive for higher consciousness.

With regards to asanas, Swami Kriyananda stated that Patanjali was describing the stages of withdrawal and absorption, and not specific yoga practices. The absorption that Patanjali talks about is the absorption of our consciousness with God's Consciousness.

All who would unite their souls with God must follow that same path: **Yama** and **Niryama** (right action), **Asana** (firmness of posture, and keeping the spine straight to enable the energy to flow freely through it), **Pranayama** (control over the energy of the body), **Pratyahara** (interiorization of the mind), **Dharana** (one-pointed concentration), **Dhyana** (absorption in deep meditation) and **Samadhi** (oneness). This known as the **Eightfold** (more literally, the eight-limbed **Ashtanga**). **(R 271)**

Those that truly follow the Eightfold Ashtanga above are more of what I consider a true Yogi.

Although meditation is the ultimate tool to help us reach that state of Samadhi or Divine absorption, many if not most systems will only bring the practitioner to the beginning or intermediate depth of meditation. Although at this level, it may create outstanding health benefits, Divine absorption remains out of reach. Although many meditators have much mastery for meditating for many hours, many or most will not experience that Cosmic absorption that Swami Kriyananda, Paramahansa Yogananda and Patanjali wrote and talked about.

The meditation system that brings us to that God-realization and Christ Consciousness include Kriya Yoga that was taught to many great masters by the great avatar, Babaji and it was brought to the west by Yogananda. Incidentally, it is believed by some spiritual masters that Babaji taught Jesus Kriya Yoga. Other practices may include Tibetan Dzochen Meditation and kundalini or chakra meditation practices.

U.U.M.M. (discussed in Chapter 9) is a more recent system that the Universe gave to me to be shared with all of humanity to give everyone an equal opportunity to experience God in the most intimate ways.

Most people think that Yogis only come from India and are Hindus, but all who follow the path of the Truth and live a Christ Conscious God-realized life can also be considered a Yogi. There are Christian, Catholic and Buddhist Yogis who have transcended the limitations of religion and have gone on to understand the greater and Divine Universal Truth and Wisdom that unites all of us. Many of these individuals have become Yogis or Mystics. It is my understanding that some Catholics even practice Zen meditation or Kriya Yoga in private to reach higher consciousness and ultimately to have that communion with God.

According to Swami Kriyananda, spiritual seekers in any religion, if they pray and meditate sincerely, may rightly be termed Yogis. (R 272) I believe a Yogi is an individual who has dedicated himself or herself in the search of Truth, God-realization and Christ Consciousness. The individual has some type of ritual, spiritual practice or devotional practice that is dedicated to daily prayer and meditation and is fully dedicated to the Light and Divine Love of God. The Yogi does deep meditation to establish communion and oneness with God and seeks to have harmony within the Self and in their outer reality. The Yogi is filled with God's Cosmic Light, Love and Consciousness and acts out of love, compassion, mercy, forgiveness and kindness.

The Yogi seeks to serve, give and heal others. When the Yogi becomes fully realized, he or she will become a God-Realized and Christ Conscious Being where there is no longer a veil between the Yogi and God. The Yogi may work in the inner realms alone or with other Yogis and enlightened beings to send healing energies to humanity and Mother Earth. The more of us Yogis there are on the planet, the greater the power of change and transformation will manifest through our collective consciousness.

The Yogi acts and thinks not from the context of me versus them mentality but in terms of us (all of creation, Mother Earth, the Universe and God's Consciousness, Light, Love and Energy is all part of a whole and all exist as one). Us being one Divine expression of Divine Consciousness. The Yogi sees all realities as expressions of God's Consciousness but realizes he or she is that Consciousness and God in action in this physical plane. He or she lives, acts, manifest, and thinks like God and always has this oneness with God's Consciousness and allows God's Consciousness, Light and Love to always illuminate and radiate from them to others.

The Yogi becomes one in Holy Communion and Holy Matrimony with God or Source in all aspects of their lives, especially during meditation. Therefore, the Yogi acts in service to help others learn how to end their suffering and live in harmony with themselves, Mother Earth and the Great I Am.

The path of a Yogi is not an easy one but the rewards can lead to our ultimate liberation and freedom from the matrix we have co-created and lead us to our Ascension or salvation. The journey is focused on one's dharma while also gaining mastery in spiritual practices in preparation for his or her Ascension.

During the last year of the Yogi's life, he or she will most likely have mastered the art of living and with his or her many years of meditation, spiritual practices and virtuous and righteous behaviors will also master the art of dying. Different spiritual sects have different spiritual methods of Ascension or mastering the art of dying. However, there is a common thread to all of them that we can incorporate into our final year, month or days to help us to master the Art of Dying and help us with our Ascension. We will explore that further in the next chapter.

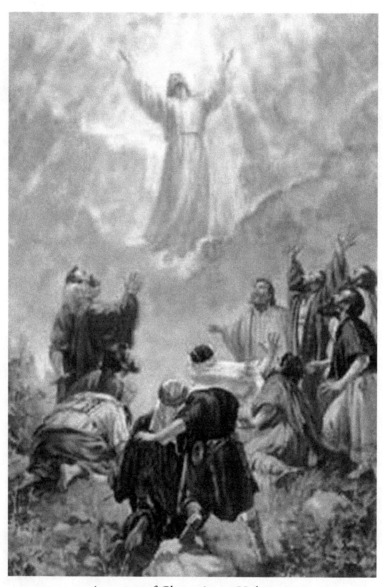

Ascension of Christ, Artist Unknown

CHAPTER 18

ASCENSION

Death as we currently know it in duality is the separation of our Soul/Spirit from the blessed physical form (body temple) that we have been gifted with for our journey upon Earth, and its return to the realm of Light to continue our evolution in form or not. In our journey of bringing Heaven to Earth through us, the manner in which we experience our transition out of form can be upgraded from a time of fear and grief, to one of rejoicing and embodying our mastery to an even greater level.

My first book, *Dare to Imagine,* is about the art of living and the path to enlightenment. My second book, *Beyond Imagination*, is about spiritual mastery and the communion with God. This book is about assisting humanity in ending much of its suffering, awakening them into their true and Divine Nature so that we may all create heaven on Earth and within, and guiding humanity on how to transcend the laws of karma and attain liberation or Ascension. The book goes on to give the wisdom and tools to facilitate everyone in living an empowered and enlightened life of a modern-day Yogi or Mystic.

The path of the modern-day Yogi and Mystic is about living a God Conscious and Christ Realized life full of harmony, Divine love, high attainment and spiritual mastery. Part of the realization and spiritual mastery is the preparation for our own spiritual Ascension which may or may not be through the "death" of our physical body.

I have been around death throughout my life. I have seen people die, attended many funerals and even lived near a mortuary. I could hear the funeral marching band march around the neighborhood practically every weekend when I grew up in San Francisco.

I witnessed my grandmother's listless body in bed after she died of heart failure when I was a young man, was at both my parents' and mother-in-law's death beds until they transitioned and was even there for two of my canine family members during their last hours of life. My wife, daughter and I supported our canine family members and gave them lots of love and comfort until their very last breath, in all cases holding space and witnessing as their spirit left the body and returned to the Realms of Light.

I have talked with people who had NDE (Near Death Experience) and even experienced my father visiting me a couple of times after his death as I have written in *Dare to Imagine*. These experiences occurred twice on the day of his funeral and then a year after he passed away. I also wrote about Near Death Experiences in *Dare to Imagine* and know people who have had such experiences.

One of my former colleagues was involved in an accident that put her in a coma. She had severe brain damage. As she was dying, she saw her soul levitate above her body. She could see the doctors and all who were present. She could even hear everyone's conversation. As she was departing away from life and her body, something caught her attention; it was the extraordinary amount of love from friends and family present. That love gave her the strength and reason to come back. She eventually woke up after a long coma and did extensive rehab. She now miraculously lives a relatively normal life. Her experience only validates the soul phenomenon and the power of love.

In addition, I have witnessed a ghost in a three- dimensional form at a rehab facility, felt the negative energies of negative entities and even a demonic entity. I have also received messages from deceased relatives and friend's parents while in a state of meditation. I have seen a vision of my soul and souls of others travelling back to Earth to fulfil our Dharma during this embodiment. Hence, I have no doubt about the afterlife and know a thing or two about death and dying. However, what I experienced with my mother-in-law's and mother's process of dying was quite extraordinary and amazing.

Being Present

As previously shared, I was fortunate to have had the privilege of being a part of one of the most beautiful ways of dying I have ever witnessed. I observed and supported my mother-in-law, Encarnacion, with her transition. The love of all her children, relatives and in-laws was something that I have never witnessed before; I found it quite extraordinary, healing and comforting to Encarnacion and to all of us who were there. What I learned from our many hours together is something I feel that we can all learn from and utilize in assisting others and ourselves during these major transitions.

Many people take for granted people who are in a coma and think they are not aware or listening. Though they may be in a coma, they can still hear and perceive through their senses. This truth is well documented.

After Encarnacion suffered a massive stroke, she fell instantly into a coma. This was the second stroke that she had within seven months. While she was in this coma, family members, friends and relatives came from all around the world to visit her. They all addressed her as if she were awake. Her children would give her daily massages, groomed her, painted her nails and would even talk to her regularly despite her inability to respond verbally. The family began taking over the many of the responsibilities of the nurses and even helped to clean and change Encarnacion towards the end. She was always surrounded by the love and support of her family, friends and relatives. She was never being left alone, especially when her death was pending.

During the final hours, each family went to her and privately said their last words of respect, love and support. Those of us who were spiritual would pray for her smooth transition. My soul sister **Marissa Beltran** is a Reiki practitioner and worked on clearing Encarnacion's energy in preparation for her transition. I prayed for her graceful release as well. I meditated and merged my consciousness with hers to offer my support with helping her to transition peacefully. As her death began to draw near, her closest children and family members drew even closer to her and offered their ongoing love and support.

When the moment of her transition arrived, she gracefully gave out her last breath and departed peacefully. She was in much peace and tranquility as she transitioned. We all cried at her final moment of life but were eventually comforted by how peaceful and serene she was at the moment of her physical death. All of us felt at peace with her departure and with ourselves because we all were able to make our amends with her before she departed.

After this extraordinary experience, I have come to realize how great and wonderful Encarnacion's process of releasing her spirit from her physical body truly was, and how this is possible for everyone. Yet, I have also come to realize how we can further perfect the dying process to an even higher level. I had no idea that a year later, I would be utilizing everything I learned and more for my own mother.

On November 1st, 2018, (All Saints Day) I received a call from my sister that my mom was admitted to the hospital and the doctor said she was dying. I was overcome with grief and burst out crying in front of my client. I excused myself and quickly drove from Walnut Creek to Pacific Medical Center ER in San Francisco. While driving I asked my sister to tell my mom that I was on the way and to please wait for me.

My sister told me that the street parking by the hospital was extremely bad and that I had to park in the garage. I made a decree and prayer for a space nearby so I could get to my mom on time and when I arrived near the hospital, a car just started to pull out of a space that was across from the hospital. The nearest parking lot was 2 blocks away where all my relatives had parked. I was so thankful the Masters allowed my decree to manifest during this crisis.

When I arrived in my mother's room, I was greeted by mom's weak and rapidly deteriorating body. She was wearing an oxygen mask that was delivering about 12 liters of oxygen which is extremely high. She tried to take off the oxygen a few times and was getting somewhat uncomfortable. My daughter is a registered nurse and saw the discomfort and distress and quickly notified the nurse to contact the doctor for an I.V. morphine to help my mom breathe better and decrease any pain associated with all the apparatus attached to her. After a few minutes my mom was calm again.

Her blood pressure was low and her heart was being elevated to a more normal range by a Pacer, a mechanical device to shock the heart and keep up the heart rate from going dangerously low and quitting altogether.

I immediately went to mom and talked with her. I held her hand and massaged it. I spoke kind and loving words and telling her how much I loved her. My brother, sister and cousins came and offered my mom love and support as well. Eventually my mom was transferred from the emergency room to a larger room upstairs to the hospice ward which was much quieter and more conducive to creating the perfect milieu for my mom's eventual liberation.

Shortly after mom was settled in at the hospice ward, the Pacer was removed as well as the oxygen. I knelt by mom's side and just massaged her head by her third eye point reassuring her that everything was OK. Initially, she had some tension on her forehead from some discomfort but that began to dissolve after my continuous massage and reassurance to her. I surrounded her with God's Love, Light and Energy. As the time grew near, I suggested to my brother and sister to say or express their last words or actions of love to mom, which they did.

I began making a decree to God to calling for clearing all mom's karma from all lifetimes and to set her spirit free. "I am the presence of God clearing away all karmas from all lifetimes and setting Lily free to ascend."

Mom's breathing began to slow down gently more and more until she reached a Zen state of oneness with the Universe and then she peacefully let out a gentle breath of completion of a perfected life and death. She departed with dignity and great bravery demonstrating her trust in the transition process. Her transition was completed in such a short time, setting her spirit free.

The days and week after her transition were nothing less than mystical. She began manifesting to me in the inner realms quite regularly the first week after her death. She was always comforting me and letting me know that she was OK and that she was there for me.

She also appeared to Peter Mt. Shasta and a friend of mine Mardi. She is a famous artist, visionary and Mystic. After Peter Mt. Shasta found out that my mom transitioned, he called me right away to offer me support. As we talked, he was able to tune in to my mother's consciousness and saw that she was ok and told me how proud she was of me. He was even able to see her wearing her favorite red dress.

Mardi tuned into my mother's consciousness within a week after she passed away. She could see the red dress my mother was wearing although she had never met her before or seen any of her pictures. One of mom's favorite dresses was a red one. In fact, the funeral picture of my mother has her wearing a red dress. Mardi told me that my mother was hugging me and comforting me. She told me that my mom wanted me to get the red blanket to wrap around me so that I could feel support and security from her in a metaphorical way.

I didn't know what red blanket she was talking about until I went to my mom's apartment a week later and found it in her storage room. When I opened the door to her storage room, I was flabbergasted that there it was, a small red blanket waiting for me to take it. It is perfect because it is a personal blanket that keeps me so warm. When I wrap myself with it, I feel somehow more connected to my mom. Mardi also stated that my mom was protecting me from the other side.

My mom also appeared to her favorite caregiver and friend, Claudia. She was always very fond of her and loved her dearly. After my mom died, she had multiple dreams about my mom. A week after my mom transitioned, she appeared in Claudia's dream. Claudia stated that my mom was very happy and was waiting for her turn. She mentioned to her that everything is going to be fine. Both Claudia and I felt she was referring to her excitement and optimism about going to Heaven.

In another dream, she could hear my mom laughing near her baby's bassinet. Shortly after, her baby woke up as if by my mom's laughter. Then a year later on my mom's death anniversary on 11/1/2019 (All Saints Day), she visited Claudia again in the astral plane. She introduced her to her brother, my uncle, a woman and a young child. When my mom was living in China, she had a young brother who died at a young age and that younger brother may be the one she introduced to Claudia. The woman may possibly be my grandmother. Claudia stated, "She was so happy with her relatives."

Those of us who are fortunate to be alive are given an amazing gift. This gift is an opportunity to master the art of dying. Many people see a terminal diagnosis as a death sentence and automatically give up. Our attitude, perception and how we cope with our experience will either harm us more or further prepare us to deal with it more gracefully.

I see major illnesses as a wakeup call from the Universe to begin the search within that will lead us back home to God's Love, Peace and Harmony. I see a terminal diagnosis as the Universe's last attempt for us to wake up and embrace Life in this lifetime. We either wake up and gracefully navigate our way through the dying process or we can become angry, anxious or depressed and close our door to the world and to our own salvation. One way will lead to our salvation and liberation while the other will keep us a prisoner of the karma we have created for ourselves and lead us to more suffering.

There are phases many of us go through when confronted with the knowledge of our body's imminent death. According to Elizabeth Kubler Ross, there are five stages of grief:

- Denial
- Anger
- Bargaining
- Depression
- Acceptance

However, if we have lived a fulfilling and enlightened life, we may go through those phases much more gracefully. **(R 273)**

Obtaining Support

It is very important to get a support group when we are gravely ill. If we are not spiritual by now, this is the time to do so. We may find more comfort by aligning ourselves with a spiritual or religious group we resonate with.

Principles for Ascension or the Art of Dying

Begin **searching within**, to understand who you really are, and know why you are here. This is the time we must re-evaluate our lives and be **introspective**. It is a time to reflect on how we have lived our lives and how we have affected others by our actions, words, emotions and life.

Find joy in reflecting on those memories of the people you have influenced positively in this lifetime. Be aware of the people you may have hurt intentionally or unintentionally. If you are aware of any of these people, forgive yourself what you did and pray for forgiveness from the person you hurt; it is also important that you apologize to the person as well, if possible.

Forgive yourself for the wrongs you have done to others.

Forgive those who have done wrong to you even though you may think you are right. This is time to let go of your pride and ego and to fully set yourself free.

Forgive yourself and others over and over again until all have been forgiven. Learn to receive God's Grace, Unconditional Love and Forgiveness through visualization, prayer and through U.U.M.M.

Apologize to all you have done wrong in this lifetime or previous lifetimes. It is ideal to do so in person, and if not, pray that the individual or individuals forgive you for what you have done. You could even pray that you apologize to all sentient beings from the beginning of time that you have harmed in any way. You may say,

> *I apologize for all the wrongs I have done to all sentient beings and all creatures great and small I have come across since the birth of creation. I thank you for being a part of my journey and helping me to see the consequences of my actions and helping me to be who I am today.*
>
> *I Am the Presence of God blessing you and your ancestors with infinite love and blessings along with the gift of the awareness of God's love and consciousness within you and your family or species. I Am the Presence of God cutting off all karmic ties, cords or links that we may have been co-created between us. I Am the Presence of God's Grace, Love and Forgiveness and set you, your families, friends, ancestors and species to be free to evolve and find your way back home as well. The Truth will set all of us free!!!*

Although the body temple that you came in is no longer supporting your spirit staying embodied, realize that you are only a passenger in it and have existed before it was created and you will continue to exist after it is recycled back to Mother Earth.

Our Souls are eternal and are ever evolving. We just need to realize that and learn to **connect to that Cosmic Love and Presence** within which is anchored within our heart or center of our being. Thereafter, we must learn to **merge our Consciousness with our Creator.**

Practicing U.U.M.M. will help us to experience that I AM Presence and that oneness with God.

Practicing meditation such as U.U.M.M. daily will assist in illuminating the Light of God within our heart and fill the Universe within and without with that Love. In addition, practicing how to circulate our kundalini energy, achieving stillness of thoughts and merging our consciousness with the mind of God through U.U.M.M. and other related meditation methods will help us better prepare for the final moments of transition. It will also allow us to exit the crown chakra much easier.

Remember, you are not the body and yet it is a sacred temple that allows you and your Presence to journey, learn and be of service upon Earth. Daily gratitude to and for your Earth body is part of that service to Life.

We must **live each moment with great mindfulness** and allow our thoughts, emotions and actions be filled with love, compassion, mercy, forgiveness, and kindness. We must learn to serve others by our prayers, gentleness and active presence when with others. **Live in the moment and not in the past or future.** This moment is what matters most especially at this time.

Take time to make amends with friends and family members. Take time to say words of love, edification and wisdom to those around us. It is very important to learn to **accept ourselves** as we are and learn to relinquish judgement on ourselves and others. We accept the fact that our earthly life is only transient and the vessel we travel in has an expiration date.

Begin giving all your material things away. This will help us realize that material things are not important and what is important is the love of the self, others, Mother Earth and God.

Realize that God's Consciousness is in all form, all of the elements, and in all of creation in the Universe and that **we are all beautiful expressions of God's Consciousness.**

Realize that all material things that we have and all of our material reality that we have experienced are **finite and have an expiration date.**

Realize that we are not the elements that comprise us and that we exist beyond the earth, water, fire and air elements that make us up.

Realize that our current life is only an illusion and is **only temporary** in the bigger cosmic scheme of things.

Though it may appear that we are losing ourselves, our vessel, material things and material reality to death, we are actually expanding our reality and consciousness beyond the confines of our senses, perceptions, body and time and space in our rebirth to a higher level of consciousness.

At the time of our transition, it may also appear that we are being separated from our loved ones. We are actually more connected to them more than ever before at a Soul level that transcends time and space.

Our Soul is part of our I AM Presence, connected to God and to our loved ones. Realize that the process that humans call death cannot and does not disconnect the energetic connections we have with one another regardless of where we are in time, space and dimension. We are all One, in the body and in our light forms.

Practicing the yogic breathing exercises will help to minimize the fear and anxiety we may feel.

The closer we get to our transition, the more we should **fill our entire being with the Love, Light and Energy of God.**

We must choose to focus on the positive parts of our lives and relinquish all the negative things.

Realize that our loved ones, the Creator, Ascended Masters are waiting to receive, surround and embrace us with their love.

Purify the body, mind and spirit through daily prayer, meditation, mantras, visualization exercises and yogic breathing.

Following the Eight Buddhist Precepts especially during the last few years of life (or whenever you are ready) may be very helpful with our ascension but I feel some of the precepts could be updated or clarified further for the modern day and age. Some sources list 10 precepts but I would like to focus on the eight I feel are important to me. I will list the precepts and my perceptions and recommendations. (Realize that there are differences in all religions and that includes Buddhism. There are many branches of Buddhism as well and they differ in their teachings.)

They are as follows:

1. To abstain from being harmful to living beings.
2. To abstain from stealing.
3. To abstain from all sexual practices. Tantra practices that focus on spiritual energies may be an exception. Spiritual discernment is necessary for determining right action here.
4. To abstain from uttering lies.
5. To refrain from intoxicating drinks and drugs which lead to carelessness.
6. To abstain from eating after noon time (only if your body can tolerate it and it is not against medical advice due to some type of medical condition like diabetes or related illness).
7. To abstain from listening or playing music, songs, wearing flowers, jewelry and other ornaments. I believe listening to spiritual and inspiring songs are an exception and listening and watching motivational programs are recommended.
    Jewelry that has spiritual significance could be included as well as those that have special sentimental and spiritual value. Any jewelry worn for decorative or festive purposes, however, should be minimized or not be worn.
8. To refrain from sitting or lying on high and luxurious places (only if you are medically able to without incurring health related issues).

For all who are seeking to enrich their spiritual practice, personal guidance and intention are important in how to incorporate these principles in full alignment with their I Am Presence and their particular circumstance.

Those who are devout Buddhists are expected to follow the precepts strictly. **(R 274, 275)**

The Art of Dying is about purifying ourselves from toxic thoughts, emotions and actions; instead, we replace all that with Cosmic Love, Peace, and Harmony.

Do not watch TV or read about anything that creates fear and anxiety. Instead, read books like *Life After Life* by Raymond Moody, *Dying to Be Me* by Anita Moorjani and books by Elizabeth Kubler -Ross.

Listen to calm and relaxing music.

Avoid drinking coffee but, instead, drink therapeutic teas like Spring Dragon, Chamomile and Lavender tea.

Pray to your Ascended Masters and God for guidance to help you navigate through the portals of consciousness or bardos with grace.

Allow your last thoughts that you have to be completely full of Love, Bliss and Joy before you disengage from your physical reality.

During the last hours of death, have your loved ones create a milieu of love, peace and ascension. Joshua David Stone, Ph.D. wrote about 15 steps of preparation for the exact moment of death. **(R 276)** He included:

1. The burning of orange light in the room. He felt it stimulated the brain centers which caused the kundalini to flow upwards.
2. He recommended burning Sandalwood since it is the incense of the first or destroyer ray. The scent of the sandalwood has the metaphysical effect of breaking down the old energies.
3. The dying person must be guided to merge with the clear Light of God and to not focus on anything else.
4. Death-bed confessions to a friend, family member, or priest may be valuable. As much as possible of one's personal karma should be resolved to insure the highest passing.
5. The body should face eastwards because the spiritual current is the strongest when facing in this direction. (This direction is also recommended for meditation). The feet and the hands should be crossed.
6. Prayers should be made to God and Masters for help just prior to death.
7. All drugs should be avoided just prior to death. Drugs can cloud a person's consciousness to the point where he or she might possibly miss the opportunity to merge with the clear Light of God.
8. If the last thought on the person's mind before death is of God, that is where she or he will go.
9. Everybody should have been forgiven.

10. The Chanting of mantras or the repetition of the name of God by the person dying is valuable.
11. Loved ones should have been bidden farewell so the soul extension is ready for the next step on its journey.
12. Spiritual Music in the background is helpful
13. The playing of an actual bardo tape especially designed for the dying process is of particular value. The Mystery School of Astara (Earlyne Chaney) has one. **(R 277)**
14. Guidance should be provided to the soul extension so that it will exit through the crown chakra when it leaves.
15. Make sure a will is complete and all affairs of estate are in order to ease the dying person's mind of material concerns.

According to **Darshan Baba,** the following are important for moksha or liberation:

- Become aware and realize that the body exists as part of a whole.
- Systematically work to align the actions and efforts of the body, speech, and mind to be in Harmony with, and Service as a contribution to the Whole.
- All "spiritual" practices or methods of internal cultivation will be ineffective or limited without Loving Kindness and Compassion or the simple realization that we are a part of and One with the Whole of Life.
- Any practices which are undertaken as an effort to be of greater service to, in alignment with, and a function to the Harmony of the Whole will be most effective.

"Love or the realization and expression of All Life as One is the key to miraculous longevity and light body attainment."

"This Love is the very Life force within all beings.
It is the presence of *Super Intelligence, Omniscience, and Divinity.*
Love All Life as One." *Darshan Baba*

"The Siddha Bogar, who was also known as Lao Tzu, attained the secret 'Amrit Sanjeevani Kaya Kalpa' elixir because of an overwhelming compassion to save all beings from death and disease. Because he wasn't seeking only for himself or to attain for selfish interests the knowledge was given to him. "Ramalinga Vallalar had attained an alchemical transmutation of his fleshly body into one of pure light even while still on the Earth. This body could not be harmed by weapons, disease, elements or by nature, and required no sustenance. However, Ramalinga Swami said that if the force of Loving Compassion were to leave the body that he would be dead.

"In similar fashion Ramalinga Vallalar easily attained miraculous powers practices simply through his Love for all Beings."

According to **Savannah Brooke**, Ascension Guide, Shaman, Pranic Healer, writer and speaker, "in order to fully experience the ascension process and become one with our higher spirit we must remember that it is, in fact, a oneness journey. This includes the process it takes to evolve mentally, spiritually, physically, and metaphysically across and throughout many timelines, dimensions, and realms. It has been documented that we have the ability to attain the Rainbow Body and to be and exist as pure light here on Earth.

Currently the shifting cosmic energies and linear timeline we are in allows more of us to tap into this quantum space and exist as a being of light. To bring the higher-self into the body requires more **focus** and much **isolation for self-reflection** and **truly letting go of the lower vibrations** that keep us in between dimensions.

Just because we are practicing mindfulness or yoga on a daily basis will not breed the environment to become in union with and harness the higher-light spirit within our body. It begins with the purification process within the mind, body, and soul in order to allow the descent of the higher spirit into the physical body in lower dimensions. In the beginning when you are connecting with your higher spirit, you simply exist separately in different dimensions, and in unity at the same time. As your mental consciousness expands so does your inner soul awareness. As we become more deeply connected to our inner world there is a lot of inner work that needs to be seen, known, and healed as the experiences of our past across this lifetime, past lifetimes, ancestral and DNA wounds all tie into our soul blueprint." (Note: I work regularly on past life healing and integration during my meditation system and have incorporated ancestral karmic healings and integration).

"These experiences carry energy, as all things, and some are denser rather than light. The soul must achieve levels of purity in light form to evolve as a fully composed light being within.

The soul purification process includes ridding yourself of dark and scary fears that show up like entities or demons, which also are just soul lessons in disguise. Working with the violet flame, and high vibrational light from cosmic and astral planes throughout the process is essential for clearing and elevating in the physical realm too.

By creating and bringing in more light from the cosmos within the soul, we can achieve this ascension which would assist the transformation of our carbon-based DNA to Crystalline structures.

Additional effort is required to evolve by making changes to our outer bodies. Since we are HU-man-beings, our minds seek to understand some practical tips that allow you to achieve the light-body connection. Purification, as mentioned above, is key for ascension and maintaining the light-body evolution. Outer world purification is very important in supporting us on our journey to Ascension and they include: **getting more sunlight, salt water, pranic/reiki/quantum healing, nutrition** and implementing **physical exercise to embody the light consciousness**."

Savannah stated that we should get sun light on a daily basis and that it increases our moods, our serotonin levels and vitamin D for immune health. "It has so many amazing properties and has the energy that we need for ascension." It also brings in high vibrational diamond radiant rainbow energies within your body and chakras.

Salt water is a valuable tool for purification of the aura, chakras, energy, and physical body. You can bathe in it, use the ocean, create your own salt water bowls to intentionally send energy from your inner and outer body as a means of absorption of negative or dense energies. For outer energy bodies pranic/reiki/quantum healing are beneficial for expanded healing. Nutrition is critical, and honoring the soul's calling to fast or restrict certain foods when your intuition strikes. Finally, implementing physical exercise to move energy and embody the light consciousness.

Next, or foremost, **intuition is the key (Note:** or what I refer to as the I AM Presence or Divine Presence within) Your intuition is the key to unlock all of your codes to your personal transformation. You have the plan inside and each soul has a different route and path that will bring them closer to their light body. When your true intuition speaks, listen and honor it even when it is upsetting to the ego/mind with devout higher vibrational energies such as love and joy to transmute or clear the lower fields. Remembering that karma plays a huge role in the ascension. Learning how to continually **self-reflect** and take responsibility to rise above the lower dimensions of emotions and physicality, or the mental box. **Identify your mental triggers** and use them as tools to navigate the lower world to achieve ultimate heaven in your oneness. **Pay attention to the inner-child for deep transformation and life cycle trends.** Finally, additional characteristics that will assist you in using your intuition to purify your mind-body-soul and allow for spirit to descend, are the power of your **true intention, dedication to evolution, discipline, and patience.**

Intention speaks to the universe greater than action, so you will be continuously tested to trust that you are on your highest path in this lifetime over and over again. Remember, in your hologram everything is merely a dimension for lessons to achieve the higher place within.

Ultimately, once you surrender completely and give yourself to God and attain union, you can experience the spirit tuning process where the spirit leaves the physical body, goes to higher heaven realms, and come back after tuning the Spirit-Soul-Baek where you will be given a new purpose to obtain."

With regards to attaining a Light Body, Savannah stated that the actual process may include a series of yogic movements, breathwork, and other movements in combination with cosmic activations through vibrational attunement of the soul-energy body may help to successfully launch the spirit into its Light Body

The important thing she would do during an Ascension is to tune into her **intuition** on what more she needs to do to help her with a successful attainment of a Light Body. She further mentioned that acts of service, surrendering self to the divine oneness and prayer before Ascension is important. Lastly, she stressed the importance of enlisting the assistance of the Ascended Masters to guide and help you through the process.

* * * * *

The following methods are techniques that may be of assistance to your liberation, Ascension and moksha:

As your vessel begins to disconnect from its senses or when you are guided to leave this Earthly reality, begin to focus your consciousness within to the familiar place of peace within your heart.

Imagine it filling up with all the unconditional love of Mother Earth, our Heavenly Mother/Father/God, Sun of God, all of your family members into the center of your being. Allow that Love to illuminate brightly and purify your heart, mind, Soul and the five organs (lung, heart, kidneys, liver and spleen) and the rest of your bodies (physical, emotional, mental and causal bodies). Intend that you merge your consciousness and awareness with your I AM Presence and you may decree, "I AM the Presence of God setting my soul and consciousness free to ascend and be liberated from the laws of karma." Those who have other sacred mantras may chant it at this time. **The Tibetan 100 Deities Mantra** is a powerful mantra to chant. It is as follows:

Om Ah Hum (*It is pronounced as Hung.*)
Bodhicitta Mahasukha
Jnana, Dhatu Ah
Om Ah Hum

The meaning of these words are as follows:

"Invoking the All Encompassing and All-Pervasive Essence, bringing focus and resolve to the energy of purification, aspiring to the transcendent bliss of the enlightened mind, may the understanding of the skillful means for purifying, releasing and transforming the constituent elements of being be present. Let it be so!" **(R 278)**

Guru Padmasambhava said, "This is a very special and supreme teaching, as one can attain liberation by simply hearing it – attaining enlightenment without practice, and attaining Buddhahood in a split second. It is the most profound method of attaining the perfect enlightenment, and also a method for freeing one of all negative karma created through wrongful actions. One who hears this teaching will not fall into the dark realms. It is a teaching only revealed to sentient beings who have accumulated great merits through their past practice. Upon hearing the teaching, one will receive great blessings and instantaneously attain Buddhahood."

It is a hidden teaching (terma) transmitted by Guru Padmasambhava, not revealed to those without merits. It is generally unheard of by most people. But once you hear it, you will have the seed of Buddhahood planted within your being. You ought to know that Guru Padmasambhava is someone who spoke of the true speech – the vajra speech. **(R 279)**

Thereafter, focus on visualizing your heart, lung, kidneys, liver and spleen illuminating an intense radiating Light of perfect Divine Light, Love and Consciousness. Visualize this light and consciousness merging together and descending down to your first chakra. Focus your consciousness there for a moment or two and visualize a Merkaba forming around it. Allow all the Love, Light and Energy to fully activate your first chakra. Then consciously release your kundalini shakti energy 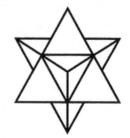 by allowing it to spiral up the spinal channels. As it is spiraling up each chakra, imagine seeing the dominant color of each chakra activated and spiral up each chakra as it opens like a rainbow following the **Merkaba Shakti Star.**

Allow your kundalini energy to continue to spiral up each chakra and fully activating and opening each chakra as it continues to go through your crown chakra and goes up towards the Rainbow Body above your body. Allow your kundalini energy and the Rainbow Light to become one with your Rainbow Body. Surrender yourself to it and allow it to direct you to your Creator and loved ones as you begin your journey to the next level of consciousness and reality.

During this **first phase of your death process or bardo** (The gap or intermediate state between death and rebirth), there will be the brilliant Light of God that awaits you. Release all fear and surrender yourself to merge your consciousness with this Light. It is extremely important that during this phase, there is an absence of fear, regret, attachment or any negative emotions. The theme emotion during this time should be a surrender to love in its entirety. We must embrace the Light of God and enter it in the way we know best.

If you are anxious, learn to focus on your breath to release it or pray that your Ascended Master guides and overlighting angels assist you on how to navigate through the portals of realities or consciousness as you head towards your Ascension, freedom, salvation. Focus on merging your consciousness to the pure Light of God's Love lifting you to your salvation. Regular practice of U.U.M.M. will assist your ascension process, making it more automatic and easier. In fact, Padmasambhava appeared to me around April 13, 2020, and told me that it is through discipline and regular practice of spiritual techniques and meditation that makes our journey into liberation much more automatic.

Those of you less skilled with doing this or prefer an alternate method, you may just focus on the heart chakra or center of your being. Focus on allowing Divine Love to fill the reservoir of you heart and entire being. Allow an energetic whirlpool of love to attract all the love around you. Allow the love of your loved ones, friends and colleagues to be sucked into the center of your being.

Allow all that love to expand and fill your entire being and be one with it. Surrender your consciousness with the love and consciousness of God and pray that God and the Ascended Masters will help guide you through the portals of consciousness and then let go of all attachment to your senses, body and emotions and allow yourself (Consciousness) to prepare to levitate and leave behind the confines of your ship, shell or temple you have been trapped in for all these years.

Begin to allow your consciousness to experience the bliss of freedom, peace and harmony that comes from full surrender to God's Love and Consciousness. Next begin to ascend up your spiritual highway and exit out of your crown chakra. Continue up until you merge with your Rainbow Body. Surrender yourself to it as you allow it to direct you to your Creator and loved ones as you cut the silver cord that connects you to your physical body. Then go through the bardos as you were instructed from above or through the guidance of your Ascended Master/s. (*For a spoken Bardo ritual you might go to the Astara.org website.*)

I believe that after you physically die, there may be a pause in consciousness between bardos, depending on your readiness to ascend to higher consciousness. At this bardo (in between first or second bardo), your emotions of fear, anxiety and attachment to this physical plane may keep you trapped between dimensions. Those of you who fight it and resist it strongly may find yourself gravitating back to the earthly plane. While in this state of consciousness, you may still be living in denial and ignorance of your own death and continue existing as a ghost as if nothing ever happened. However, for those of you who have spiritually prepared for this journey or surrender to the process and embrace the light with open arms, you will quickly go into the Light of God and become one with his Light, Love and Consciousness. While going into this transition you may experience a temporary loss in consciousness. Thereafter, you may go through intermittent turbulence of consciousness as you are adjusting and slowly awakening from this new realm of reality, perception, awareness and consciousness.

Those of you who are less prepared may hesitate in this Ascension Process and may be distracted by the sights of various Lights and Colors or hear various Sounds. Fear not and embrace it and realize that they are only emanations from your own Light, Consciousness and Energy. Embrace the process and proceed as a Light of Consciousness with a more enlightened state of consciousness as you finally merge yourself with God's Light to complete your Ascension process. This may be considered the second bardo.

After you have merged more fully with the Light of God Consciousness and Light, you will enter into a new dimension or reality. This will be the next phase or bardo. This is the third phase of the bardo and is called by Joshua as the "valley of judgement." It is not an ego judgment but rather a review of one's life.

Once you have reached this next higher level of consciousness, realm or bardo, open your heart and mind to experience the love and warmth coming from your Ascended Masters, guides, angels, animal companions and the relatives and friends that have left before you as you now reunite with them. Take time to soak in the heavenly bliss and love that surrounds you. When you are ready you will begin to review your previous life times

This bardo or state of consciousness is similar to that state of consciousness during your dream state and parts of U.U.M.M. but perceptions, awareness and clarity of consciousness in this bardo is heightened significantly with regards to the interactions with your loved ones and the Ascended Masters.

Tibetan Buddhism also teaches that there are 3 bardos that we go through when we die. I believe that how we go through it depends on your belief system, spiritual lineages, religion, level of spiritual maturity and consciousness.

After things have settled and you have met with your spirit guides, Ascended Master or God, you have a choice to come back for a noble cause in another embodiment, choose to explore other realities, choose to help humanity raise its consciousness further or choose to go between dimensions. Your choices on where you go in the astral or earthly planes depend on your level of spirituality on Earth and any remaining karmic debt you have accumulated. The higher the spiritual mastery, the higher the realms one can enter into.

While in your current astral plane, you are no longer bounded by the time and space continuum. Visiting your family and loved ones is only a thought away. Think of them and there you will be. *Dare to Imagine* is no longer a creative abstract but a tangible reality. We can manifest and create whatever we desire within this realm including creating heaven or hell.

Realize that your human body temple, organs, and vessels only contained you and limited you from experiencing your full conscious potentials. Although some of you may have experienced less limitations due to your advanced spiritual mastery, the majority of humanity is still limited by it especially those who are attached and guided by their ego and those who are still mentally and emotionally immature. Once we attain ascension, we are no longer bound by our body, organs and duality. When we finally reach this high state of elevated consciousness, we finally have clarity to our true nature and realize that we are now pure Love, Light and Consciousness unadulterated by our previous body temple, senses, perceptions, emotions and subconsciousness limitations. It is here where we experience reality as it is and create and manifest whatever we want and live in oneness and alignment with God's Consciousness. However, as wonderful as it sounds, this spiritual transitory level is only temporary even if it last 100 years; we can go even higher in consciousness. The Ascension process is not a one stop final destination but a continuous process. Even Ascended Masters are on a journey to higher consciousness. On July 31, 2020, I was meditating and my consciousness was at my heart chakra and suddenly my Consciousness expanded beyond the confines of my heart chakra, body temple, emotional body and auric body and into the Cosmic Universe where there was complete severance of my body, emotions, senses and worldly connections. I existed as Pure Consciousness and the Universe. I began to think in Cosmic proportions with no concerns with my personal earthy desires or spiritual ambitions. I began creating more balance and harmony in the Universe through my Consciousness with no emotions or attachment to outcome. I was formless but yet omnipresent. It was an incredible transcendental experience that was Divine, Sublime, Beautiful, Holy, Pure and Perfect. I and God existed as one Pure Consciousness in the absence of duality. As my "self" began to emerge, I tried to connect with my human perceptions and feelings but found it difficult. It was easy for me to just relinquish my body (mental, emotional and physical) and continue in this Divine expression of Pure Consciousness but eventually God guided me and assisted me back to being able to return to my heart chakra and getting me grounded with Mother Earth. I have achieved Samadhi many times before but never like this. It was a true blessing and a reminder of what awaits us in our evolutionary Ascension Process. I am humbled by God's lesson of Ascension.

As humans, we have had to search deep for the Divine Spark of Light. When we have achieved our initial Ascended status of Consciousness, we become a fully realized Living Light of God Consciousness that is ready to serve others and explore the greater beauty and splendor of the Universe. Welcome to the Great White Brotherhood (and Sisterhood) of Light! It is here where you now have become an active ambassador of God's Love, Light, Energy and Consciousness. As you were guided to your freedom, set others free as well and teach all sentient beings who are hungry and thirsty for spiritual knowledge and truth. However, we must not let the illusion of being an Ascended Being or Master stop us from evolving further. Through great spiritual practice, devotion, mastery, awareness, enlightenment and surrender, we all have an opportunity to transcend beyond the limitations of our beliefs and even spiritual aspirations.

Blessed are those of you who have chosen to return on Earth to further serve humanity. Blessed are you for taking on such a noble cause and to re-experience the limitations of the vessels you have traveled in until your re-awakening.

Those of you who have chosen to reincarnate in this physical reality for a noble cause may have glimpses of memory of your soul travelling back into another embodiment in your rebirth. This is something I clearly remember later in life as I had a clear vision of my soul as well as those of others descending upon Earth in preparation of our next embodiment. I was formless, conscious and bounded together in some form of energy. I was coming back to Earth to help humanity end much of its suffering. My books are the fulfillment of my Divine mission and plan.

Those who are interested in learning more about Ascension, and all the various planes or dimensions of reality may get more detailed information from *The Complete Ascension Manual* by Joshua David Stone, Ph.D. (**R 280**) and *Live in Love – A Life Handbook for the New Golden Age* by Mikaelah Cordeo, Ph.D. (**R 281**)

I hope by now all of you are much more positive and excited with your Ascension and next phase of awakening. Release all fear and anxiety and fully embrace God's Love and Light for that will ultimately set you free.

Fear not my dearly beloved one for the kingdom of God is within your grasp. Seek ye first the kingdom of God and all these things shall be added onto you.

Those of you who are interested in attaining more advanced Tibetan Rainbow Bodies, may want to study Tibetan Buddhism, Togal and Dzogchen Meditation and practices.

Although there is so much we can do on our own for achieving freedom or liberation, it helps to have support groups, spiritual groups, Yogis, arahants, spiritual masters or teachers, friends and family surround us with love, prayer and support.

Compiled around 800 A.D., *The Tibetan Book of the Dead* or *Bardo Thodol* teaches how a person, under the guidance of a priest or Mystic, can attain spiritual liberation at the moment of death. The secret of spiritual liberation from the cycle of rebirth is for the dead entity to follow the white light wherever it goes and not to mind any other vision no matter how grotesque or heavenly. (**R 282**)

The most important thing with the ascension process is our very last thought or emotion at the moment of death. Master or Venerable Panyavro Vachira also emphasized the importance of our very last thoughts and emotions with regards to the afterlife. What it is will affect our journey in whether we are successful with our Ascension.

According to Buddhist teachings, the last thought before death is crucial and is therefore extremely powerful. This thought may determine whether one is to be reborn in the Pure Land or to reenter the samsara. **(R 283)**

If this thought is peaceful and calm, then one will be reborn as a human being. If one believes in God and the last thought is praying to God, one will be able to communicate with God and be reborn in heaven in Oneness with God.

At this juncture of life and death, our thoughts should be full of love, light and gratitude to facilitate a graceful transition. A full surrender and oneness to God's Love and Light is the ideal way to let go of our earthly dimension. We just need to surrender to God's Light, Love and Consciousness to guide us through the bardos and into our Ascension.

When Encarnacion was in a coma, we all did our part to help her allay her anxiety and fear of death. We flooded her consciousness with lots of love to dissolve the imbalance of emotions of sadness and anxiety. The massage and human contact we did with her further assisted her in receiving the love at a deep level. When she finally passed away, we continued to gather as a family to pray for her soul to transition with greater grace. As part of the Catholic tradition, the family prayers, rituals and gatherings were done for nine days.

When one of my clients passed away, his Buddhist's wife promised him that she would go and stay at the Buddhist temple for 30 days to meditate for his soul for a good transition and help him with his liberation.

What we do when a person is dying is very important but the prayers, mantras and rituals we do after death is also very important. I believe the first three days to a week are the most crucial.

Those who are too ill or in a coma will need help from family, friends, clergy, Mystic, Yogi or spiritual masters to guide and support them on their journey. We can visualize an energetic ball of love around the person and guiding their consciousness to their I AM Presence and to God's

Consciousness. We can also chant the sacred mantras and invoke powerful decrees to set the individual free.

Helping others to discover their true nature and helping them navigate their way to their awakening, self-realization and liberation is the ultimate act of love, compassion and kindness. By uplifting ourselves into greater Light and Love, we in turn assist others to be uplifted. By assisting others and ourselves, we become whole again with our Creator and Supreme Consciousness.

The act of Ascension may seem like the ultimate goal for all or many spiritual aspirants; however, it is only a gateway to another dimension of higher consciousness and Energy. It is like a spiritual bus stop to a whole new world. Enlightenment and Ascension are ongoing and ever evolving as long as we continue to gain mastery with opening our hearts, mind and souls to serving God and others and continue to identify with the oneness with God, the Universe and all creation that is seen and unseen.

Attaining liberation in one lifetime is possible and highly encouraged to raise the energy and consciousness of Earth and the Universe to help end its suffering. Those that choose to go through life on autopilot blindly will more than likely return to Earth in another embodiment with a clean slate memory. Those who have caused much suffering to others may go into a lower astral plane or possibly reincarnate as a creature other than a human.

Reincarnation

Master Relica once talked about a very abusive alcoholic person who reincarnated as a dog. The dog had some of the same eating behaviors as he did when he was a human. He liked eating mango with spicy sauce and seemed to remember where he kept important things. Although he was a dog during an incarnation, he still had his abusive emotions and behavior and continued to attack those he attacked in his previous lifetime. Eventually, he had to be given away since he was so aggressive but got killed in an accident and surprisingly enough, he returned again as another dog. Lifetimes will repeat over and over again until we can learn the lessons that are created from our karmas.

This recycling of life and reincarnation is samsara and will continue to perpetuate suffering of the individual as well as with others. Hence, it is very important to do our best to follow the path that leads to God and our true nature and live an empowered God-Realized life full of Divine Light, Love, Energy and Consciousness. We can then be set free and help set others free as well so we can all return home from whence we came to help end all sufferings.

When you have fulfilled your final earthly mission, or dharma, in this lifetime, may you enjoy your Ascension to the heavenly realms as you transcend the laws of karma into your liberation, be set free from the bondage of the endless birth and rebirth cycle and evolve into a noble, empowered and enlightened being of Light, Love and Consciousness of God that can be of even greater service to humanity, God and the heavenly hosts.

Let us explore how we can create the optimal scenario where we live in our true Divine and Enlightened Nature on a path towards Ascension that includes supporting those in our lives, in our city, country and planet. The planet is going through phases of ascension and many of us are ascending with her to higher energy and consciousness. However, there are many who are suffering and have suffered many lifetimes including our human and non-human friends. We must support Mother Earth, all of humanity and all creature great and small with navigating through life and attaining an eventual ascension in a much more graceful way and help end the great suffering of many. By helping others, we help ourselves in our own salvation, liberation and ascension.

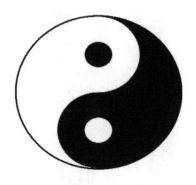

CHAPTER 19

WORLD PEACE AND HARMONY

Once we have reached great mastery with meditation, prayer, visualization, I AM decrees, gratitude and other practices, it may seem like all that remains to do is bring about the healing and harmony that we have attained for others, including Mother Earth. Although there is much merit in what we can do in solitude, we can be even more effective if we can reach out to others, develop ourselves further and learn a little about how others see the world. We can also further expand our consciousness, understanding, compassion, energy, unity and global oneness. We can begin building bridges, tearing down walls and begin to pave the way for more of an enlightened society where love, peace, harmony and respect prevail.

It is important that we join or be a part of groups that share our vision of unity, peace, love, compassion and global oneness. As we unite with groups when we feel a heart connection, our concerted efforts can have a very powerful effect on our community, country and Earth.

I have been a part of S.O.P.P. (Symphony of Peace Prayer) for about 4 years. It is a group that is based in the Fuji Sanctuary in Japan. Each year the group invites dignitaries, spiritual and religious leaders from all around the world during May to unite and pray that peace May Peace Prevail on Earth. All around the world, local groups also set up a gathering to invite spiritual and religious leaders from the community to be a part of this global prayer group.

In the Bible, Jesus states that "for where two or three are gathered together in my name, there am I in the midst of them". Matthew 18:20 **(R 284)**

Can you imagine how strong the presence of God would be in this worldwide group of religious and spiritual leaders which include many enlightened beings of varied backgrounds? What if Yogis, arahants and Mystics were to be a part of such a group? The collective energy and love of God would be so powerful in bringing greater harmony onto the planet.

What makes the event even more powerful is that the main event that is held at Fuji Sanctuary is located at a powerful energy vortex. Praying at a vortex amplifies the prayer and intentions exponentially.

Praying and meditating at sacred places and mountains like Mount Shasta, Mt. Kailash, Mt. Banahaw and Mt. Fuji can be so powerful and transformative. Places in India like a Linga or Dhyanalinga can have profound spiritual effects on one. It can also accelerate your spiritual awakening and evolution.

The Fuji Sanctuary is the headquarters for the group called Byakko, meaning The White Light. The head of this group is Masami Saionji. She is a scholar, spiritual leader and is the direct descendent of the Royal Ryukyu family in Okinawa.

She is also the chairperson of three world peace organizations and she and her daughters have done so much to bring peace and unity to our planet.

Their group is very spiritual and teaches its members how to access their I AM Presence or what they call Divine Spark of Light. What is unique to this group is that they teach the In Mudras activation. They are mudras done to activate the Divine Spark of Light within all of us. I practice the most recent In mudra and it has been helpful with my spirituality as well. It helps to bring peace to ourselves, to others and to the world.

All are welcomed to learn the In Mudras that the group has shared with so many people. You can order a booklet from the Fuji Sanctuary on how to do it.

Masami Sensei even teaches her members to say you are a Divine Being to 10,000 people. I believe this is a good exercise to help instill in our mind that we are all sacred and Divine Beings that should be treated with love, compassion and kindness.

The members are taught to give respect and gratitude to all manifestations of God and believe that ultimately God is Love. This includes the mountains, rivers, trees, humans, plants, animals, oceans - all elements and kingdoms of Nature. This is a beautiful organization to support and help because their mission is to help humanity reestablish their awareness of their Divine Nature and help restore harmony, unity and peace on our planet.

When more groups like this begin to collaborate with the community and world leaders and they all unite in prayer, meditation, In mudras and visualization, our planet's energy will experience an even greater shift in consciousness, energy and unity.

It is also important to collaborate with local and international Mystics, Yogis, arahants during difficult times in our planet. I have worked with Mystics during challenging times to help bring more balance on neutralizing some of the toxic energy on this planet.

Besides the spiritual stuff we can do alone or with a group, there are other ways we can help perpetuate peace and harmony on the planet and help dissolve much of the toxic ideations, emotions and memes generated from our collective disharmonious ego. Here are some principles that will help create greater oneness, harmony and peace in our planet.

1. Practice the 9 virtues of living in harmony:
   a. Love (love unconditionally to all sentient beings)
   b. Compassion
   c. Forgiveness and Mercy
   d. Nobility
   e. Service
   f. Kindness
   g. Integrity/ Honesty
   h. Humility
   i. Reverence for all life (Ahimsa - the practice of non-violence for all sentient beings)

2. **Guide the children.** Those of you who have children, nephews or nieces must take time to guide them when they are very young about the Divine Spark of Light in all of creation and all of humanity. The more children realize that all life is sacred, the less likely they are going to take away their own life or the lives of others. We must show the young ones the beauty they possess inside. If we do not have children directly in our lives, we can be a big brother, sister, father or mother to those in need - being a guide to helping them discover the greatness within. Being a brother, sister, father and mother does not have to be biological. Being a mother figure or father figure is just as important.

3. **Feed your body, mind and soul only those things which are in the best interest of your higher self** and that will support your Divine Spark in allowing it to create an inner Universe of Love, Peace and Harmony. Listen to calm, nurturing and positive music or audios.

4. **Avoid condemning what food people eat and what religions they practice.** Instead, hold space, pray and decree for everyone to be lifted into harmony with the Divine Plan including having reverence for all of Life. People do what they do because of where they are in their consciousness and spiritual evolution. As people begin to reach higher consciousness they will automatically begin to eat in more harmony with the planet and their own inner Universe. They will also begin to learn how to transcend the limitations of religions and see the great Truths that are in common in all religions that are predicated upon God's Divine Love. Instead of judging or condemning others and being self-righteous, we should be supportive, compassionate and loving towards others and pray daily for others to wake up from their spiritual coma or sleep. We can always enlighten and educate others, but we must never condemn.

5. **Learn to sever the tie with money and spirituality.** So many new age self-proclaimed gurus are making a business out of spirituality. There is nothing wrong with money because it is how many sustain themselves but then what happens to those people who have limited money and resources? Are they not welcomed to

the kingdom of God? Some spiritual teachers charge from $150.00 to $400.00/ hour for spiritual services; meanwhile there are those who charge $800.00/hour for spiritual guidance. It all depends on the experience and expertise of the spiritual teacher, master or guide and the services being rendered.

i.   Then there are those who are on the extreme side who charge $1,000.00 to $20,000.00 for a healing session. I can understand the lower ranges of $150- $400.00/hour but $800.00, $1000.00 and $10,000? There are many false prophets and charismatic self-proclaimed gurus who are making much money off innocent people and promising them things that would lead them further away from their true nature and more towards their ego. Spirituality is the path to all God's children.

ii.   Money should never be a limiting factor for helping God's child discover the greatness within. Jesus said, "Let the little children come to me, and do not hinder them, for the kingdom of heaven belongs to such as these." Matthew 19:14. Though this Bible verse is in reference to little children it applies to all of us as well since we are all children of God. It is downtrodden and need help. I do it out of pure love and as guided by the Ascended Masters. The point that I am trying to make is that I understand that we all have to make a living but after we have enough, it is blessed to help those who are in need and are less fortunate. Many I helped gratis are now living happy and fulfilled lives and that has also positively affected their friends and families. It's a ripple effect that will come back.

iii. The spiritual community at Mount Shasta have discussed this delicate topic and there is no easy answer but some have come up with some creative solutions like bartering and time banking; it is a reciprocity-based work trading system in which hours are the currency. It is a form of community currency, which enables a person with one skill set to trade hours of work with someone with another skill set, without any money changing hands) and sliding scale according to Kathryn Shanti Ariel. (R 285)

6. **Find ways of serving others.** Blessed are those who help the poor, the needy, the elderly and the youth. We can volunteer at a hospital, nursing home or ashram. Volunteering or Seva is the ultimate expression of love. There is nothing more beautiful than serving others out of pure love. The moment we learn to serve others is the moment we begin to truly live and become God in action.

7. **Be more conscious and mindful where you spend your money.** You should support those businesses and companies that are eco-friendly, environmentally conscious, charitable, practice fair trade, and do not use toxic chemicals in their food or products.

8. **We should practice Social Media and TV fasting regularly.** Abstinence from it will create more space in your life for peace, contemplation and self-cultivation. If you find yourself checking your Social Media hourly or daily then I highly recommend you to practice the fasting. Instead of all the junk you watch in TV, watch quality TV programs found in PBS (public broadcast service) like KQED or pick quality movies to watch from Netflix or other apps.

9. **Practice random acts of kindness.**

10. **Donate-** donate regularly to those in need of the material things you have like clothes, books, toys, furniture, cars, etc. Donate your time to educate, empower, heal and liberate online, in your community or private practice.

11. **Practice seeing the greatness in everyone and in all creatures great and small.** When we look at someone say Namaste silently and realize they are a Divine Being deep within.

12. **Practice forgiveness on a daily basis.** Forgive yourself on what you have done to keep you further away from your true nature and God. Forgive the wrongs you have done to others and forgive what others have done wrong to you.

13. **Always be grateful and count your blessings.** Learn to see the good in every situation. Try to always seek the lesson that it is to be learnt even in difficult times.

14. **Learn to see the good in every situation.** Try to always seek the lesson that it is to be learnt even in difficult times.

15. **Help those who are in need**. Help in whatever capacity you can. If you are rich, share your wealth. If you are wise, share your wisdom. If you are well connected, share your contacts. If you are a healer, send healing energy and prayers. If you have much time, share your time and talents.

I once helped a homeless lady find work. She was practically living in her car. I gave her work off and on and even gave her referrals to support her new business. Eventually she got back on her feet and found regular work. The good news is that she is no longer homeless and is now able to sustain herself.

I have helped many people that I have met over the years. The wife of one of my clients had called me and told me that her husband had passed away, but that he thought of me fondly even during his last hours of life. After he passed away, his wife was tossed into a new reality she was unfamiliar with which caused her much anxiety, stress and sadness. Her husband apparently had done everything for his wife and hence she was completely lost when he was gone like many other widows whose husband took care of everything.

When she contacted me about the sad news and her overwhelming situation, I immediately jumped into action to help her systematically get her life back. I coordinated with my nephew and my daughter's boyfriend to help her physically move out of her apartment. I later guided her on what to do with her insurance, finances and how to live again.

I gave her support and gave her guidance on how to navigate her way to finding meaning in her life. I even drove her to her husband's military cemetery to show our last respect to him. His last wishes were that his wife and I would be there at his military funeral service. I prayed for his soul as well as his wife while we were at his grave site and offered her support throughout her grieving period. I never once asked for money or expected anything in return. I did it out of pure compassion for this grieving child of God.

She is now living happily with her long-lost son (separated and abducted when he was a baby) and relatives in Thailand. She still appreciates all I have done for her and calls me her brother.

Earlier in the book, I wrote of an individual I helped in India. Besides helping her to break through the psychic blockage she had in her head, I gave her emotional and spiritual support and guidance. Although she was flat broke and could not offer to pay me, I did it because my I AM Presence guided me to help her. Now she is doing well mentally, emotionally and spiritually. In fact, now she has become a shaman and hypnotherapist and is helping others heal.

We should never judge and always help those who are in need. We never know how great the impact of our love and healing is to others. Love without action is dead and stagnant. When we learn to serve others selflessly out of love, compassion and kindness, the effect can be quite healing and transformative for both the giver and the receiver. Once we act out of love, our actions begin to create waves of love, compassion and kindness which build up and are contagious and healing.

Below are some suggestions on how we can further help create Heaven on Earth and oneness on this planet. (Select those that resonate with you.)

1. **Listen to inspiring speeches and lectures** and watch programs that foster your spiritual, mental, emotional and physical well-being.

2. **Eat and drink things that support your health,** such as organic, non-GMO, soy-free and gluten-free products, food and drinks. It's helpful to minimize processed food and drinks that contain high sugar, sodium, cholesterol, preservative, food coloring, etc. Make sure that your food, drink, vitamin, supplement or medication is supporting the harmony within your body, mind and spirit.

3. **Share your gifts and talents to contribute to the flow and harmony of Mother Earth's Elements.** The Earth, too, is made of earth, air, fire and water elements. We must stop our deforestation and insatiable appetites for our animal-based diets. We must stop our technology from polluting our air. More affordable electric cars must be made in order for the average person to afford one. We must stop out dependency on fossil fuel. We must develop technology for solar panel and systems that are long lasting and cost effective. We must support those scientists who have developed free energy for the benefit of humanity. We must send more love

to Mother Earth and all of humanity while purifying it with the Violet Consuming Flame for all the toxic and unhealthy energies that are preventing many from awakening and evolving. We must protect our seas from plastics, microbeads, chemicals, radiation and oil spills. We must learn to recycle and avoid plastics.

4. **Prioritize the education and awakening of humanity** about what is going on in the world. Share with your friends the lists of videos listed on the **Game Changer reference**. Tell as many people as possible to read this and all my other books to empower humanity to reclaim our Divine Nature and Presence on this planet.

5. **Devotion**-Read sacred teachings daily to be uplifted and inspired. We could recite or read the teachings of the Dalai Lama as often as we can especially the one titled *A Precious Life* and *The True Meaning of Life.* Scrolls of those Divine teachings can be found at most Tibetan or Nepalese stores. It is very important to have a regular devotional practice that includes prayer, reading, chanting and meditation. **Master Mun** has appeared to me on several occasions from July to August 2020 and has stressed to me the importance of a regular devotional practice and that it is through regular faithfulness to it that allows me to have more mystical experiences and connections with him. **El Morya** appeared to me on August 6, 2020. He told me how important my devotional practice was and explained to me how it is spiritual food for my soul. Through regular practice, it helps to keep me focused on my spiritual path, increases my spiritual mastery, and keeps me spiritually protected. Through a commitment to devotion, I have been visited and guided by many Ascended Masters on a more regular basis and live in greater Love, Light and harmony.

6. **Value travel** - travel to as many foreign lands as possible and learn about their food, language, culture, religion, philosophy, etc. Those of you who are unable to travel physically can travel vicariously through reading books about other countries. The more we learn about other countries, the more likely we are to have greater tolerance and respect for those who are different than we are. Some of the most intolerant people I have met have never been

anywhere out of the country let alone out of their state. Conversely, some of the most broadminded and fascinating people I have met have travelled all around the world or at least have made friends with people from all around the world.

7. **It may be helpful to learn a couple of new languages** or ways of how to greet people and/or learn how to say I love you and thank you. Language controls our perception and how we relate to people and see the world. The more languages we learn, the more our minds will be connecting with people out of respect and the more open our minds will become with understanding the world. When we do that, others will respect you as well and will be more open to learning about you since you took the effort to learn about them.

8. **Learn about at least two other religions** other than your own. By learning how others find peace and comfort, you will learn how to evolve further in your spirituality. Remember, Jesus was not a Christian, Buddha was not a Buddhist, and Mohammed was not a Muslim. The great Truths are in all religions that are based in God's Love. Learning about the other religions will begin to help you better understand spirituality and will help you relate more to others who are different. Focus on the Universal teachings that unite us.

9. **Encourage** unity through interfaith prayer, meditation, singing, dancing, entertainment and even dining.

10. **Practicing U.U.M.M. daily** will shift your awareness from being an ego conscious being to becoming more a Divine Being of Light, Love and Energy. In other words, you will become more like a God-realized Being. You will no longer hunger or thirst but be satiated by the fullness of God's Love, Grace and Blessings. Practicing U.U.M.M. will begin to shift the energy within your inner Universe to your house, community, Mother Earth and the Universe to be full of love, gratitude, harmony, and peace. You will become a very illuminating Light of God to heal those who need healing and to guide those who need guidance. Though U.U.M.M. you will begin to see how the Universe is within and without us. You will learn to see how our body, chakra system and

consciousness is also on Earth, the Universe and Universes. Our micro Universe is connected to our macro Universe and beyond.

11. Through U.U.M.M. meditation, you will realize that there is no boundary or limit of time and space with your prayer, visualization and intentions of healing through love and compassion. Through your journey through this system, you will realize that creating health and harmony starts with the self but extends to others; however, it must extend to Mother Earth and to all sentient beings on this planet and the Universe and Universes. Through mastery of the U.U.M.M. Meditation, you will no longer think just in terms of yourself or ego but more from a context of a God-realized and Christ Conscious Being of Light and realize that humanity, Mother Earth and the Universe and you are one. You will then start to focus more on the global state of well-being and harmony as well as a Cosmic one and will embark on a noble quest to bring about global and Cosmic oneness.

12. **How we create Heaven from within** is how we can create Heaven on Earth as well. There is no limit in how we can affect our planet and Universe especially if we create alliances with the great Ascended Masters who are part of **the Ascended Council of Light** (Great White Brotherhood and Sisterhood). I have decreed and called upon the assistance of Hotei, Saint Germain, Kwan Yin, the Violet Tara, etc. to form a powerful alliance to help create more positive energy, love, peace, harmony, etc. on the planet.

13. **Listen to sacred and uplifting music.** Here is some music that I have found quite helpful with supporting my spirituality:

   a. *Shree Bhaktamar Stotra.* The version that I like best is sung by Anuradha Paudwal. There is a mystical story behind this song written by a monk and scholar that was imprisoned by the king of Avanti, Vriddha Bjoj, so that the king could witness a miracle. The monk, Archarya was kept in a dark cell and in order for him to come out he would have to open 48 chained doors. While in prison, he meditated for three days and on the fourth day, he composed this song and began to chant it. When he chanted the chains began to come off until all of the chains

405

were gone. Through the song, all the chains that locked the doors for his exit were broken. When I listen to it, I imagine the shackles to my soul, emotions and my consciousness being unshackled and being healed and set free. **(R 286)**

b. *Gayatri Mantra* (You can watch a YouTube video with an explanation at **(R 287)**

c. *The Healing Tones* **(R 288)**

d. *Gregorian Chant*

e. *Healing music* by Steven Halpern

f. Samuel Barber's *Agnes Dei* (my personal favorite that I would like to listen to during my own Ascension)

g. Tina Turner's *Peace Mantra* (Sarvesham Svastir Bhavatu) **(R 289)**

h. Yuan Miao's *Guan Yin*

i. *The 48 Stotras* **(for blessings)**

j. *100 Deities Mantra* **(R 290)**

14. Watch and listen to **Videos/CDs** that may inspire you, such as:

a. Wayne Dyer

b. Joel Osteen

c. Deepak Chopra

15. **Promote methods that support wellness, harmony and health of body, mind and spirit through new educational and world values.** Meditation, nutrition, energy healing, and yoga should be taught in schools at all levels of education to pave the way for an enlightened and healthy civilization

16. **It is very important to activate and nurture the Divine Feminine Energy within ourselves and the collective consciousness** so we might gain greater self-mastery to love and have compassion, mercy and kindness to shift our planet towards manifesting Heaven on Earth where there is greater peace and harmony. The masculine energy has ruled our planet for way too long and has only led millions to much fear, anxiety, oppression and suffering.

17. In order for humanity to make a big impact on our planet, it helps for us to **be more mindful of who we support and where**

we spend our money. Those who embrace a new beginning of unity, peace and harmony for all are the ones we should support the most.

18. **Technology** is advancing rapidly along with A.I. (Artificial Intelligence). If we do not learn to fast and eventually unplug from technology, we will allow our freedom to slip away from us as we become slaves of the technology that the few behind the curtains of our Oz have created. After taking a break from social media and TV, I find myself living in more joy, peace, love and meaning.

19. **Be a spiritual role model and inspire change in others - Dr. Sonia-Badreshia-Bansal** is one of the most intelligent, evolved and enlightened doctors I have ever met. (She is also such a beautiful soul and caring doctor) She once told me that **"inspiring for change is our biggest duty to the world!"** I totally agree and add that inspiring others through God's love is the ultimate goal of all Yogis and Mystics.

Pax Navitus

My dear friend, Mardi Coeur de Lion, Global citizen/ champion for goodness, poet, visionary and world acclaimed artist, shared with me

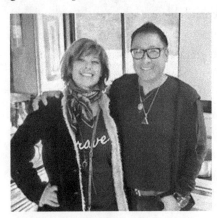

her draft of **Pax Navitus** and I find it quite inspiring and empowering. Interestingly, her grandfather was a Chief Justice in India. Her passion with local and global justice is admirable. Mardi and her family took in 40 foster children in dire need over 25 years. Most were First Nations teens who were the second generation of fallout from a severely abusive government/church residential school policy, recognized as a crime against Humanity.

Mardi Coeur de Lion (Global Citizen and cover designer) with Blake Sinclair

Inspired by her wish for a better world for her children, Mardi wrote a World School of Peace proposal that was endorsed by the Dalai Lama,

Dr. Robert Muller, founder of the United Nations University of Peace and International Olympic Committee members.

The Pax Navitus proposal, is a bold, strategic, Hermetic win/win/ win global solution that could potentially deliver world peace, power and prosperity to all of Humanity in one checkmate maneuver on the geopolitical "Grand Chessboard." Some of its components include:

1. Applicable Law - Primum, Non Nocere - First Do No Harm. This profoundly simple principle is the keystone Create a universally tenet overarching, enlightened, civilized societies, philosophies and religions - bridging myriad faiths and beliefs in the primacy of our shared acknowledgement of all living beings.

2. Declare a Global Climate State of Emergency and forming an Earth Alliance.

3. Global Diversion of 11% of the Global Military Budget to create Free Green Energy for all of Humanity. If energy cost was dramatically reduced globally, the cost of living would be dramatically reduced for everyone - potentially eradicating poverty. Products will be produced far cheaper; transportation costs will drop; manufacturing cost will drop and everyone will reap the benefits. Citizens will experience a huge economic boost. Everyone will have far more expendable income, resulting in global prosperity boom.... oil/resource wars will become obsolete. We can share resources and create great civilizations if we evolve past our barbaric, intrinsically violent, war-loving tendencies.

4. **Pax Navitus** is a Global Peace, Power and Prosperity Plan that can save us and our Paradise Planet. Visionaries, like Mardi abound - the question is, is Humanity ready to evolve past our barbaric history and addiction for war and global weapons sales - and invest instead, in creating great global civilizations...together. If you would like to support the Pax Navitus initiative, please contact Mardi at mardi@mardi.ca.

* * * * *

Creating world peace or contributing to it by becoming peaceful within is a goal of every Mystic and Yogi. Inner peace is just the beginning of enlightenment. When we begin to expand our inner peace, compassion, love and kindness to others in our actions, deeds, emotions, prayers and meditation practices, we will expand our consciousness and spiritual evolution even further. This will help bring humanity to higher level of consciousness and to a greater degree of enlightenment.

Besides doing our sadhana or spiritual practices, we must also educate humanity about the causes of our suffering that we have co- created through the collective ego. We must learn to realize the Divine Presence within all of us and that all of Creation is in a constant flow of creating harmony within our inner Universe as well as the Universe without us but it is being hampered by our current way of collective ego-driven life by how we fill our physical, emotional, mental and spiritual bodies as well as the physical, emotional, mental and spiritual bodies on Earth and in space. We are truly one and interconnected.

Planetary Chakras

We have chakras within as well as on Earth. The first chakra of Earth is Mount Shasta; second is Lake Titicaca Peru; the third is Uluru in Australia; the fourth is in Glastonbury, Somerset, Shaftesbury, Dorset; fifth is in the Great Pyramids near Mt. Sanai and Mt. Olives; sixth is in Western Europe and the 7th is in Mt. Kailash, in the Himalayas. **(R 291)**

Mikaelah Cordeo, Channel and Messenger for the Ascended Hosts of Light, reported new information (received from Mother-Father God of the Multiverse) on the Planetary Chakras and other key energy sites on Earth in her book, Live in Love. **(R 292)** She also observed that there was, and still is, a great deal of diversity of opinion on which planetary locations are so identified. All the published lists appear to have some major differences with one another.

Her channeled information indicated several things. Unlike human chakras, these appeared to be "managed" by higher Divine sources. and were: 1) able to be shut down or made partially operational, 2) able to be moved to new locations, and 3) even operate at human created structures such as the great pyramid in Egypt and the standing stones at

Stonehenge in England. She points out that "this implies that they serve as technologically managed, electro/magnetic receivers and transmitters, or at least something that can magnify higher consciousness thought waves. Her channeled information suggested that all but Mount Shasta were either fully shut down and relocated or only partially active. Mount Shasta is temporarily acting as the primary planetary receiver of energies and these were then redirected as needed.

* * * * *

Interestingly enough, one of the most important movements of one of the planetary chakras happened in Northern California in the sacred and mystical town of Mount Shasta. This is home of many spiritual masters and enlightened beings. Thousands of seekers come from all around the world each year in search of the Truth in this little town, including Swamis, Buddhist Monks, Lamas, and other enlightened beings. Many people go here as part of their spiritual pilgrimage. I was no exception. This is where Saint Germain first appeared to Guy Ballard aka Godfré Ray King in the early 1930's. This is where I first met Peter Mt. Shasta and many of the Ascended Masters including the Maha Chohan, Saint Germain, Jesus, Kwan Yin and Mother Mary. The details of that event were documented in my second book in the Golden Book Series, Beyond Imagination. **(R 293)**

While Mikaelah lived in Mount Shasta, she learned that a group of Tibetan monks had arrived and gone up the mountain to leave certain ancient, sacred artifacts, to offer ceremony and basically 'move' and/or anchor certain energy fields from Tibet to Mount Shasta - exact details were not given. (Incidentally, it was after my visit to a Tibetan Stupa in Mount Shasta when my relics of Buddha multiplied miraculously in a sealed container.)

* * * * *

The bottom line is that only one planetary chakra, Mount Shasta, is reported as being fully functional, and is now serving as the planetary Crown Chakra.

This means that all energy coming to the planet goes first through Mount Shasta and is then redirected to the other planetary, major and minor, chakra points as is appropriate and from there transmitted to the rest of the planet. *(For more information on the Planetary Chakras and other key energy centers around the world, Mikaelah is placing the entire chapter from her book **Live in Love** on her website https://MikaelahCordeo.com.)*

According to Mikaelah's higher sources, the inner plane Shambhala was also relocated in the Mount Shasta area at about the same time.

One interesting synchronicity about another planetary chakra is Mount McKinley in Alaska. It was identified as the new Root Chakra in Mikaelah's book, and it was noted that its original Native name, Mount Denali, was better able to hold the new frequencies that it now carried and needed to be changed back. Several years later, the mountain was indeed renamed Mount Denali. All of this reflects the enormous changes happening on every level on Earth.

Even as this is being written in 2020, Great fires have raged across Australia, first the Chinese borders were closed due to quarantine of a new "Super-virus", rapidly followed by a never-before-recorded planetary "lockdown" by almost all world governments – not to mention, a mountain of plastic in the oceans as big as a continent and the sudden die-off of whole species of a magnitude not seen since the demise of the dinosaurs.

Mikaelah observed that "a variety of signs suggest that these are the prophesied "end times". That is, the End of an Era (Astrologically, the end of the Piscean Age of the last 2,000 years, and beginning of the Aquarian Age); a transition to "Heaven on Earth"; return to Eden Consciousness; and planetary Ascension to the 5th Dimension.

"The bottom line is – the planetary energy field is being raised every day and seemingly, faster and faster. All that is denser energetically cannot remain and is coming up to be cleared – old karma, core issues, pain, suffering, disease and death. Relationships that aren't working must be upgraded or released."

Mikaelah recounts that she once asked Jesus, with reference to world changes, "What is going on?" - a very simple question; His profound answer: **"All the bonds that are less than Love are being broken."**

She reports that almost everyone she knows is in the midst of major upheaval right now, either their own health, work or relationship issues or family and friends with major issues, such as death of a parent or child. Think of all those who lost loved ones, jobs and homes in the recent fires all over the Western U.S. and Australia and the anguish over the global pandemic and its health, education, work, travel and economic impacts as other examples.

Mikaelah remarks, "Topics such as planetary chakras and shifting to a new dimensional reality may be way outside your belief system – or not – but the many great suggestions covered in this book provide help in this time of transition and transformation:

- Take care of your health.
- Pray for yourself, one another and the world.
- Choose Love and focus on the positive vision you hold for the future.
- Release all that no longer serves you to make way for your far superior, higher frequency, next steps.
- Clear regularly with Violet Flame (for forgiveness and the transmutation of negativity).
- Find balance in your life – physical, emotional, mental and spiritual.
- Breathe in Light, Life, Health, Hope and Love.
- Breathe out All that no longer serves."

Honoring the Earth and the Journey Home

The lungs of the planet are its forests and especially the Amazon; the oils are Earth's blood; the core of Mother Earth contains the I AM Presence of the planet; the mountains and land are Mother Earth's body; the wind and air are like her breath; the ocean are like the large body of fluids in our body.

Abusing our body temple, Mother Earth and space with contaminants of toxins, junk and toxic and negative energies we have created will lead to greater suffering of millions for many years to come. (Note: There are many people and entities that thrive on the negative emotions we generate like anger, anxiety and fear.)

When one suffers, we all suffer; when one succeeds, we all succeed. Hence, the modern-day Yogi must also be a teacher, spiritual warrior, educator and healer to be of greater assistance to humanity and the Ascended Council of Light. By living a God-Realized Christ Conscious life, we can help awaken, heal, educate and empower thousands and million around the world to begin creating an Earth Alliance that will pave the way for an enlightened civilization as we begin heading towards a new Golden Age of oneness and enlightenment.

In Summary: Thank you for joining me on this amazing and extraordinary Journey to the W.E.S.T. (Wisdom, Enlightenment, Salvation and Truth) especially those who have read all three books of this Golden Book Spiritual Trilogy series. Congratulations to those of you who have been guided and assisted in finding your way back home to your true and Divine Nature! Much information was shared to help you and others navigate out of much of your suffering that we have co-created collectively. You must remember to be mindful what you put in your mind, body and soul. Whether it is TV, music, movies, social media, food, beverage, vitamins, minerals, herbs, medicine or anything you inhale, inject or put on your skin, hair, body or face, make sure you find out what you are putting into yourself, know what it is made of and pay attention to see if it is creating more harmony within you and others or more chaos, disharmony and illnesses.

If it causes disharmony or illnesses then you may consider that something else might be better suited for you in supporting your I AM Presence to promote greater wellness. Always listen to your body, your I AM Presence and do you own homework and research.

Although I have given you much info and resources on what to buy, take and do to attain health, harmony and wellness, it seems there are a lot of things to purchase. The plethora of things shared with you will help our current Consumer Conscious Civilization in many different circumstances. However, 2020 is a transformative year and is an invitation for us to evolve further into a God Conscious Civilization by going within and being one with God, Mother Earth humanity and the Universe.

We must get back to basic to heal ourselves and humanity by living in harmony with ourselves, others, Mother Earth and the Universe and becoming much more aware of living a sustainable life. We can begin living this way by planting a vegetable and fruit garden and eating what you planted which is not tainted by chemicals and outside forces trying to manipulate its purity and nature. Receiving God's gifts (fruits, vegetables, herbs, spices and water) in its organic and true form is what our bodies really needs. Supporting your local farmers is a good way to support your community and eat healthy and fresh fruits and vegetables as well. Planting fruit bearing trees in homeless areas may be a great one to supply them with a good source of minerals, fibers and nutrients.

If we meditate, exercise regularly, get enough sunshine, eat and drink healthy, enjoy life, live happy, rest enough, serve others, laugh often, pray, practice daily devotion with our Creator and live in alignment with God's Love, we can minimize our need for excessive vitamins and supplements. Unfortunately, until we learn to stop exhausting our soil and Mother Earth's resources, we will most likely need some form of supplementation to help us navigate through our lives with more grace. Therefore, you must go forth and educate and create more awareness for others about the collateral damage (the physical, emotional, mental and spiritual suffering) of the ego perpetuated reality we have co-created. Teach and guide others in helping them end their suffering as well. The matrix we have been living in is growing thin as more people are awakening from their spiritual coma and sleep.

This book was written at a time where humanity's suffering has reached an all-time high with millions and millions of people suffering all around the world and dying prematurely. The complexities of the various types of sufferings are growing in numbers and are leaving many experts scratching their heads as to the etiology of many illnesses and diseases. Shamans, traditional Chinese Medicine practitioners, Ayurvedic Medicine practitioners and other holistic healers have long understood the importance of the interplay of the body, mind, emotion and spirit for creating harmony, wellness and health. They and many others are also aware of the many effects that the advancing technologies have on our health, especially from the radiation that is constantly bombarding us. It is up to us to stand up for what we need in terms of a healthy environment. It is up to us to collectively encourage the development of advancing technologies that are in alignment with the harmony and wellness of all life on Earth.

It is more important now than ever before that we work towards creating greater health and wellness within and expanding our consciousness and spiritual awareness.

There are many theories of the origin of the virus that has captured the attention of the world in 2020. However, it is not the time for us to live in fear, but to move forward with full confidence that we will navigate through this crisis more gracefully with all the knowledge I have shared with you. Through the great wisdom contained within this book and through your partnership with your physician especially a Holistic physician or practitioner, you will attain greater health, harmony and wellness. You will also weather through 2020 more triumphantly especially with the help of God, his or her Angels and Ascended Beings and Masters around us.

It is especially important to know that this is a very critical time in our lives; how we handle this cleansing and transformational period will affect our lives and future in how we live and create greater harmony in the planet. We are living in a very pivotal time in the history of humankind.

I hope you are beginning to see a pattern and realize that the root cause of many of our woes, sorrows and illnesses are due to our separation from God and our Divinity; instead, many of us are strongly attached, enslaved or addicted to the ego-perpetuated matrix we have co-created.

It is the perfect time for us to go within to reflect and open our minds and hearts to being that change we want to see in the world. We must meditate to gain more awareness and insight on what is going on in the world. We must use all the tools in the book to assist all of us in raising our energies and consciousness and that of Gaia to further empower and protect all of us.

We are living in a time where the veil and maya is growing thin as more enlightened beings are waking up from the matrix. However, many more of our brothers, sisters, families and friends near and far are still blind, lost and asleep in this illusory dream we live in. You, in turn, are called to help them.

We can help them pierce this illusory veil by imparting knowledge and wisdom to as many people as we can reach through social media, radio, and through all the people we meet.

You have been given many great tools and secrets to empower yourself in living a Christ Conscious, God-realized life full of God's Love, Light

415

and Consciousness. With great power comes great responsibility! However, if we continue to live in power, fame, fortune and ego we will continue to be trapped in the Matrix. This cannot continue in the new rising frequencies of humanity. All life on Earth and Gaia herself (the Divine Consciousness of our planet) are currently undergoing an evolution into an enlightened civilization. And all that can no longer be sustained must be cleared and released.

Those who live in Oneness with God and humbly serve others through God's love, mercy and compassion will be given the key to eternal life.

I hope you realize by now that you and God co-create the inner Universe and Heaven within yourselves as well as around you. You should also know that in a Divine state of consciousness there is much more you can do to affect the future of humanity and Mother Earth especially when we collaborate with the noble angelic beings known as the Ascended Masters who are all part of the **Ascended Council of Light** (Great White Brotherhood and Sisterhood).

During meditation, I have seen much dark energy around Mother Earth and humanity that keeps many people divisive, blind, ignorant and asleep in a spiritual slumber or even coma.

Although there has been some degree of dark energy in the planet for many years, there has been an increasing amount that has spread throughout the planet especially during last 100 years or more. We have all watched the Wizard of Oz but who would have guessed that there are a lot of truth in that movie.

Little does humanity know that it is behind the curtains of our Oz where scenarios of fear, chaos and divisiveness are created, devised and mastermind by a few to keep the collective consciousness asleep for their own gain. Should we fear? Absolutely not! We must embrace the unity of our consciousness with God, Mother Earth, the Ascended Council of Light and humanity to empower us to be the pioneers of change to save our planet and humanity.

We currently live in a very sophisticated matrix that has been feeding and fueling our egos and creating much fear, divisiveness, anger, anxiety, jealousy, discontentment, sorrow, greed, lust, desire and hatred. Those who are still asleep continue to perpetuate the tsunami of negative emotions on our planet. As bad as it is, it serves as fuel for entities, demonic beings and a certain small percentage of humanity and who seem to thrive and delight in chaos and negative energies. The matrix system was designed to keep us ignorant and asleep but glitches (inconsistencies between what we read or hear versus what we have already read, heard, seen, discovered or know as the truth) in the system has started to awaken many to its illusions and deceptions.

Despite the toxic and negative energy throughout the planet, the planet is undergoing a shift in consciousness and cleansing. More people are awakening all around the world and are making their voices heard and known. People from all around the world are beginning to protest to the injustice and discrimination they see and are angered by the system that is broken and is slow to change. We can change it through unity, love and peaceful protest!

I also see many great enlightened beings, Mystics, Yogis, spiritual warriors, light warriors, Rainbow Warriors, and benevolent extra-terrestrial beings, etc. who are actively working towards bringing more light, love, unity, compassion, respect, wisdom and peace to the world.

This is the perfect time for us to collaborate with one another and put our differences in dogma and ideology aside for the greater good of our civilization and planet. We must realize that we are all beautiful expressions of God's Consciousness to various degrees, light, awareness and illumination. Religion, dogmas and ideology can limit your spiritual evolution and experiences. Moving beyond that, you can find that it is the intersection of all religions and mysticism where the Truth exists.

We must also collectively be mindful of how we are treating Gaia or Mother Earth. We must choose to stop polluting the ocean, rivers, lakes and land. We need to make choices to minimize pollutant emissions in the air. We must stop deforestation and our over-reliance on fossil fuel. Instead, we should learn to harness the free energy that was once discovered by Nikola Tesla.

We must learn to be good stewards of Mother Earth, humble servants of God, and not be enslaved by the technology that we have created.

We must realize and accept that Mother Earth is a living and conscious planet and give her the love and respect she needs. We must learn to see beyond our inner Universe. Besides purifying our inner Universe, learn to also purify the planet and beyond by invoking the presence of God and the various members of the Ascended Council of Light to help with that Cosmic clearing of Mother Earth and beyond with the Violet Flame and Divine healing Light, Love and Energy of God. Realize that we are the living Light of God that has the power to change our future as we learn to step into the sovereignty of our Divine Presence.

Learn to see the common thread that connects all great wisdom and teachings that unite us. Realize that we the people are 7.8 billion people strong, and we can start a global movement through our increasing interest in health, wellness and longevity. It can actually lead us to a deeper understanding of our spirituality, divinity and God. We are called to assist in the awakening of millions and billions to their true nature and begin the necessary change to create Heaven on Earth full of enlightened and empowered beings of God's Light, Love and Consciousness.

I see humanity stepping into the sovereignty of our Divine Nature and being the cosmic change we are seeking. The only limit we have with what we can or can't do is our imagination.

Many of you may view the author as a highly evolved spiritual being of Light who was born that way. If that were the case, that would have been too easy for me and I wouldn't have been able to empower you with real life experiences and wisdom. Those of you who read my first book, ***Dare to Imagine: 18 Principles for Finding Peace, Happiness and True Success***, will realize how I was born into the most toxic and unhealthy environment. I endured much hardship and many disappointments in life but all that catapulted me into finding myself and embarking on my incredible spiritual journey which led me to my awakening and connections with God and the Ascended Masters.

I incarnated here to show all of you what is possible. I was not born into a spiritual family nor lived in an ashram. I had no guidance on my spiritual journey during most of my life and as a result made many mistakes and suffered from depression, anxiety and much stress for many years. Fortunately, my path to enlightenment led me to living in love, peace, happiness and joy through oneness with God's Love.

God has put many challenges in my life so I could learn from it and overcome it, so that I could share the wisdom and experience with all of you. So, you too can be free from suffering and live in harmony with others and God.

I am no different or better than any one of you. What I have achieved and have done, can be done by anyone of you; in fact, many of you will do even more than what I did and may all glory be given to God.

We must allow our numbers and diversity to dissolve all that toxic energy on Earth and help us restore that oneness with God, Mother Earth and humanity. It is time for us to become Modern Day Yogis and Mystics who will save humanity and Mother Earth from destruction with our collective love, mercy, kindness, compassion and healing energies.

Remember, we need to stop looking for answers and solutions outside of ourselves. We need to stop being spoon fed deception, lies and toxic and divisive information from the creators of the matrix that many are still enslaved to. We need to be proactive and feed and drink from the nectar of God's Love, Light, Energy and Wisdom.

We need to remember that all we need lies within us in the center of our being – that I AM Presence, Magic Presence, Spark of Light, our G.P.S. (Gods' Presence/Source consciousness). When we align ourselves with this infinite love and consciousness, it will guide us on what we should do and who we should meet. It will empower us to do and manifest the impossible. Our reality is only limited by our beliefs and imagination. Ultimately, it will set us free to be infinite beings of Love, Light and Consciousness and bring us home from whence we came.

Know ye that you are Gods and Goddesses, individualized aspects of the Supreme Consciousness.

The planet has been going through significant shifts and changes and the dawning of the Golden Age is upon us. It is a beautiful time to be alive.

Let's step into the sovereignty of our Divine Nature and be the cosmic change we are seeking. The only limit we have with what we can or can't do is our imagination. Therefore, let us work together to create Heaven on Earth and may God's will be done on Earth as it is in Heaven.

Wishing my beloved brothers and sisters,
Infinite love and blessings!

Blake Sinclair

419

Namaste
Sat Sri Akal
Allah-u-Abha
God Bless All Life.
Om Mani Padme Hum
May Peace Prevail on Earth!
Om Shanti, Shanti, Shantihi!

.-- .-- --. .---- .-- --. .-
.-. .--. .----

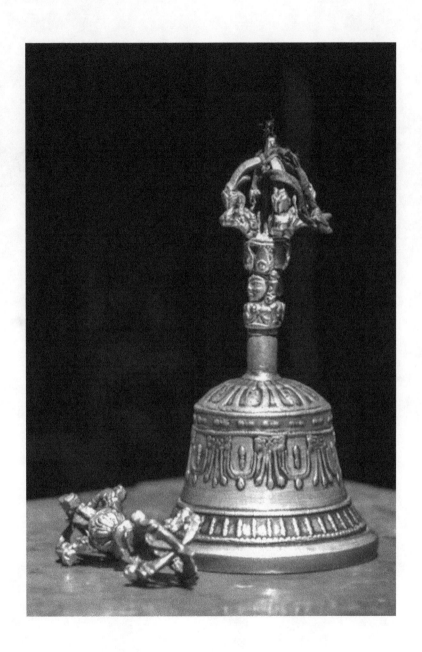

APPENDICES

AUTHOR'S NOTES AND CODES

GLOSSARY

---

*= Sold at Valley Health Mill
IS= Immune Support
R= Reference
***= Author's favorite

Adaptogen: special plants, which have unique properties. These have natural, biologically active substances or "organic chemicals" which protect the body from stress. Adaptogens were classified by the ancient Chinese as the most effective plants to increase physical and mental capacity, reduce fatigue, improve resistance to diseases, and extend lifespan.

Amrita: is a Sanskrit term that is literally translated to mean "immortality." It is also sometimes referred to as "nectar." In fact, it is linked to the Greek word, ambrosia, and has a similar meaning as it is also a drink that confers immortality upon those who consume it.

Analgesic: relating to, characterized by, or producing <u>analgesia</u> - relieving or lessening pain without loss of consciousness. Ginger, a member of the same plant family as turmeric, contains anti-inflammatory compounds and volatile oils that show analgesic and sedative effects in animal studies. Anahad O'Connor.

Antioxidant: a substance (such as beta-carotene or vitamin C) that inhibits oxidation or reactions promoted by oxygen, peroxides, or free radicals.

APOE Gene: Apolipoprotein E (ApoE) is one of the proteins the body uses to transport fats (lipids) in the bloodstream from one tissue or cell type to another. It is essential for healthy metabolism of cholesterol and triglycerides, two important types of fats the body has to deal with regularly.

The relationship between ApoE and heart disease has been studied quite intensively in recent years. Furthermore, the association between a subtype of ApoE called ApoE4 has received much attention because of its correlation with increased risk of Alzheimer's disease.

Arahant: In Theravada Buddhism, an **arahant** is a person who has eliminated all the unwholesome roots which underlie the fetters - who upon their death will not be reborn in any world, since the bonds (fetters) that bind a person to the samsara have been finally dissolved.

Ascended Master: These are Individuals who were once embodied on Earth and learned the lessons of Life in Their embodiments. They transcended human limitations and **Ascended** into Divine Freedom. They gained Mastery over the limitations of the matter planes, balanced at least 51% of negative karma, and fulfilled Their Dharma (Divine Plan).

Ascension: by definition, is elevating your vibration through spiritual practice, meditation, receiving codes of awakening, light, and DNA activations. **Ascension** allows you to access spiritual energetic upgrades to rise above the experience of duality, transcend negativity, know oneness with Mother-Father God and live as an awakened divine being in physical form.

Ayurveda: a form of <u>alternative medicine</u> that is the traditional system of medicine of India and seeks to treat and integrate body, mind, and spirit using a comprehensive holistic approach especially by emphasizing diet, herbal remedies, exercise, meditation, breathing, and physical therapy.

Autoimmune disease: an illness that occurs when the body tissues are attacked by its own immune system. The immune system is a complex organization within the body that is designed normally to "seek and destroy" invaders of the body, including infectious agents.

Bardos: Stages of transition and choice following death.

Bellows Breathing: Bhastrika, otherwise known as **bellows** breath, is a form of pranayama and is considered one of the most important and beneficial yogic **breathing** techniques. The name is derived from the Sanskrit word for "**bellows**" because the abdomen pumps the breath like the **bellows** used by a blacksmith.

Chakra: any of several points of physical or spiritual energy in the human body according to yoga philosophy. The human body has more than 88,000 points of physical or spiritual energy according to yoga philosophy, each known as a *chakra*. In Hinduism there are seven major chakras, and in Tantra (practices outlined in later Hindu or Buddhist scriptures) there are four, each associated with a color, shape, sense organ, natural element, deity, and mantra. The most important are the heart chakra, the chakra at the base of the spine, and the chakra at the top of the head.

Chi (QI): vital energy that is held to animate the body internally and is of central importance in some Eastern systems of medical treatment (such as acupuncture) and of exercise or self-defense (such as chi gong or tai chi).

Contraindications: something (such as a symptom or condition) that makes a particular treatment or procedure inadvisable. For doctors, an *indication* is a symptom or circumstance that makes a particular medical treatment desirable. Serious anxiety, for example, is often an indication for prescribing a tranquilizer. A contraindication, then, is a symptom or condition that makes a treatment risky, such as taking certain other medications at the same time. Drugs and conditions that are *contraindicated* for a medication are listed on its label, and reeled off at high speed in TV ads. Patients can guard against the dangers of drug interaction by reading labels carefully and making sure their doctors know what else they're currently taking.

Dantian: dan t'ian, dan tien or tan t'ien is loosely translated as "elixir field", "sea of qi", or simply "energy center". Dantian are the Qi Focus Flow Centers, important focal points for meditative and exercise techniques such as qigong, martial arts such as t'ai chi ch'uan and in traditional Chinese medicine. It is located in and around the navel. Dr.Mantak Chia considers this area and the associated Mesentery to be the Second Brain.

Darshan: Darshan is derived from the Sanskrit, darsana, meaning "sight," "vision" or "appearance.". In Hinduism, darshan is the act of beholding a deity, divine person, sacred object or natural spectacle, especially in a physical image form. Darshan also refers to the six Hindu philosophical systems: Samkhya, Yoga, Nvaya, Vaisheshika, Mimamsa and Vedanta.

Decrees: (Prophetic or Spiritual)

The Ascended Masters teach that the Science of the Spoken Word is a step-up of all prayer forms East and West.

It combines prayer, meditation and visualization with what are called dynamic decrees, placing special emphasis on affirmations using the name of God—I AM THAT I AM.

Decrees differ from regular prayer because they have been taken from the words of the saints and masters of East and West. Because these enlightened ones have reached the highest levels of intimate communion with God, their words are like ropes that we too can use to sustain a strong spiritual connection. They are sacred formulas for the release of God's power.

The ascended masters say that decrees as a form of devotion are the most effective method known today for spiritual resolution, the balancing of karma, and soul advancement. (Summit Light House)

Dystonia: any of various conditions (such as Parkinson's disease and torticollis) characterized by abnormalities of movement and muscle tone.

Earthing: a movement that taps into the electrical energy of the earth. A form of grounding, in earthing, it is believed that Earth's electrical field transfers to the body if some part of the body touches the earth or touches an object that can conduct Earth's electrical field.

With this connection to Earth, the body takes in free electrons, which are believed to serve as antioxidants. Antioxidants are molecules that block oxidation of other molecules, preventing the development of free radicals, which harm the body.

Fasting: is voluntarily not eating food for varying lengths of time. Fasting is used as a medical therapy for many conditions. It is also a spiritual practice in many religions.

Feldenkrais Method: The Feldenkrais method is an educational system that allows the body to move and function more efficiently and comfortably. Its goal is to re-educate the nervous system and improve motor ability. The system can accomplish much more, relieving pressure on joints and weak points, and allowing the body to heal repetitive strain injuries. Continued use of the method can relieve pain and lead to higher standards of achievement in sports, the martial arts, dancing and other physical disciplines.

Pupils are taught to become aware of their movements and to become aware of how they use their bodies, thus discovering possible areas of stress and strain. The goal of Feldenkrais is to take the individual from merely functioning, to functioning well, free of pain and restriction of movement. Feldenkrais himself stated that his goal was, "To make the impossible possible, the possible easy, and the easy, elegant."

Fibromyalgia: a chronic disorder characterized by widespread pain, tenderness, and stiffness of muscles and associated connective tissue structures that is typically accompanied by fatigue, headache, and sleep disturbances.

Glutathione level: Glutathione (GSH) is an antioxidant in plants, animals, fungi, and some bacteria and archaea. It is capable of preventing damage to important cellular components caused by reactive oxygen species such as free radicals, peroxides, lipid peroxides, and heavy metal

Homeopathy: a system of medical practice that treats a disease especially by the administration of minute doses of a remedy that would in larger amounts produce in healthy persons symptoms similar to those of the disease. Like heals like. The active ingredients used in *homeopathy* are traditionally plant, animal or mineral-based.

Hotei: in Japanese, one of the Shichi-fuku-jin ("Seven Gods of Luck"). This popular figure is depicted frequently in contemporary crafts as a cheerful, contented Buddhist monk with a large exposed belly, often accompanied by children.

I AM Presence: There are three figures represented in the "Chart of Your Divine Self", (a painting originally commissioned as a teaching tool by Guy Ballard for the Saint Germain Foundation and since recreated for various Ascended Master schools. A google search will show the details). The upper figure represents the **I AM Presence (the I AM THAT I AM) - the unique individualization of God's presence for every son and daughter of the Most High.** The Divine Monad consists of the I AM Presence surrounded by the spheres (color rings) of light that make up the body of First Cause, or Causal Body.

The middle figure in the Chart represents **the Mediator between God and man, called the Holy Christ Self,** the Real Self or the Christ consciousness. This Inner Teacher over-lights the **lower figure** (shown surrounded by the Violet Flame of Forgiveness and Transmutation of Negativity). This represents the soul evolving through the four planes of Matter using the vehicles of the four lower bodies—the etheric (higher mental) body, the mental body, the emotional (desire) body, and the physical body—to balance karma and fulfill the divine plan. The goal being reunion with the I AM Presence and release from separation, expressed by Jesus with the words, "I and the Father are One."

Kundalini: is considered to occur in the chakra and nadis of the subtle body. Each chakra is said to contain special characteristics and with proper training, moving Kundalini through these chakras can help express or open these characteristics. Kundalini is described as a sleeping, dormant potential force in the human organism.

Laser diodes: a laser in which a semiconductor is the light-emitting source, used in many medical procedures.

Lightworker: an awakened spiritual being in physical form who has reconnected with their soul plan and mission crafted prior to their birth. **Lightworkers** commit internally to be a shining light in the world; to serve humanity, Earth, and the unfolding ascension.

Medical Intuitive: A **medical intuitive** is an alternative medicine practitioner who uses their self-described **intuitive** abilities to find the cause of a physical or emotional condition. Other terms for this practice include **medical** clairvoyant, **medical** psychic or **intuitive** counselor. Another component in the multiple talents of the **medical intuitive** is the ability to link illness to an individual's thoughts and emotions. It is a fact that emotional triggers cause dis-harmony in the energy body and then filter down to the physical body.

Merkaba: is another name for one's Light Body. Part of full consciousness, when spiritual, astral and physical bodies are integrated. The **Merkaba** allows self to shrink to baseball size and to travel anywhere, instantly. The alternate spelling **MerKaBa** is also used and refers to two intersecting tetrahedrons – a spinning structure of light.

Mesentery: One or more vertebrate membranes that consist of a double fold of the peritoneum and invest the intestines and their appendages and connect them with the dorsal wall of the abdominal cavity.

Myofascial release: A type of soft tissue therapy used in osteopathy to **release** physically restricted musculoskeletal groups. It is believed that chronic tension and trauma cause the fascia, which envelops muscle, to become fixed in a particular position, known as a **myofascial** restriction.

Mystic: a person who seeks to gain religious or spiritual knowledge through prayer and deep thought: someone who practices mysticism and often has knowledge beyond normal human understanding.

Mudras: (gyan mudra is the one with thumb and forefinger touching.) A **mudra** is a symbolic, ritualistic gesture used in yoga, Buddhism and Hinduism. The word is Sanskrit meaning "gesture," "mark" or "seal." **Mudras** are most commonly known as hand positions in yoga and meditation, which are believed to affect the flow of energy in the body and to unblock chakras. There are numerous types of **mudras**.

Neuropathy: Damage, disease, or dysfunction of one or more nerves especially of the peripheral nervous system that is typically marked by burning or shooting pain, numbness, tingling, or muscle weakness or atrophy, is often degenerative, and is usually caused by injury, infection, disease, drugs, toxins, or vitamin deficiency Each of the drugs for treatment comes with a long list of possible nasty side effects, ranging from liver and kidney damage to pancreatitis and neuropathy in the limbs. In the condition known as diabetic neuropathy, there is a gradual deterioration of peripheral nerves that generally affects older patients and initially causes a painful burning sensation in the hands and feet.

Nerve conduction: the transmission of an impulse along a nerve fiber.

Occupational Therapist: therapy based on engagement in meaningful activities of daily life (such as self-care skills, education, work, or social interaction) especially to enable or encourage participation in such activities despite impairments or limitations in physical or mental functioning.

Opioids: 1: any of a group of endogenous neural polypeptides (such as an endorphin or enkephalin) that bind especially to opiate receptors and mimic some of the pharmacological properties of opiates — called also opioid peptide. 2: a synthetic drug possessing narcotic properties similar to opiates but not derived from opium.

Oxidation: is a process in which a chemical substance changes because of the addition of oxygen. The reaction between magnesium metal and oxygen involves the **oxidation** of magnesium. When exposed to oxygen, silicon undergoes **oxidation** and forms silicon dioxide. Considered to be one of the theories of the cause of aging.

Parasympathetic nervous system: the part of the autonomic nervous system that contains chiefly cholinergic fibers, that tends to induce secretion, to increase the tone and contractility of smooth muscle, and to slow heart rate, and that consists of a cranial and a sacral part.

Prana: is an ancient concept and is referred to in many Hindu scriptures and texts, such as the Upanishads. These texts state that prana originates from Atman. From the Sanskrit, an, meaning "movement" and "to breathe," and pra, meaning "forth," prana means "breathing forth," and refers to the idea that vital or life force energy is always dynamic.

Pranayama is the formal practice of controlling the breath, which is the source of our prana, or vital life force.

Prebiotics: a substance and especially a carbohydrate (such as <u>inulin</u>) that is nearly or wholly indigestible and that when consumed (as in food) promotes the growth of beneficial bacteria in the digestive tract Prebiotics are naturally found in certain fruits, vegetables, and herbs, including artichoke, asparagus, bananas, chicory, garlic, and onions.

Probiotics: a microorganism (such as lactobacillus) that when consumed (as in a food or a dietary supplement) maintains or restores beneficial bacteria to the digestive tract; also a product or preparation that contains such microorganisms.

Qi (or Chi): vital energy that is held to animate the body internally and is of central importance in some Eastern systems of medical treatment (such as acupuncture) and of exercise or self-defense (such as tai chi).

Reiki: is a form of alternative energy therapy developed in 1922 by Mikao Usui of Japan. It is a form of hands-on healing therapy that combines the use of touch and energy channeling to promote a sense of deep relaxation and healing.

Rolfing: also called Rolf **therapy** or structural integration, is a holistic system of bodywork that uses deep manipulation of the body's soft tissue to realign and balance the body's myofascial structure. **Rolfing** improves posture, relieves chronic pain, and reduces stress.

Spect-Scan: (Single-photon emission computed tomography) Single-photon emission computed tomography (**SPECT**, or less commonly, SPET) is a nuclear medicine tomographic imaging technique using gamma rays. It is very similar to conventional nuclear medicine planar imaging using a gamma camera (that is, scintigraphy), but is able to provide true 3D information. This information is typically presented as cross-sectional slices through the patient, but can be freely reformatted or manipulated as required.

Sri Yantra - is a mystical diagram, mainly from the Tantric traditions of the Indian religions. Sri Yantra is said to represent the microcosmic level of the Universe as well as the human body.

Stem Cells: One of the human body's master **cells**, with the ability to grow into any one of the body's more than 200 **cell** types. **Stem cells** are unspecialized (undifferentiated) **cells** that are characteristically of the same family type (lineage). They retain the ability to divide throughout life and give rise to **cells** that can become highly specialized and take the place of **cells** that die or are lost.

Superlumious: having a very high luminosity

Telomere: the specific DNA–protein structures found at both ends of each chromosome, which protect the genome from degradation, repair, and interchromosomal fusion. Telomeres play a vital role in preserving the information in our genome. As a normal cellular process, a small portion of telomeric DNA is lost with each cell division. When telomere length reaches a critical limit, the cell undergoes senescence. Shorter telomeres have been associated with increased incidence of diseases and poor survival. The rate of telomere shortening can be either increased or decreased by specific lifestyle factors. Better choice of diet and activities has great potential to reduce the rate of telomere shortening or at least prevent excessive telomere attrition, leading to delayed onset of age-associated diseases and increased lifespan.

Voo breathing: This is a breathing exercise comparable to an "Om" in yoga. The vibrating waves created by making a deep, fog horn like projection of the sound "**Voo**" over

Yoga: 1. a school of Hindu philosophy advocating and prescribing a course of physical and mental disciplines for attaining liberation from the material world and union of the self with the Supreme Being or ultimate principle. 2. Sanskrit definition of yoga. Yoga means 'union' or 'connection'. In Sanskrit, the word 'yoga' is used to signify any form of connection. Yoga is both a state of connection and a body of techniques that allow us to connect to anything. Conscious connection to something allows us to feel and experience that thing, person, or experience.

Glossary References: Webster's Dictionary, Yogapedia, Wikapedia, Medical online dictionary, Summit Lighthouse

A NEW BEGINNING REFERENCES

Introduction

(1)   (John: 1:1) Bible Gateway, King James Version, Public Domain, https://www.biblegateway.com

(2)   *Re: AUM, Ananda, The Yogic Encyclopedia;* https://www.ananda.org/yogapedia/aum/

(3)   (Exodus 3:14) Bible Gateway, https://www.biblegateway.com

CHAPTER 1

(4)   Ganga Nath and Tara Leela, *Herbs for Spiritual Development,* Universal Fellowship of Light Publishing, 2017, p 64.

(5)   (John 10:34; John 14:12). Bible Gateway, https://www.biblegateway.com

CHAPTER 2

(6)   https://en.wikipedia.org/wiki/Peter_Singer

(7)   *Re: "Full Debate – Animals Should be Off the Menu"; The St. James Ethics and Wheeler Center* https://www.youtube.com/watch?v=mNED7GJLY7I

(8)   https://www.thebetterindia.com/76587/jagdishchandra-bose-indian-biophysicist-radio-plant-physiology/

(9)   *Re: The Backster Affect;* https://en.wikipedia.org/wiki/Plant_perception_%28paranormal%29

(10)   *Re: "Marcel Vogel Rational and Scientist"* https://www.autodesk.com/products/eagle/blog/marcel_vogal/

(11)   Brian Scott Peskin, BSEE-and Robert Jay Rowen, M.D. *PEO Solutions Conquering Cancer, Diabetes and Heart Disease with Parent Essential Oils,* Pinnacle Press, 2015.

(12)   *Re: How much protein;* https://www.facebook.com/
       medicalmedium/videos/1239420652859777

(13)   *Re: soy suspect increasing risk for breast cancer; https://www.hsph.
       harvard.edu/nutritionsource/soy/*

(14)   *Re: soy and senile dementia connection;*

(15)   https://www.onegreenplanet.org/vegan-food/vegan-sources-of-
       protein/ https://www.healthline.com/nutrition/iron-rich-plant-
       foods

(16)   https://www.organicfacts.net/health-benefits/fruit.

(17)   *Re: Vegetables are a source of many nutrients;* https://Healthyeating.
       org

(18)   https://www.savorylotus.com/5-reasons-to-stop-cookin
       g-with-olive-oil/

(19)   *Re: Mary Vance NC, How to Choose the Healthiest Olive Oil;*
       https://www.maryvancenc.com/how-to-choose-the-healthies
       t-olive-oil/

CHAPTER 3

(20)   https://en.wikipedia.org/wiki/Masaru_Emoto

(21)   Jon Dunn, *Family Guide to Naturopathic Medicine,* Naturopathic
       Health Care Inc, 2010.

(22)   https://www.globalhealingcenter.com/natural-health/
       how-safe-is-fluoride/

(23)   *Re: What is in our water supply?* https://articles.mercola.com/
       sites/articles/archive/2010/09/11/alkaline-water-interview.aspx

(24)   https://www.findaspring.com

(25)   Dr. Masaru Emoto, *The Hidden Messages in Water,* Atria Books,
       2011.

(26)   *Re: Crystal Vault, Vogel Crystals Explained;* https://www.
       crystalvaults.com/vogel-crystals-explained

(27)   *Re: Wave Q water alkalinizer;* https://www.kangenwaterionizers.
       com/K8.html

(28)   *Re: MMP-9090 Water Ionizer by Tyent;* https://www.tyentusa.
       com/mmp-9090t-ssbl.html

(29) *Re: Dr. Mercola on water alkalinity;* https://articles.mercola.com/sites/articles/archive/2010/09/11/alkaline-water-interview.aspx

(30) Dr. Barbara Hendel and Peter Ferreira, *Water and Salt: The Essence of Life, The Healing Power of Nature.* 2001

(31) https://www.webmd.com/oral-health/features/oil-pulling

(32) https://us.foursigmatic.com/mushroom/mushroom-coffee

(33) https://www.slenderkitchen.com/article/how-to-calculate-how-much-water-you-should-drink-a-day

CHAPTER 4

(34) https://www.medicalmedium.com/blog/heavy-metal-detox

(35) Anthony William, *Medical Medium*, Hay House Publishing, Pages 43-45.

(36) https://www.healthline.com/health/mercury-poisoning

(37) https://www.globalhealingcenter.com/natural-health/10-health-dangers-of-bromine/

(38) https://www.nourishingplot.com/2014/08/30/detoxing-fluoride-bromine-and-chlorine-naturally

(39) https://www.healthline.com/nutrition/iodine-rich-foods

(40) https://www.foxnews.com/health/dangers-of-formaldehyde-lurk-in-everyday-products

(41) https://www.indoordoctor.com/health-hazards-plug-air-fresheners/

(42) Anne Steinemann, *Air Quality, Atmosphere and Health* 9(8)· October 2016.

(43) https://www.nextavenue.org/the-potential-health-dangers-of-air-fresheners/

(44) http://naturestreasures.com.au/Microwave-ovens.html

(45) https://www.mercola.com/article/microwave/hazards2.htm

(46) *Re: Juicing and wellness film "Fat, Sick and Nearly Dead".*

(47) https://www.healthline.com/health/iodine-poisoning#symptom

(48) https://www.verywellhealth.com/thyroid-disease-and-the-heart-1746112

(49) https://www.globalhealingcenter.com/natural-health/uses-for-iodine/

(50) https://www.webmd.com/balance/guide/what-is-chelation-therapy#1

(51) https://www.wellandgood.com/good-food/benefits-of-spirulina-buying-tips/

(52) https://www.healthline.com/nutrition/benefits-of-chlorella#section2

(53) https://drjockers.com/selenium-detoxify-mercury/

(54) *Re: signs of selenium toxicity;*https://www.ncbi.nlm.nih.gov/pmc/articles/PMC3225252

(55) https://www.healthline.com/nutrition/selenium-benefits#1

(56) *Re: Geoengineering and Chemtrails;* https://www.riseforwar.com/2017/02/25/10-natural-ways-to-detoxify-from-chemtrails/

(57) Andrew Hall Cutler, *Amalgam Illness*, Andy Cutler Publishing, 2000.

(58) Brian Scott Peskin and Robert Jay Rowen, M.D., **PEO Solution**, Pinnacle Press, 2015.

(59) https://draxe.com/vitamin-b12-benefits/

(60) https://www.thestar.com.my/lifestyle/health/2014/05/25/vitamin-e-could-protect-you-from-radiation/

(61) https://www.xray-protection.com/x-ray-protection.html

(62) James Colquhoun and Laurentine Ten Bosch, *Ditch the Diets, Conquer the Cravings, and Eat Your Way to Lifelong Health,* Permacology Publishing Party, 2015.

(63) https://www.healthline.com/health/food-nutrition/benefits-vitamin-d

(64) https://draxe.com/magnesium-supplements/

(65) https://www.globalhealingcenter.com/natural-health/types-of-magnesium/

(66) https://www.everydayhealth.com/type-2-diabetes/diet/diabetes-magnesium-deficiency-you-need-more-this-mineral/ and http://purelife-bio.com/magnesium-taurate-supplements-benefits/

(67) https://gundrymd.com/supplements/lectin-shield/

(68) https://www.globalhealingcenter.com/natural-health/link-between-depression-anxiety-and-gut-health/

(69) https://blog.paleohacks.com/probiotic-foods

(70) https://draxe.com/nutrition/probiotics-benefits-foods-supplements/

(71) https://www.betternutrition.com/checkout/prebiotic-probiotic-foods-lists

(72) https://thriveprobiotic.com/a-thriving-lifestyle/

(73) https://www.sovereignlaboratories.com/what-is-colostrum.html

(74) *Re: Colostrum 6*; https://anovite.com

(75) *Re: More information on protecting the gut;* Viome.com or https://Thegutinstitute.com.

(76) https://www.marywillnourish.com/post/minerals-the-body-s-spark-plugs

(77) https://www.organicfacts.net/health-benefits/oils/properties-of-coconut-oil.html

(78) https://www.getholistichealth.com/78198/soy-unfit-human-consumption-industry-lies

(79) https://www.carriesexperimentalkitchen.com/foods-for-depression/

(80) https://www.pyradyne.com/collections/essential-supplements/products/shou-wu-chih

(81) *Re: NAD;* https://f1000research.com/articles/7-132/v1

(82) https://www.verywellhealth.com/the-benefits-of-haritaki-88828

(83) https://www.banyanbotanicals.com/info/blog/the-banyan-insight/details/getting-to-know-your-herbal-allies-haritaki/

(84) https://www.healthline.com/nutrition/12-proven-ashwagandha-benefits

(85) Kulreet Chaudhary, *The Prime: Prepare and Repair Your Body for Spontaneous Weight Loss,* Harmony Books, 2016

(86) https://chopra.com/articles/the-benefits-of-triphala

(87) https://www.healthline.com/nutrition/benefits-of-chlorella

(88) https://www.healthline.com/nutrition/mct-oil-benefits#section2

(89) https://www.bulletproof.com/diet/keto/mct-oil-keto-benefits

(90) *Re: Constipation;* https://www.mensfitness.com/nutrition/what-to-eat/10-best-sources-of-fiber/slideshow

(91) *Re: Vitamin E and tocotrienols;* https://www.sciencedirect.com/topics/biochemistry-genetics-and-molecular-biology/tocotrienol

(92) http://www.cnn.com/2009/HEALTH/expert.q.a/12/04/cancer.radiation.vitamins.jampolis/index.html

(93) http://thechart.blogs.cnn.com/2011/10/28/does-diet-really-matter-in-breast-cancer/

(94) *Re: Can foods protect you from cancer?* "Pharmacological Research," Volume 130, April 2018, Pages 259-272.

(95) *Re: tocotrienols prevent/inhibit growth of different cancers;* https://www.sciencedirect.com/science/article/abs/pii/S1043661173146039 Pharmacological Research J., Volume 130, April 2018

(96) https://organixx.com/turkey-tail-mushrooms-cancer/

(97) *Re: Tones to heal the body further;* https://foreverconscious.com/sound-healing-528hz-the-frequency-of-love-and-miracles and https://www.youtube.com/watch?v=hdmvMc7TZn0

(98) https://draxe.com/cancer-fighting-foods/

(99) *Re: Kelley Eidem's Protocol;* https://www.healingcancernaturally.com/habaneropeppers-garlic-oilcure.html

(100) *Antonio Jimenez, M.D. on Laetril;* https://www.youtube.com/watch?v=pZwJJxIvNos

(101) *Re: Selenium and Brazil nuts;* https://www.medicalnewstoday.com/articles/325000

(102) https://gerson.org/gerpress/the-gerson-therapy/

(103) *Re: Ty Bollinger cutting edge info on cancer. First episode* https://www.youtube.com/watch?v=KqJAzQe7_0gandt=15s

(104) https://hope4cancer.com/about-us/why-hope4cancer/

(105) *Re: High-intensity focused ultrasound for Alzheimers;* https://stanfordhealthcare.org/stanford-health-care-now/2017/hifu-q-a.html

(106) https://www.mdanderson.org/publications/cancerwise/the-keto-diet-and-cancer--what-patients-should-know.h00-15922 3356.html

(107) https://www.diabetesselfmanagement.com/blog/is-cinnamon-good-for-diabetes/

(108) https://www.plantbasednews.org/lifestyle/doctor-takes-42-diabetics-off-medication-nfi-protocol

(109) https://www.betternutrition.com/features-dept/supplements-for-heart-health

(110) https://articles.mercola.com/vitamins-supplements/coq10.aspx

(111) https://lpi.oregonstate.edu/mic/vitamins/vitamin-C

(112) Dr. Dean Ornish, *Reversing Heart Disease*, Ivy Book, an imprint of Random House Publishing, 1990, 1996.

(113) https://www.ornish.com/undo-it or https://www.amazon.com/Ornishs-Program-Reversing-Heart-Disease/dp/0804110387

(114) https://www.dailymail.co.uk/news/article-5644745/Dementia-suffering-mother-REGAINmemory-thanks-Mediterranean-style-diet.html

(115) https://www.drwhitaker.com/lithium-for-brain health

(116) *Re: Danish study, lithium in drinking water;* https://www.ncbi.nlm.nih.gov/pubmed/28832877

(117) *Re: link for Super Brain Yoga;* https://www.youtube.com/watch?v=KSwhpF9iJSs

(118) *Re: For more complete info, please visit Dr. Lipman's link at:* https://drfranklipman.com/2019/05/27/10-ways-to-protect-your-brain-and-keep-alzheimers-at-bay/

(119) Dale E. Bredesen, M.D. *The End of Alzheimer's,* Best Journals, 2019.

(120) Joanne Koenig Coste, *Learning to Speak Alzheimer's: A Groundbreaking Approach for Everyone with the Disease,* Houghton Mifflin Harcourt Publishing Company, 2003.

(121) https://www.sciencealert.com/astonishing-new-study-treats-alzheimer-s-in-mice-with-a-light-and-sound-show?fbclid=IwAR24010yB0e3VeVjCZE-sW1K5 _awvd24MOfwk MYwNSmgeHKVRTZtLKwvrRs

(122) https://picower.mit.edu/news/brain-wave-stimulation-may-improve-alzheimers-symptoms

(123) *Re: Sa Ta Na Ma Meditation benefits*; https://agelessartsyoga.com

(124) https://scottjeffrey.com/decalcify-your-pineal-gland/

(125) https://medicinal-foods.com/decalcify-pineal-gland/?fbclid=IwAR3zHA9-NEhR87OQCTOJJGH0 uk8Mzcc5EpZjR puoe1W3Lvuc4qhZqm6TMI

(126) *2017 Physician's Desk Reference* by PDR staff, (71st edition) (it has all the possible side effects and might be too much for the lay person) or *The Pill Book* (15th Edition), Mass Market Paperbacks, (which is much more user friendly.)

(127) *Re: APOE gene and foods that affect disease;* Pamela McDonald, NP, Integrative- Medicine Nurse Practitioner, *Perfect Gene Diet. Hay House, Inc, 2007,2010.*

CHAPTER 5

(128) https://www.healthline.com/health/types-of-pain#chronic-pain

(129) https://www.mayoclinic.org/diseases-conditions/prescription-drug-abuse/in-depth/tapering-off-opioids-when-and-how/art-20386036

(130) https://www.healthline.com/health/opiate-withdrawal

(131) https://feldenkraisfoundation.org/

(132) https://www.healthline.com/health/rolfing-chronic-pain#1

(133) https://products.mercola.com/earthing-mat/

(134) https://www.healthline.com/health/boswellia#research

(135) *Boswellia: Stop 5-LOX Inflammation,* 2017, pp. 1-2. (part of In-Depth Booklet series "Terry Talks Nutrition" by Terry Lemerond)

(136) *Re: Sombra Gel*; https://ncmedical.com

(137) https://medium.com/@josephbinder_98743/natures-strongest-pain-killer-is-probably-growing-in-your-backyard-and-is-more-effective-than-e04b174ae175

(138) https://www.healthline.com/nutrition/msm-supplements#section1

(139) https://shop.kyani.net/en-us/products/category/5/kyani-nitro-family

(140) *Re: Can Be Done Topical Salve;* https://www.goodcommon sense.com

(141) https://resonantbotanicals.com/pages/about-us

(142) *Re: Uno Roller*; https://www.addaday.com/collections/originals

(143) https://www.synergystone.com/heat-wave/

(144) https://bioflexlaser.com/products/

(145) https://www.verywellhealth.com/what-is-ultrasound-therapy-2564506

(146) https://www.spine-health.com/treatment/pain-management/cold-laser-therapy-pain-management-treatment

(147) https://www.silkntherapy.com/

(148) https://thedermreview.com/lightstim/

(149) https://www.tennantbiomodulator.ca/products/instruments/tennant-biomodulator-plus and https://senergy.us/tennant-biomodulator/

(150) *Ref: Vibroacustic Apparatus VITAFON-T User Guide.*

(151) *Re: Chakra Sweep PEMF (Pulsed Electromagnetic Field)—Shealy-Sorin Gamma PEMF available at:* https://normshealy.com/

(152) Robin McKenzie, *Treat Your Own Back*, Penguin Group, 2011.

(153) *The Back Pain Help Book* by various health professionals.

(154) Kathryn Shanti Ariel, *Holistic Emergency Care and Trauma Recovery for Animals*, Earthwise Institute, 2015.

(155) https://resonantbotanicals.com/collections/all-products/products/ neuro-soothe-neuropathy-fibromyalgia-relief-lotion

(156) https://www.pyradyne.com/collections/pyramids/products/pyradome-24kgold-plated-headgear-pyramid-to-detox-brain-relax

(157) *Re: do not take glutamine if you are diabetic;* https://www.livestrong.com/article/530466-glutamine-and-your-blood-sugar/

(158) https://nccih.nih.gov/health/catclaw#hed1

(159) *Re: cat's claw;* https://www.nccih.nih.gov/health/cats-claw

(160) *Re: Enerex;* https://enerex.ca/collections/all

(161) *Re: acetylglucosamine and children with Crohn's*; https://ncbi.nlm.nih.gov/pubmed/11121904

(162) *Re: Vitamin D and Crohn's;* https://ncbi.nlm.nih.gov/pubmed/26837598

(163) *Re: Vitamin B12 deficiency and Crohn's Disease;* https://healthline.com/health/crohns-disease/herbs-supplements#1

(164) https://enerexusa.com/articles/serrapeptase.htm

(165) https://enerex.ca/products/serrapeptase-120-000su?fbclid=IwAR1u9692yTd8VnB9dwW5bFV4SdaL 1ePpIXXRjUX8ADg UMlzT0O1wLrMVCwU

(166) https://www.mayoclinic.org/tests-procedures/cortisone-shots/about/pac-20384794

(167) Anthony William, *Medical Medium*, Hay House Publishing, 2015

CHAPTER 6

(168) https://worldpopulationreview.com/countries/suicide-rate-by-country/

(169) https://afsp.org/about-suicide/suicide-statistics/

(170) *Re: 9 Types of pain;* https://www.higherperspectives.com/emotional-pain-1461050437.html

(171) Louise Hay, *You Can Heal Your Life, ay* House Publishing, 1984, 1987, 2004, pp. 202-203

(172) Karol Truman, *Feelings Buried Alive Never Die*, Olympus Distributing, 1995 – 2005.

(173) Mantak Chia and Dena Saxer, *Emotional Wisdom: Daily Tools for Transforming Anger, Depression, and Fear*, New World Library, 2009

(174) https://atfacevalu.com/the-history-of-face-reading/

(175) https://www.easterncurrents.ca/for-practitioners/practitioners'-news/eastern-currents-news/2018/04/25/chinese-face-reading

(176) https://www.rebeccakim.com

(177) https://www.daocloud.com/pro/janet-doerr and https://www.facebook.com/TheIntuitiveNutritionista/

(178) Blake Sinclair, *Dare to Imagine, 2014*and *Beyond Imagination, 2015, Golden Lotus Books.*

(179) *Ketamine and PTSD;* https://www.medicalnewstoday.com/articles/302663#therapeutic_uses

(180) *Re: Dr. Daniel Amen, Spect Scan;* https://www.amenclinics.com/

(181) *Re: 4-7-8 Breathing;* https://www.medicalnewstoday.com/articles/324417

(182) https://www.artofliving.org/us-en/yoga/breathing-techniques/alternate-nostril-breathing-nadi-shodhan

(183) https://www.mcdowellsherbal.com/human-conditions/nervous-system/319-rescue-remedy)

(184) http://www.bachflower.com/rescue-remedy-information/

(185) Kathryn Shanti Ariel, Holistic Emergency Care and Trauma Recovery for Animals, Earthwise Institute, 2015.

(186) https://www.anaflora.com/essences/index.html

(187) *Re: John Gray on Lithium Orotate;* https://www.youtube.com/watch?v=5wWtFBvl1fw

(188) *Re: Lithium orotate for Alzheimer's - Robert McMullen, M.D.* https://www.youtube.com/watch?v=vRmuBrO9rUM

(189) https://www.greatplainslaboratory.com/articles-1/2016/2/22/lithium-the-cinderella-story-about-a-mineral-that-may-prevent-alzheimers-disease

(190) https://www.webmd.com/vitamins/ai/ingredientmono-329/st-johns-wort

(191) Anthony William, ***Medical Medium***, Hay House Publishing, 2015.

(192) https://rapideyetechnology.com/

(193) https://www.thetappingsolution.com/what-is-eft-tapping/

(194) https://psych-k.com/about/4

(195) https://science.howstuffworks.com/science-vs-myth/extrasensory-perceptions/hypnosis2.htm

(196) https://exemplore.com/paranormal/Psychism--7-Signs-Youre-an-Empath

(197) Mikaelah Cordeo, Ph.D., *Live in Love - A Life Handbook for the New Golden Age*, 2nd ed., 2013, Golden Rose Publishing.

(198) https://www.italiaoliver.com/uncategorized/grounding-crystals-for-empaths\

(199) Eckhart Tolle, *The Power of Now*, Namaste Publishing, 1999.

CHAPTER 7

(200) https://www.grandsecretsofspiritualmysteries.com/decrees.html

(201) Matthew 18:20, https://www.biblegateway.com

(202) Peter Mt. Shasta, *Adventures of a Western Mystic,* Church of the Seven Rays, Book 1, 2013, Book 2, 2010-2016.

(203) www.healdocumentary.com

CHAPTER 8

(204) *Re: Deepak Chopra on Meditation;* https://youtu.be/hxRpvEk KzTA

(205) https://amma.org/groups/north-america/projects/iam-meditation-classes

(206) *Re: Vipassana Meditation information*; https://www.dhamma.org.

(207) *Re: Peter Mt. Shasta, Getting started with Vipassana Meditation*; https://www.youtube.com/watch?v=qrj8f1rEZ38

(208) *Re: Kriya Yoga;* https://yogananda.org

(209) Babaji's Kriya Yoga Satsang, 165 de la Gauchetiere W. #3608, Montreal, Quebec, CA H2Z1X6.

(210) *Re: Wayne Dyer's I AM Wishes Fulfilled Meditation*; https://youtu.be/RAtKO2vcXfc

CHAPTER 9

(211) https://drsarahallen.com/7-ways-to-calm/

(212) https://brennanhealingscience.org/the-human-energy-field-and-chakras/

(213) https://2empowerthyself.com/what-is-the-dan-tien/

(214) https://www.psypost.org/2019/07/study-provides-evidence-that-dmt-is-produced-naturally-from-neurons-in-the-mammalian-brain-54051.

CHAPTER 10

(215) https://my.clevelandclinic.org/health/articles/10881-vital-signs

(216) https://en.wikipedia.org/wiki/Pursed_lip_breathing

(217) *Re: Voo Breathing for Trauma with Dr.Peter Levine;* https://www.youtube.com/watch?v=G7zAseaIyFA

(218) https://www.yogaoutlet.com/guides/how-to-practice-alternate-nostril-breathing-in-yoga

(219) https://www.yogameditation.com/reading-room/why-hold-your-breath/

(220) Wim Hof VIP experience November 4, 2019 San Francisco

CHAPTER 11

(221) https://www.healthline.com/nutrition/water-fasting#section

(222) Anthony William, *Medical Medium,* Hay House Publishing, 2015, P. 273. *(Juice Fasting)*

(223) https://www.healthline.com/nutrition/intermittent-fasting-guide#what-it-is

(224) *Re: Help for gut support during intermittent fasting;* https://rskoso.com/pages/cleanse?fbclid=IwAR15LZRw GFgHUYODrEoAXI6mU5qPgVv09pwi0_-3xlXu-| ura5z3TY0N3lBk

CHAPTER 13

(225) https://www.universalfellowshipofllight.com/

(226) https://www.emfanalysis.com/basic-steps/

(227) hibiscusmooncrystalacademy.com/crystals-lower-emf-risks/

(228) *Re: A Nuclear Receptor;* https://www.pyradyne.com/

(229) *Re: EMF Solution - a tool that neutralizing negative EMF effects;* https://Iconnect2all.com/products/metaforms/

CHAPTER 14

(230) Robert Tennyson Stevens *Conscious Language, Mastery Systems International, 2007-2014.*

(231) Godfré Ray King, *Unveiled Mysteries,* 1934 and *The Magic Presence,* 1935, Saint Germain Press.

(232) *Re: Patricia Cota Robles;* https://eraofpeace.org.

(233) Re*: The Yellow Emperor;* https://www.shenyun.com

CHAPTER 15

(234) Ganga Nath and Tara Leela, *Herbs for Spiritual Development - Ganga's Adventure in the World of Tonic Elixirs,* Universal Fellowship of Light, 2017.

(235) https://draxe.com/astaxanthin-benefits/

(236) https://blog.radiantlifecatalog.com/bid/39522/What-is-Glutathione-and-why-do-we-need-it

(237) Dr. Lester Packer and Carol Coleman, *The Antioxidant Miracle,* John Wiley & Sons, Inc., 1999.

(238) Ganga Nath and Tara Leela, *Herbs for Spiritual Development - Ganga's Adventure in the World of Tonic Elixirs,* Universal Fellowship of Light, 2017.

(239) *Re: Deepak Chopra - to stimulate the Vagus Nerve;* https://www.youtube.com/watch?v=LK3dQdj8YWQ

(240) *Re: Mantak Chia activates the dantien;*https://www.youtube.com/watch?v=kaefdiE4ovk

(241) *Re: Dr. Andrew Weil as he demonstrates 4-7-8 Breathing process;* https://www.youtube.com/watch?v=gz4G31LGyog

(242) https://fractalenlightenment.com/14950/spirituality/sun-gazing-why-you-should-be-doing-it

(243) fasting https://www.youtube.com/watch?v=VWtaLLjJzn4)

(244) Susan Shumsky, *Ascension Connecting With the Immortal Masters and Being of Light,* Career Press, 2010, p. 104.

(245) Hatha Yoga Pradipika

(246) https://medium.com/@krishmuralieswar/what-is-kayakalpa-yoga-871f62111a47 and https://www.kayakalpa.com/

(247) *Mystic Masters Lecture* from Romarishi Siddha (Ganga Nath) and Tara Leela, 5/12/2019 in San Francisco.

(248) *Re: Stem Cell Therapy;* https://repairstemcell.wordpress.com/?fbclid=IwAR3HdXJQqn73qCygIiWxgDM6pREoyjP6KC82vtvgW-nTDX4viFR35-QOV5c

(249) Pamela McDonald, N.P., *The Perfect Gene Diet,* Hay House Publishing, 2010, p. 10.

(250) Pamela McDonald, N.P., *The Perfect Gene Diet,* Hay House Publishing, 2010, p 54. (More information on medical providers can be found at htttps://www.ThePerfectGeneDiet.com.)

(251) https://normshealy.shop/collections/the-five-rings/products/shealy-sorin-biogenics-ring-of-water

(252) Ron Teeguarden, *The Ancient Wisdom of the Chinese Tonic Herbs,* Warner Books, Inc. 1998, pp. 61-62.

(253) https://www.whats-your-sign.com/symbolism-of-water.html

(254) https://medlineplus.gov/ency/article/001982.htm

(255) Ron Teeguarden, *The Ancient Wisdom of the Chinese Tonic Herbs,* Warner Books, Inc. 1998, p. 46.

(256) https://www.amazon.com/AIRMEGA-Smarter-Purifier-Covers-560/dp/B01C9RIACG/ref=sr_1_3?keywords=coway+airmegaandqid=1573441142andsr=8-3h

(256.5) Purifying Plants, Prime Time Health William Sears, MD page 123

(257) https://www.health.harvard.edu/staying-healthy /precious-metals-and-other-important-minerals-for-health

(258) Ron Teeguarden, *The Ancient Wisdom of the Chinese Tonic Herbs,* Warner Books, Inc. 1998, pp. 59-60.

(259) https://daolabs.com/blogs/the-way/your-tongue-why-its-so-important-in-chinese-medicine

(260) *Re: Mantak Chia's Second Brain activation exercises* https://www.youtube.com/watch?v=kaefdiE4ovk

CHAPTER 16

(261) *Re: books by Saraydarian and Fojas recommended for Protection: Battling Dark Forces:* Torkom Saraydarian, *A Guide to Psychic Self-Defen*se, 2011 and *The Eyes of Hierarchy, 1998 The Creative Trust.*

(262) Felix Fojas, *The Supernatural and Beyond,* University of Arizona Libraries, 2017

(263) https:// www.summitlighthouse.org

(264) *Re: Mohan Ji's Prayers for Protection;* https://open.spotify.com/album/1Up8HEMfBIVbrlJTZvQ52l

(265) https://www.holographichealth.com/ecommerce/delete.html

(266) https//www.originalbotanica.com/blog/steps-for-spiritual-bathing/

(267) *Re: Smudging;* https//youtu.be/XwZFoTrES78

(268) *Re: Oxytocin – a key hormone for empathy, generosity and orgasm;* hhttps://www.psychologytoday.com/us/basics/oxytocin

(269) https://Iconnect2all.com/products/iconnect/

(270) *Re: Aura cleansing videos;* https://www.youtube.com/watch?v=w6sbrmcrSuo

CHAPTER 17

(271) *The Essence of the Bhagavad Gita* explained by Paramahansa Yogananda, as remembered by Swami Kriyananda, Crystal Clarity Publishers, 2006, p. 154.

(272) *The Essence of the Bhagavad Gita* explained by Paramahansa Yogananda, as remembered by Swami Kriyananda, Crystal Clarity Publishers, 2006, p. 119.

CHAPTER 18

(273) https://en.wikipedia.org/wiki/K%C3%BCbler-Ross_model

(274) http://en.dhammadana.org/dhamma/practice/8_precepts.htm

(275) http://www.sfzc.org/about-zen-center/principles-governance / ethics/ethical-principles/the-ten-essential-precepts

(276) Joshua David Stone, Ph.D., *The Complete Ascension Manual,* Light Technology Publishing, LLC, 1994, pp. 81-82.

(277) https://www.astara.org/death-bardo

(278) http://mybuddhadharma.blogspot.com/2010/10/100-deities-jang-chog-prayer.html

(279) http://spiritscienceyoga.com/blog/2017/1/3/tibetan-buddhist-mantra-for-purification-and-liberation.

(280) Joshua David Stone, Ph.D., *The Complete Ascension Manual,* Light Technology Publishing, LLC, 1994,

(281) Mikaelah Cordeo, Ph.D., *Live in Love – A Handbook for the New Golden Age*, 2ⁿᵈ Edition, 2013, Golden Rose Publishing, pp. 125-140.

(282) The Tibetan Book of the Dead or Bardo Thodol, Compiled around 800 A.D.

(283) http://www.nonahz.org/home_eng/LastMind.htm

CHAPTER 19

(284) http://biblehub.com/matthew/18-20.ht

(285) https://timebanks.org/what-is-timebanking/ and https://www.investopedia.com/terms/t/time-banking.asp#:~:text=Time%20banking%20is%20a%20bartering,to%20supplement%20government%20social%20services

(286) http://www.jaintirthankars.com/bhaktamarstotra.html

(287) *Re: Gayatri Mantra:* https://www.youtube.com/watch?v=SarlTxrAbIYandt=79s.

(288) *Healing Tones:* https://www.youtube.com/watch?v=4Tno4L-6vP4

(289) *Re: Tina Turner's Peace Mantra;* https://www.youtube.com/watch?v=6XP-f7wPM0A

(290) *Re: 100 Deities Mantra;* https://www.youtube.com/watch?v=mFCWqLHoarRI

(291) https://gostica.com/aura-science/chakras-earth-7-amazing-places-filled-powerful-energy/

(292) Mikaelah Cordeo, Ph.D., *Live In Love - A Life Handbook for the New Golden Age*, 2ⁿᵈ Edition, 2013, Chapter 15- Planetary Chakras.

(293) Blake Sinclair, *Beyond Imagination*, Golden Lotus Books, 2015.

BIBLIOGRAPHY

Ariel, Kathyrn Shanti, *Holistic Emergency Care and Trauma Recovery for Animals,* Earthwise Institute, 2015.

Chia, Mantak and Saxer, Dena, *Emotional Wisdom: Daily Tools for Transforming Anger, Depression, and Fear*, New World Library, 2009.

Chaudhary, Kulreet, *The Prime: Prepare and Repair Your Body for Spontaneous Weight Loss,* Harmony Books, 2016.

Colquhoun, James, Laurentine Ten Bosch and Mark Hyman, **Hungry for Change: Ditch the Diets, Conquer the Cravings, and** *Eat Your Way to Lifelong Health*, Permacology Publishing Party, 2015.

Cordeo, Mikaelah, Ph.D., *Live in Love – A Life Handbook for the New Golden Age*, Golden Rose Publishing, 3rd Ed. 2013.

Cutler, Andrew Hall, *Amalgam Illness*, Andy Cutler Publishing, 2000.

Dalai Lama, *A Precious Life* and *The True Meaning of Life*. (Scrolls of those Divine teachings can be found at most Tibetan or Nepalese stores.)

Emoto, Dr. Masaru, *The Hidden Messages in Water*, Atria, 2011.

Fojas, Felix, *Supernatural and Beyond,* University of Arizona Libraries, 2017.

Ganga and Tara, *Herbs for Spiritual Development*; Universal Fellowship of Light Publishing, 2017.

Hay, Louise, *You Can Heal Your Life*, Hay House Publishing, 2004.

Hendel, Dr. *Water and Salt: The Essence of Life: The Healing Power of Nature*. Natural Resources Inc, 2003.

Kubler Ross, Elizabeth, *On Death and Dying,* Scribner, 1969

Kulreet Chaudhary, author of *The Prime: Prepare and Repair Your Body for Spontaneous Weight Loss* Harmony Books, January 2016, McDonald, NP, Pamela, *Perfect Gene Diet,* Hay House, Inc, 2010.

McEnzie, Robin, *Treat Your Own Back,* Penguin Group, 2011 (I have used some of exercise tips with great relief.) Another book is *The Back Pain Help Book* by various Health professionals.)

Moody, Raymond, *Life After Life, Bantam Books 1975. 2015,*

Moorjani, Anita, *Dying to Be Me* Hay House, 2014.

Mt. Shasta, Peter, *Adventures of a Western Mystic;* Church of the Seven Rays, Vol 1, 2013, vol. 2 2010; *I AM the Violet Tara*, Church of the Seven Rays,2019.

Peskin, Brian Scott and Rowen, Robert Jay, M.D., *PEO Solution*, Pinnacle Press, 2015.

Saraydarian, Torkom, *The Eyes of Hierarchy,* Creative Trust, 1998.

Sears, William, M.D. and Sears, Martha, R.N., *Prime-Time Health.* Little, Brown Spark Hatchett Book Group, 2010.

Sinclair, Blake, *Dare to Imagine: 18 Principles for Peace, Happiness and True Success*, Golden Lotus Books, 2014 and Beyond Imagination: A Path to God and the Divine Realm, Golden Lotus Books, 2015.

Singer, Peter, *Animal Liberation the Life You Can Live*, Harper Collins Publishers, 1975-2009.

Tennyson Stevens, Robert, *Conscious Language*, Mastery Systems International, 2007-2014.

Stone, Joshua David, Ph.D., *The Complete Ascension Manual*, Light Technology Publishing, LLC, 1994

Teeguarden, Ron, *The Ancient Wisdom of the Chinese Tonic Herbs*, Warner Books, Inc. 1998.

Truman, Karol, *Emotions Buried Alive Never Die*, Olympus Distributing, 1995 – 2005.

William, Anthony, *Medical Medium*, Hay House Publishing, 2015

Yogananda, Paramahansa, Autobiography of a Yogi, -Self Realization Fellowship, 1994 -2002.

The Tibetan Book of the Dead or *Bardo Thodol* Compiled around 800 A.D. Bantam Books, 1994

GAME CHANGERS

Health Resources

1. Dr. Daniel Amen, MD - http://danielamenmd.com/ **(Brain wellness)**
2. Dr. Josh Axe - https://draxe.com/
3. Grandmaster Mantak Chia - https://www.mantakchia.com/ One of the Top Healers in the world. Time magazine voted him as Qi Gong Master of the Year and one of the 100 Most Spiritually Influential People in the world.
4. Dr. Deepak Chopra - https://www.deepakchopra.com/
5. Wim Hof - https://www.wimhofmethod.com/
6. Dr. Frank Lipman, MD - https://www.ananda.org/yogapedia/aum/
7. Dr. Grace Liu, PharmD, AFMCP aka **The Gut Goddess** - https://thegutinstitute.com/about **(Gut Health)**
8. Dr. Joseph Mercola, MD - https://www.mercola.com/
9. Brian Scott Peskin, BSEE-MIT - https://brianpeskin.com/ **(Parent Essential Oil)**
10. Dr. Robert Jay Rowen, MD - https://drrowendrsu.com/ He is considered the doctors doctor.
11. Dr. William Sears, MD - https://www.askdrsears.com/- health, wellness and longevity.
12. Dr. Sonia, EliteMD, World Class Plastic Surgery and dermatologist, elitemdspa.com
13. Dr. Andrew Weil, MD - https://www.drweil.com/
14. Anthony William, Medical Medium - https://www.medicalmedium.com/

Special Guests

1. Alexis, Medical Intuitive - contact author at blakesinclair.org
2. Darshan Baba, Yogi, Author, Spiritual Mentor, Subtle Energy Healer, and Teacher of Online Subtle Energy & Meditation Courses - https://mokshagyan.webs.com/
3. Bella, CEO and Founder of Metaphysical Medium, Master Hypnotherapist, Life Coach, Holistic Health Practitioner and Reiko Master - https://themetaphysicalmedium.com/
4. Marian Brandenburg, a body healer, an intuitive massage therapist, Chi Nei Tsang Practitioner, and Ajna and Neuro Light Practitioner - www.threecornerstoneswellness.com
5. Dr. Mikaelah Cordeo, Ph.D - Spiritual Teacher, Healer and Messenger for the Ascended Host of Light - https://mikaelahcordeo.com/
6. Rebecca Danbe - Kim, Feng Shui Practitioner, Face Reading, Personal Energy Clearing- https://www.rebeccakim.com
7. Lisa De Witt, Healer - contact her through messenger on Facebook
8. Janet Doerr, Intuitive Nutritionista - https://www.facebook.com/TheIntuitiveNutritionista/
9. Dr. Alex Feng, Traditional Chinese Medicine Doctor (Voted as one of the top ten Traditional Chinese Medicine Doctor), Acupuncturist, Qi Gong Master and Daoist Master - http://thetaoistcenter.com/
10. Felix Fojas, veteran spiritual warrior, Mystic, lecturer, teacher, Reiki Master and healer - contact Blake for any inquires at www.blakesinclair.org
11. Patty Gee, Massage Therapist and Holistic Health Practitioner - contact Blake at www.blakesinclair.org
12. David Granovsky, Stem Cell expert or advisor- https://repairstemcell.wordpress.com/
13. Lori Guidinglight - contact Blake at www.blakesinclair.org
14. Dr. Paul Hannah, M.D., Intuitive Keynote Speaker- https://hannahsholistichealing.com/
15. Dr. Steve Jackowicz, Mac, Lac, PhD- sjackowicz@bridgeport.edu
16. Joanna Marie, Reiki Master- contact me for any inquires at www.blakesinclair.org

17. Tai Monique - http://taimoniquekristjansen.arbonne.com.
18. Flenje Oaferina, Doctorate Candidate for Physical Therapy - contact Blake at www.blakesinclair.org
19. Dr. Hector Oksenendler, DC and Physical Therapist - contact Blake at www.blakesinclair.org
20. Star Santos - www.stargazer.ph/
21. Dr. Sonia, EliteMD, World Class Plastic Surgery and dermatologist, elitemdspa.com
22. Andrei Volhonttseff, Nutritionist - https://www.myyp.com/Pleasanton,CA/Valley-Health-Mill/profile
23. Dr. Paul Wang, Doctor of Acupuncture and Chinese Medicine and Wu Shu Master -www.daocenter.com
24. Zhang Yuan Ming - www.qigongmaster.com

Spiritual Resources

1. Darshan Baba - https://mokshagyan.webs.com/
2. Dr. Mikaelah Cordeo-https://mikaelahcordeo.com/
3. Dr. Alex Feng, Ph.D., O.M.D. L.Ac. (He is also a spiritual leader, master of healing, Qi Gong Master and Daoist Master. - https://thetaoistcenter.com/
4. Romarishi Siddha (formerly known as Ganga Nath) and Tara Leela, authors of Herbs for Spiritual Development, Yogi and spiritual teachers - http://www.universalfellowshipoflight.com/?fbclid=IwAR1z-6fiOg8dAlbsyI5J_9KKVQu8Kd0qysJ-pWAmUdTWKKt837clU9u8K68
5. Masami Saionji, Spiritual Leader and Chairperson of Byakko Shinko Kai - https://byakko.org/
6. Peter Mt. Shasta, author of many spiritual classics, apprentice to Saint Germain, spiritual master and teacher and Mystic - https://www.i-am-teachings.com/
7. Blake Sinclair, author of Dare to Imagine, Beyond Imagination and Eat, Drink, Meditate and Pray your way into Being a Modern Day Yogi, Internationally Recognized Blogger, Health and Wellness Optimizer, Spiritual Teacher and Mystic - http://www.blakesinclair.org/

Alternative Health Practitioners

1. Traditional Chinese Medicine Doctor
2. Acupuncturist
3. Herbalist
4. Ayurvedic Medical practitioner
5. Reiki Master
6. Cranial Sacral Therapist
7. Hypnotherapist
8. Psych-K Practitioner
9. Chiropractic Medicine
10. Naturopathic Doctor
11. Homeopathic Doctor
12. Osteopathic Doctor
13. Functional Medical Practitioner
14. Massage Therapist
15. Shamans
16. Medical Intuitive and Mediums
17. Ajna Light Practitioner
18. Neuro Light Practitioner

Herbal Tonic Elixirs
1. https://www.dragonherbs.com/

Ergonomic help for structural health

1. Shoulder, wrist and hand issues may be related to poor ergonomics. Additional info about ergonomics can be found at
   a. https://www.mayoclinic.org/healthy-lifestyle/adult-health/in-depth/office-ergonomics/art-20046169.
   b. http://www.heldtite.com/ergonomics.html

2. Places to purchase equipment for better ergonomics include:
   a. https://www.alimed.com/office-ergonomics/
   b. https://www.amazon.com/HUANUO-Escritorio-ordenador-almohadilla-integrada/dp/B07SM57QTM/ref=sxbs_sxwds-stvp?cv_ct_cx=ergonomic+laptop&dchild=1&key

words=ergonomic+laptop&pd_rd_i=B07SM57QTM&pd_
rd_r=b5da7cab-2344-4a53-8b69-9e6d0b5c1099&pd_rd_
w=xS8rM&pd_rd_wg=V2Tmc&pf_rd_p=183579a1-f0e6-
4556-8e39-8fe08e8f8141&pf_rd_r=F33A7PFQWMVK
SP71Z3GF&psc=1&qid=1589417726&s=hpc&sr=1-3-dd5817
a1-1ba7-46c2-8996-f96e7b0f409c

c. https://www.amazon.com/s?k=ergonomic
d. https://ergonomicshealth.com/best-ergonomic-products/#md-navigation-section-3

Quality Vitamins and Supplement Stores in The Bay Area

Valley Health Mill Pleasanton, CA 94588; 925.462.9354 (they take telephone orders and ship). https://www.myyp.com/Pleasanton,CA/Valley-Health-Mill/profile

Superfood or Nutrients

1. **Purium Superfoods-** According to Bella, CEO and Founder of Metaphysical Medium, Board Certified Holistic Health Practitioner, Master Hypnotherapist, Life Coach, and Reiki Master, they are the best superfood products on the market.

Purium is the only superfood brand that she uses because it is organic and non-gmo. She stated that they have all the essentials to cleanse and reset our bodies overall. You can use the Ultimate Lifestyle Transformation (ULT) Kit as your "daily Core 4 products" for vitamin and mineral needs, or you can use the same Core 4 products + the Super Cleans-R (parasite formula) + cut out inflammatory foods like gluten and dairy etc, and use it as an intense juice cleanse which can help reset your body in terms of chronic fatigue and autoimmune illnesses. She personally uses the ULT as a powerful detox/cleanse 4 times per year, coupled with colon hydrotherapy. She uses the Core 4 as a daily regime to provide all the nutrients, minerals and energy she needs to keep her body in a constant state of optimization, and therefore does not have to take any multivitamins or other supplements.

Follow the link below to access Purium's Ultimate Lifestyle Transformation Kit, and use the following discount code for exclusive savings: **MetaphysicalMediumDetox**

https://www.theholisticjusticeleague.com/ultimatelifestyletransforma tion?fbclid=IwAR1g0dXSgCqcaHaY6lR6gXN-XyNEwPrwTPLgkM QJZj0HAoONpahhhKL1URc

According to Bella, CEO and Founder of Metaphysical Medium, Master Hypnotherapist, Life Coach, and Reiki Master, they are the best superfood products on the market.

It is the only one that she uses because it is organic and non-gmo. She stated that they have all the essentials to cleanse and reset our body overall. You can use this kit as your daily 4 for vitamin and minerals needs or you can use the same 4 products and cut out inflammatory foods like gluten and dairy etc and use it as an intense juice cleanse which totally resets your body in terms of chronic fatigue and autoimmune illnesses. She personally uses this as a powerful detox cleanse 4 times per year. She uses these 4 as a daily regime to provide all the nutrients, minerals and energy she needs to keep her body in a constant state of optimization.

2. **Kyani Products** - I love their products! It has helped my family and clients, colleague and I with our various health issues. You can order it at https://GoldenLotus.kyani.com.
3. **Puradyme.com** - Digestive enzymes, cleansing products and probiotics. Their website is https://www.puradyme.com/.
4. **Pyradyne.com** - minerals, vitamins, Shou Wu Chih and metaphysical jewelry designed by Dr. Fred Bell (descendant of Alexander Graham Bell; the inventor of the telephone). Their website is https://www.pyradyne.com/collections/vitamins-minerals.

My Top 24 Wellness Products

1. Body Care Studio's PEO oil
2. Kyani products (NitroExtreme, Sunrise, Sunset) IS
3. Pathogen Assassin IS***

4. Echinamide IS***
5. Thrive Probiotic IS***
6. Empirical Labs Liposomal Vitamin C IS***
7. R's Koso
8. Green Barley
9. Royal Hawaiian Spirulina
10. Chlorenergy
11. Camu Camu Vitamin C IS***
12. Black Cumin Seed Oil (100% pure cold-press) IS***
13. The Eight Immortal Herbal Tonic Elixirs
14. Vital Earth Minerals, Fulvic Minerals
15. Magnesium Taurate
16. GanoMax and ShroomZoom (Reishi and Cordycep) IS
17. Juice Plus -IS
18. Humic Acid IS***
19. Sunfood Super foods Ocean Alive 2.0
20. XLEAR Nasal Spray (clears nasal infection fast) IS***
21. Thorne Quercetin Photosome + EGCg IS***
22. Zinc Glycinate IS***
23. Cinchona Officinalis IS***
24. RespirActin Deep Lung Cleanse IS***

Note: *** Author's favorite pick for Immune Support.
IS = Immune Support

Health, wellness and Beauty Products
1. **Arbonne**-http://taimoniquekristjansen.arbonne.com.
2. **Honest**.com

Healthy Food
1. Vitalchoice.com- healthy source of food (wild salmon and grass-fed beef). Recommended by Dr. William Sears.

Essential Oils
1. https://www.saje.com/essential-oils/
2. youngliving.com/

BOOK RESOURCES

Health

The Ancient Wisdom of the Chinese Tonic Herbs by Master Herbalist Ron Teeguarden

The End of Alzheimer's by Dale E. Bredesen, M.D

Heart Health- Reversing Heart Disease by Dr. Dean Ornish

Herbs for Spiritual Development by Ganga and Tara

The Lost Book of Herbal Remedies by Dr. Nicole Apelian.

Life After Life by Raymond Moody, *Dying to Be Me* by Anita Moorjani and books by Elizabeth Kubler -Ross.

Medical Medium by Anthony William (Auto Immune Diseases and other illnesses-)

Prime-Time Health by William Sears, MD and Martha Sears, RN

Acupressure Potent Points by Michael Gach

Mayo Clinic Natural Healing (Effective therapies and techniques)

Monthly Health Letters

1. UC Berkeley Wellness Letters
2. UCLA Healthy Ways
3. Harvard Men's Health Watch
4. Harvard Health Letter
5. Mayo Clinic Health Letter
6. Cleveland Clinic Men's Health Advisor
7. Duke Medicine Health News
8. Massachusetts General Hospital Mind, Mood and Memory

9. Icahn School of Medicine at Mount Sinai Focus of Healthy Aging

Comments: My former client is a 96 years young and is in great mental, emotional and physical shape. He subscribes to all of the above newsletters and reads all of them. He sums up the secrets for a youthful brain and good health to include three things- "movement, nourishment and rest." "That cultivates creativity and flexibility. It shows empathy and is well-connected and is authentic." He was a Nuclear Physicist and a UC Berkeley Alumni. He has my deepest gratitude for sharing his list to us.

Spiritual

Adventures of a Western Mystic by Peter Mt. Shasta

Autobiography of a Yogi by Paramahansa Yogananda

The Autobiography of Phra Ajaan Lee translated by Geoffrey Degraff and originally written in Thai by Phra Suddhidhammaransi Gambhiramedhacariya

Beyond Imagination: A Pathway to God and the Divine Realms by Blake Sinclair

The Complete Ascension Manual by Joshua David Stone, Ph.D.

Dare to Imagine: 18 Principles for finding Peace, Happiness and True Success by Blake Sinclair

The Essence of the Bhagavad Gita explained by Paramahansa Yogananda and remembered and written by Swami Kriyananda

The Green Book Series- Unveiled Mysteries, The Magic Presence

and The "I AM" Discourses by Godfrey Ray King

Hinduism Scriptures & Practices by Prabha Duneja

The Holy Bible

I AM the Violet Tara by Peter Mt. Shasta

I AM Affirmations by Peter Mt. Shasta

Live in Love by Dr. Mikaelah Cordeo, Ph.D.

Tibetan Book of Living and Dying by Sogyal Rinpoche

You Are The Universe by Masami Saionji

Game Changer Movies (Must Watch!!)

1. *Heal-*http://www.healdocumentary.com/- (YouTube and Netflix)
2. *Inori: Conversation with Something Great*   https://vimeo.com/officetetsushiratori/
3. *Fat, Sick and Nearly Dead* - http://www.fatsickandnearlydead.com/-(YouTube and Amazon Prime Video).
4. *Thrive-* https://www.youtube.com/watch?v=lEV5AFFcZ-s and site is https://www.thrivemovement.com/the_movie- (YouTube)
5. *Food, Inc-* https://topdocumentaryfilms.com/food-inc/- (Amazon Prime Video)
6. *Fork Over Knives-*(Netflix)
7. *Vandana Shiva -* Bringing awareness to world problems. https://www.facebook.com/prem.keerti/videos/2267572333285843/UzpfSTEwMDAwMD
8. *The Game Changer-* (Netflix) https://www.netflix.com/title/81157840?ad=true&tctx=0%2C0%2Ccc524dd9-5768-47d5-ba8f-7c1be773801f-374164330%2C%2C&trackId=13752289

.-. .--. ..---

465

A verse from an inscription of the
Buddhist Monk Meng Jing Su's Tablet

是以至人無己先天
而御六氣列仙神
地隘宇宙而遺萬物
化

A verse painted by Kumiko that captured my attention

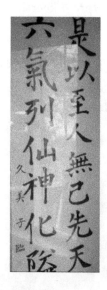

My Inspired Interpretation of the verse from an inscription of the Buddhist Monk Meng Jing Su's Tablet originally written during the Tang Dynasty

Thus, when the individual with high attainment arrives and lives in an alignment with the life of a Saint, Ascended Being or Godlike Being (an individual who is egoless, does not seek fame, fortune or recognition; who puts the needs of Heaven and Earth above his own; who relinquishes the attachment to all material things and that which is impermanent; who serves selflessly and unconditionally out of pure love and humility with no attachment of outcome; who lives in balance and alignment with him or herself, Nature, the Universe; and who lives in oneness with the Dao and follows the Way and teachings of Buddha), he or she can transcend the limitations of the six influences (Yin, Yang, Dark, Light, Wind and Rain) and attain the ranking of an immortal being who lives for the benefit of Earth and the Universe so that he or she can transmute and transform the gap that exist between the Heavens and Earth by manifesting a path that leads to the Universe, God and the Dao.

Note:
*The Verse was originally from Laozi's student Zhuangzi Xiao Yao You according to Master Yuanming Zhang and inscribed on tablets of Monk Meng Jing Su. According to Dr. Paul C. Wang, the version that caught my attention is a paraphrase from Meng Fa Shi that was painted by Kumiko. My interpretation of the Divine verse is based on the translations of various scholars, spiritual masters, translators and a Buddhist practitioner the author interviewed and through my own understanding and insights gain through my meditation practices. According to Master Zhang, the essence of the verse is about **forgetting the self** when you have **reached high attainment.** The verse is quite profound and the writing is classical Chinese which is terse, abstract and open to multiple interpretations and is based on Buddhist and Daoist teachings; hence, it is quite difficult to translate and fully comprehend. A formal translation from a Buddhist or Daoist Master and scholar can further elucidate and more accurately explain the deeper and intricate meanings of the verse. I originally saw a calligraphy painting done of this verse by a Japanese woman named Kumiko. I did not know what the verse meant but the energy of the painting was so strong and I felt so strongly connected with it and now I know why.*

Grandmaster Zhang Yuanming, Dr. Alex Feng, Dr. Paul Wang and Mary Ann Liu were contributors to interpretation of the Inscription.

AUTHOR'S BIOGRAPHY

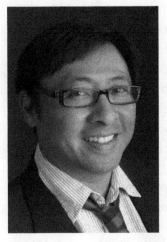 Blake Sinclair is an author of three books about spirituality, metaphysics, life and healthy living (Dare to Imagine: 18 Principles for Finding Peace, Happiness, and True Success, Beyond Imagination: A Path to God and the Divine Realm and A New Beginning: An Antidote to Civilization), a Mystic, a spiritual teacher, a life and certified Health Coach, a licensed occupational therapist (specializing in neurological and orthopedic rehabilitation), a Holistic Health Practitioner, a Reiki practitioner, a blogger, a lecturer, and an entrepreneur. He has also received formal training with clinical hypnosis, acupressure and Psych-K.

He has studied with various renowned spiritual masters, teachers and gurus including **Peter Mt. Shasta** throughout the years. After his spiritual and nutritional awakening, he began studying with various nutritionists and later successfully completed his training as a certified Health Coach from the esteemed **Dr. Sears Wellness Institute**. Dr. Bill Sears is a Harvard trained physician, an expert on health and has written 45 books on health and wellness. He has been a clinical professor at the University of Southern California School of Medicine and University of Irvine School of Medicine.

His program or wellness institute is one of the most cutting-edge in the world and the teachings are based on good scientific research and evidence. His training program is accredited and approved by many institutions including but not limited to The National Board for Health and Wellness Coaching, National Association of Nutritional Professionals, American College of Sports Medicine, etc.

Much of what Blake has written in his book is based on his experiences, extensive research throughout the years and interviews from various health experts. With regards to his certification training, he offers private coaching sessions on health and wellness. He guides his clients on optimizing their health needs and goals through guidance and support with lifestyle changes, exercise, attitude and nutrition. Some of the following services he offers include: how to optimize brain, heart, digestive and vascular support including those with dementia, heart diseases and inflammatory disorders including those suffering from pain. He also teaches his client's on how to unlock and activate their internal pharmacy (Dr. Sears calls this the fountain of youth) to support wellness and longevity. It goes beyond the scope of this book to include all the above information so he offers teachings to his clients but may write more about it in the future.

He uses his diverse background – Western and Eastern techniques and wisdom, knowledge of nutrition and health, connection to the Divine and his 30 years in the medical field to facilitate the healing process for his clients. He is also the founder of U.U.M.M. meditation system and the "I AM" Wellness Method. He has dedicated his life to sharing his spiritual secrets and cutting-edge information on wellness and spirituality. His dream is to empower as many people as possible to discover their true and Divine Nature so that they may be free from suffering and begin to live in joy, love, peace and radiant health. His goal is to help create greater peace and unity on Earth by guiding as many people as possible toward the path of enlightenment and God Realization.

His hobbies include travelling, cooking, singing, hiking, birdwatching, whale watching, earthing on the beach, star and moon gazing, listening to spiritual, classical and folk music (Indian and Japanese) as well as contemporary musicals, collecting sacred crystals, spending time in his Zen Garden and Fish Sanctuary, visiting sacred places and spending time with his family and canine family members- Hazel Reia and Coco Lakshmi, both are King Charles Cavaliers.

Besides his books and blogs, he also works at the community level at outreach programs to promote interfaith unity. He is also actively involved with the S.O.P.P (Symphony of Peace Prayer) group with its global prayer programs. Visit him at www.blakesinclair.org

Book info

1. **Dare to Imagine: 18 Principles for Finding Peace, Happiness and True Success:** Dare to Imagine: 18 Principles for Finding Peace, Happiness, and True Success is the story of one lost soul who never stopped searching. The author offers hope and actionable advice for those who want to find their own peace, happiness, and success. Read this book, and be prepared to challenge how you see yourself. You will see that miracles really do happen.

2. **Beyond Imagination: A Path to God and the Divine Realm**: In this book, Blake Sinclair describes many of his experiences on his journey of awakening. Combining innate wisdom, his connection to the Source, and the Divine Innocence that comes from a pure heart, Blake shares his excitement of the unfoldment of his awakening with his readers. The great awarenesses that came to him included the knowingness of the Divinity in all life and all things. His awakening also reconnected him with the Divine Realms which include the Ascended Masters and the Angelic Host, among others. In his great desire to be of service to the world, Blake has taken much of the knowledge that he has accumulated in his journey thus far and placed it in this book (and its predecessor Dare to Imagine) to provide for people who are now on a similar path tools to utilize. His intent for writing these books was largely to help readers make the journey more easily and in a greater state of grace. His intent is also to help bridge the gap between religion and mysticism and bring greater peace, unity, and harmony to the world.

3. **A New Beginning**: This is Blake Sinclair's final book of his Golden Book Series Trilogy. This book brings his readers to the next highest level of health, consciousness and spirituality. He takes his reader on an incredible journey of navigating through

the complexities of health, longevity and immortality in a way that makes sense, is easy to understand and follow. Blake further guides the reader in discovering our amazing body, micro universe, energy centers and Divine Presence that exist within all us as well as within our planet Mother Earth and beyond. Secrets known by Daoist Masters, Qi Gong Masters, Mystics, Yogis and healers are shared about how to optimize your health, longevity, energy and spirituality. Through Blake's own experiences, extensive research and interviews from some of the top health experts, he provides wisdom and tools to help solve many of our modern-day sufferings (mental, emotional, physical as well as spiritual). Not only are the causes of much of our collective suffering is explored, the core of it is identified to awaken us on a path of enlightenment and salvation. Ultimately, Blake guides the reader on how to step into the sovereignty of their true and Divine Nature to live a God realized life full of peace, love, harmony and radiant health so that Heaven on Earth can be created within us as well as here on Earth.

Blake video links:

1. Dare to Imagine Book Trailer- https://www.youtube.com/watch?v=DT_Kj0fdjj4#action=share
2. Dare to Imagine Extended Book Trailer- https://www.youtube.com/watch?time_continue=3&v=Cm2WEnH-ZR0&feature=emb_title
3. Beyond Imagination Book Commercial- https://www.youtube.com/watch?v=PN3EGfTRsDg#action=share
4. Mount Shasta Interview- https://www.youtube.com/watch?v=9rtIXfDhkAk&feature=youtu.be
5. This Week in America interview with Rik Bratton- https://www.youtube.com/watch?v=JU_FNi1z-Uw
6. Blake's Blog Site- www.blakesinclair.org

Blake's areas of expertise include the following areas:

1. **Physical Rehabilitation**
   a. Stroke management and Neurological Rehab
   b. General Shoulder and upper extremity dysfunctions
   c. Geriatric disabilities
   d. General rehabilitation (pulmonary, cardiac and orthopedic surgeries- shoulder and hip replacement and orthopedic repairs)
   e. Dementia management
   f. Fall prevention
   g. Home and Personal Safety and defense
   h. DME (Wheelchair, Walker, Hospital Bed, etc.) and Adaptive Devices
   i. Balance training (traditional methods as well as Tai Chi derived balance training)
   j. Fine Motor Skills
   k. Activities of Daily Living
   l. Cognitive Perceptual Deficits
   m. Long Term Placement

2. **Health and Wellness**
   a. Memory
   b. Longevity and/ reversing aging
   c. Depression
   d. Stress
   e. Anxiety
   f. Energy
   g. Optimizing heart, vascular and brain function
   h. Exercise for optimizing health and function
   i. Making Health your Hobby
   j. Living without Pain and Inflammation
   k. Moving Waste From Your Waist
   l. Activating the Internal Pharmacy
   m. Pantry Makeover
   n. Nutrition
   o. Supplements

p. Breathing

q. Meditation for Health

3. **Spirituality**

   a. Spiritual Self Defense

   b. The Art of Manifestation

   c. The Art of Living, Dying and Ascension

   d. Meditation (U.U.M.M.)- Health and Cosmic Connection

   e. I AM Wellness Method

   f. The Power of Visualization

   g. I AM Presence

   h. Journey to the W.E.S.T. (Wisdom, Enlightenment, Salvation and Truth)

   i. Connecting with God and the Ascended Masters

   j. Attaining God Consciousness

   k. Healing (personal, distant and planetary)

   l. Turbocharging Prayer and Decrees

   m. Finding purpose and meaning

   n. Discovering the True Nature

   o. Yogic Breathing Methods

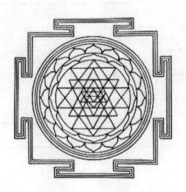

Vasudhaiva Kutumbakam

*"Let the people on Earth live like citizens -
one great empire under the pure guidance
of Supreme Divinity, the source of all life,
that connects the entire creation."*

*Chapter 6 of Maha Upanishad VI. 71-73.
Translated by
Prabha Duneja*

NOTES

GOALS

Short Term

_____
_____
_____
_____
_____
_____
_____
_____
_____
_____
_____
_____
_____
_____
_____
_____
_____
_____
_____
_____
_____
_____
_____
_____
_____
_____

GOALS

<u>Long Term</u>

_____

_____

_____

_____

_____

_____

_____

_____

_____

_____

_____

_____

_____

_____

_____

_____

_____

_____

_____

_____

_____

_____

_____

_____

_____

_____

_____

_____

_____

_____

REFLECTION

INDEX

CPSIA information can be obtained
at www.ICGtesting.com
Printed in the USA
LVHW032023290321
682891LV00010B/63